INTERNATIONAL CONGRESS AND SYMPOSIUM SERIES NUMBER 152

Editor-in-Chief: **Lord Walton of Detchant**

Fourth International Symposium on Sodium Valproate and Epilepsy

Proceedings of a symposium sponsored by
Sanofi Pharma (UK), held in St Helier, Jersey, Channel Islands,
26–28 April, 1989

Edited by

David Chadwick

ROYAL SOCIETY OF MEDICINE SERVICES
LONDON · NEW YORK
1989

Royal Society of Medicine Services Limited
1 Wimpole Street   London W1M 8AE
7 East 60th Street   New York NY 10022

These proceedings are published by Royal Society of Medicine Services Ltd with financial support from the sponsor. The contributors are responsible for the scientific content and for the views expressed, which are not necessarily those of the sponsor, of the editor of the series or of the volume, of the Royal Society of Medicine or of Royal Society of Medicine Services Ltd. Distribution has been in accordance with the wishes of the sponsor but a copy is available to any Fellow of the Society at a privileged price.

British Library Cataloguing in Publication Data
International Symposium on Sodium Valproate and
  Epilepsy : 4th 1989 St. Helier, Jersey
  IVth International Symposium on Sodium Valproate and
  Epilepsy.
  I. Title II. Chadwick, David, 1937- III. Series
  616.8'53061

ISBN 1-85315-110-6

Phototypeset by Dobbie Typesetting Limited, Plymouth, Devon
Printed in Great Britain at the Alden Press, Oxford

Contributors

Editor and President

D. J. Chadwick   *Consultant Neurologist, Walton Hospital, Liverpool, UK*

Chairmen

F. E. Dreifuss   *Professor of Neurology & Child Neurology, University of Virginia Medical Centre, Charlottesville, Virginia, USA*

P. Fenwick   *Consultant Neuropsychiatrist, Maudsley Hospital, London, UK*

L. Gram   *Medical Director, Dianalund Epilepsy Hospital, Dianalund, Denmark*

J. Oxley   *Physician, The National Society for Epilepsy, Chalfont Centre for Epilepsy, Chalfont St Peter, UK*

E. H. Reynolds   *Consultant Neurologist, King's College Hospital, London, UK*

A. Richens   *Professor of Pharmacology & Therapeutics, University of Wales College of Medicine, Cardiff, UK*

Contributors

* J. Aicardi   *Consultant Paediatric Neurologist, Hôpital Necker Enfants Malades, Paris, France*

J. Alving   *Chief Neurologist, Dianalund Epilepsy Hospital, Dianalund, Denmark*

A. R. Andersen   *University Clinic of Neurology, Rigshospitalet, Copenhagen, Denmark*

G. Anderson   *Department of Neurology, Aalborg Sygehus, Aalborg, Denmark*

D. J. Back   *Department of Pharmacology and Therapeutics, University of Liverpool, Liverpool, UK*

* J. Barre   *Assistant Director, Laboratoire Hospitalo-Universitaire de Pharmacologie, Centre Hospitalier, Creteil, France*

B. A. Bell	*Atkinson Morley's Hospital, London, UK*
Y. Berger	*Sanofi-Recherche, Montpellier, France*
H. von Bernuth	*Department of Paediatrics, Städtische Krankenanstalten, Bielefeld, Federal Republic of Germany*
D. J. Berry	*Poisons Unit, New Cross Hospital, London, UK*
* C. D. Binnie	*Consultant Clinical Neurophysiologist, The Maudsley Hospital, London, UK*
* L. D. Blumhardt	*Consultant Neurologist, Walton Hospital, Liverpool, UK*
* I. Bone	*Consultant Neurologist, Institute of Neurological Sciences, Southern General Hospital, Glasgow, UK*
A. Bowden	*Regional Neurosciences Unit, Walton Hospital, Liverpool, UK*
* M. J. Brodie	*Consultant Clinical Pharmacologist, Western Infirmary, Glasgow, UK*
* K. Budd	*Consultant in Anaesthesia & Pain Relief, The Royal Infirmary, Bradford, UK*
* N. E. F. Cartlidge	*Consultant Neurologist, Royal Victoria Infirmary, Newcastle-upon-Tyne, UK*
* W. Christe	*Klinikum Rudolf Virchow, Department of Neurology, Free University of Berlin, Berlin, Federal Republic of Germany*
P. Cleland	*Department of Neurology, Sunderland District Hospital, Tyne and Wear, UK*
R. W. I. Cooke	*Department of Child Health, Liverpool Maternity Hospital, Liverpool, UK*
* J. A. Corbett	*Professor of Psychiatry, University of Birmingham, UK*
J. A. Cramer	*Department of Neurology, Yale University School of Medicine, and Veterans Administration Medical Center, New Haven, USA*
P. Crawford	*Atkinson Morley's Hospital, London, UK*
* W. J. K. Cumming	*Consultant Neurologist, Withington Hospital, Manchester, UK*
* M. Dam	*Associate Professor of Neurology, University Clinic of Neurology, Hvidovre Hospital, Copenhagen, Denmark*
* D. L. W. Davidson	*Consultant Neurologist, Ninewells Hospital and Medical School, Dundee, UK*

* F. E. Dreifuss — *Professor of Neurology & Child Neurology, School of Medicine, University of Virginia Medical Centre, Charlottesville, Virginia, USA*

R. Duncan — *Institute of Neurological Sciences, Southern General Hospital, Glasgow, UK*

* H. M. Emrich — *Max Planck Institute for Psychiatry, Munich, Federal Republic of Germany*

* R. A. Gillham — *Clinical Psychologist, Institute of Neurological Sciences, Southern General Hospital, Glasgow, UK*

G. Groß-Selbeck — *Department of Neuropaediatrics, Städtische Krankenanstalten, Düsseldorf-Gerresheim, Federal Republic of Germany*

D. Hadley — *Institute of Neurological Sciences, Southern General Hospital, Glasgow, UK*

J. S. Hansen — *Electronics Institute, Technical University of Denmark, Lyngby, Denmark*

* H. J. Heggarty — *Consultant Paediatrician, York District Hospital, York, UK*

M. Herning — *University Clinic of Magnetic Resonance, Hvidovre Hospital, Copenhagen, Denmark*

J. M. Hochholzer — *Yale University School of Medicine, New Haven, CT, USA*

* G. Hosking — *Consultant Paediatric Neurologist, Ryegate Children's Centre, Sheffield, UK*

S. J. L. Howell — *Department of Neurological Science, Walton Hospital, Liverpool, UK*

* J. Hulsman — *Clinical Chemist, Epilepsy Centre, Kempenhaeghe, Heeze, The Netherlands*

* J. Issakainen — *University Children's Hospital, Zurich, Switzerland*

* P. Jennum — *Department of Neurology, University Hospital, Rigshospitalet, Copenhagen, Denmark*

A. L. Johnson — *Medical Statistician, MRC Biostatics Unit, Cambridge, UK*

* R. T. Jung — *Consultant Endocrinologist, Ninewells Hospital and Medical School, Dundee, UK*

K. Kellermann — *Department of Paediatrics, Städtisches Kinderkrankenhaus, Köln, Federal Republic of Germany*

F. Kotlarek — *Department of Paediatrics, Klinikum RWTH, Aachen, Federal Republic of Germany*

* P. Loiseau — *Professor and Head of Neurology, University Hospital, Pellegrin, Bordeaux, France*

B. McArdle — *Northwick Park Hospital, Harrow, Middlesex, UK*

M. McGowan — *Department of Paediatric Neurology, Guy's Hospital, London, UK*

* N. Marlow — *Consultant & Senior Lecturer, Bristol Maternity Hospital, Bristol, UK*

C. Martin — *Department of Pharmacology and Therapeutics, University of Liverpool, Liverpool, UK*

* R. H. Mattson — *Professor of Neurology, Yale University School of Medicine, and Veterans Administration Hospital, New Haven, USA*

* H. Meinardi — *Professor & Director of Epileptology, Instituut voor Epilepsiebestrijding, Heemstede, The Netherlands*

* A. J. Moore — *Senior Registrar in Neurosurgery, Atkinson Morley's Hospital, London, UK*

W. Mortier — *Department of Paediatrics, Städtische Krankenanstalten, Wuppertal, Federal Republic of Germany*

B. G. R. Neville — *Department of Paediatric Neurology, Guy's Hospital, London, UK*

R. A. Novelly — *Yale University School of Medicine, New Haven, CT, USA*

* M. Orme — *Professor of Clinical Pharmacology, University of Liverpool, Liverpool, UK*

J. Patterson — *Institute of Neurological Sciences, Southern General Hospital, Glasgow, UK*

* B. Pedersen — *Department of Neurology, Aalborg Sygehus, Aalborg, Denmark*

R. Pothmann — *Department of Paediatrics, Städtische Krankenanstalten, Wuppertal, Federal Republic of Germany*

* J. Poulton — *Hon. Senior Registrar in Paediatrics, John Radcliffe Hospital, Oxford, UK*

M. L. Prevey — *Yale University School of Medicine, New Haven, CT, USA*

* D. Price — *Consultant Neurosurgeon, The General Infirmary, Leeds, UK*

* V. Raemakers — *Department of Paediatrics, Klinikum RWTH, Aachen, Federal Republic of Germany*

* Th. Rentmeester — *Epilepsy Centre, Kempenhaeghe, Heeze, The Netherlands*

K. Rheingans — *Department of Paediatrics, Städtisches Kinderkrankenhaus, Köln, Federal Republic of Germany*

* I. G. Robertson   *Consultant Obstetrician & Gynaecologist, Sharoe Green Hospital, Preston, UK*

  U. Rubenstrunk   *Department of Paediatrics, Klinikum RWTH, Aachen, Federal Republic of Germany*

  U. Schauseil-Zipf   *Department of Paediatrics, University of Köln, Federal Republic of Germany*

  R. D. Scheyer   *Yale University School of Medicine, New Haven, CT, USA*

* G. Scollo-Lavizzari   *Professor of Neurology & Clinical Neurophysiology, Basle University Hospital, Basle, Switzerland*

* S. D. Shorvon   *Medical Director. The National Society for Epilepsy, Chalfont Centre for Epilepsy, Chalfont St Peter, Bucks, UK and Institute of Neurology, National Hospital, London, UK*

* M. de Silva   *Research Registrar in Paediatric Neurology, King's College Hospital, London, UK*

  J. A. Sorensen   *Electronics Institute, Technical University of Denmark, Lyngby, Denmark*

* G. Stores   *Reader in Psychiatry, University of Oxford, Oxford, UK*

  C. T. Swick   *Yale University School of Medicine, New Haven, CT, USA*

* R. Tallis   *Professor of Geriatric Medicine, Hope Hospital, Salford, UK*

* J. Taylor   *Chief Advisor to the Department of Transport, London, UK*

  J. Tjia   *Department of Pharmacology and Therapeutics, University of Liverpool, Liverpool, UK*

  R. Wolf   *Max Planck Institute for Psychiatry, Munich, Federal Republic of Germany*

List of Participants

(The following list is complete at 26 April 1989. We apologise for any omissions and/or errors)

UNITED KINGDOM AND REPUBLIC OF IRELAND

Dr R. Abraham
Consultant Neurophysiologist
Central Middlesex Hospital
London

Dr N. K. Agarwal
Consultant Paediatrician
Morriston Hospital
Swansea

Dr J. M. T. Alexander
Consultant Paediatrician
Pontefract General Infirmary
Pontefract, W. Yorks

Dr E. M. Allen
Consultant Clinical Neurophysiologist
Plymouth General Hospital
Plymouth

Mr G. Aplin
Manchester

Dr W. A. Arrowsmith
Consultant Paediatrician
Doncaster Royal Infirmary
Doncaster

Mr A. Aspinall
Chief Executive
British Epilepsy Association
Leeds

Mr I. C. Bailey
Consultant Neurological Surgeon
Royal Victoria Hospital
Belfast, NI

Dr R. Banks
Lecturer in Psychiatry of Mental Handicap
University of Sheffield
Sheffield

Dr R. P. C. Barclay
Consultant Paediatrician
Law Hospital
Carluke, Lanarkshire

Dr M. P. Barnes
Hon. Consultant Neurologist
Royal Victoria Infirmary
Newcastle-upon-Tyne

Dr. C. R. Barraclough
Consultant Neurologist
Midland Centre for Neurosurgery and Neurology
Smethwick

Dr D. Bates
Senior Lecturer in Neurology
Royal Victoria Infirmary
Newcastle-upon-Tyne

Mrs J. Bazley
Manchester

Mr. B. A. Bell
Consultant Neurosurgeon
Atkinson Morley's Hospital
London

Dr S. Bennett-Britton
Consultant Paediatrician
Good Hope District General Hospital
Sutton Coldfield

Dr I. Berg
Consultant Child Psychiatrist
Leeds General Infirmary
Leeds

Dr D. J. Berry
Principal Biochemist
New Cross Hospital
London

Dr F. M. C. Besag
Medical Director
Lingfield Hospital School
Lingfield, Surrey

Dr S. Bews
Manchester

Dr H. G. Boddie
Consultant Neurologist
North Staffs Royal Infirmary
Stoke-on-Trent

Mr A. E. Booth
Consultant Neurosurgeon
Walsgrave Hospital
Coventry

Dr A. R. J. Bosley
Consultant Paediatrician
North Devon District Hospital
Barnstaple, N. Devon

Dr E. Bradley
Consultant Psychiatrist
St George's Hospital Medical School
London

Dr G. P. Bray
Consultant Psychiatrist
Winterton Hospital
Sedgefield
Stockton-on-Tees

Dr D. Brickwood
Manchester

Mr M. Briggs
Consultant Neurosurgeon
Radcliffe Infirmary
Oxford

Dr S. W. Brown
Consultant Neuropsychiatrist
The David Lewis Centre for Epilepsy
Cheshire

Mrs V. Cairnie
Development Officer
Epilepsy Association of Scotland
Glasgow

Dr G. J. Calvert
Consultant Psychiatrist
Muckamore Abbey Hospital
Muckamore
Co. Antrim, NI

Dr R. Consiglio
Consultant Anaesthetist
Royal Preston Hospital
Preston

Dr M. A. Clarke
Consultant Paediatric Neurologist
Booth Hall Children's Hospital
Manchester

Dr M. J. Collins Walsh
Consultant Psychiatrist
Brothers of Charity
Limerick, Republic of Ireland

Dr N. Cookey
Paediatric Registrar
Sunderland District General Hospital
Sunderland

Dr C. W. B. Corkey
Consultant Paediatrician
Daisy Hill Hospital
Newry, Co. Down, NI

Dr R. N. Corston
Consultant Neurologist
New Cross Hospital
Wolverhampton

Dr A. J. Cottrell
Consultant Paediatrician
General Hospital
Bishop Auckland
Co. Durham

Dr I. R. Craig
Clinical Research Fellow/Geriatrics
Hope Hospital
Salford

Dr M. H. Cresswell
Consultant Paediatrician
Bedford General Hospital
Bedford

Dr A. J. Cronin
Consultant Paediatrician
Freedom Fields Hospital
Plymouth

Dr R. E. Cull
Consultant Neurologist
Royal Infirmary
Edinburgh

Dr S. Curran
Education Officer, (BEA Wales)
University Hospital of Wales
Cardiff

Dr A. A. Da Costa
Consultant Neurophysiologist
St James's University Hospital
Leeds

Dr A. Davidson
Research Assistant in Epilepsy
Dundee Royal Infirmary
Dundee

Dr R. E. Day
Consultant Paediatrician
Royal Hospital for Sick Children
Glasgow

Dr C. I. Dellaportas
Clinical Assistant/Neurology
Charing Cross Hospital
London

Dr J. S. Duncan
Registrar in Neurology
National Hospital for Nervous Diseases
London

Dr P. Eames
Consultant Neuropsychiatrist
Burden Neurological Hospital
Bristol

Dr D. Easter
Manchester

Mr P. D. Ll. Edwards
Consultant Paediatrician
Princess of Wales Hospital
Bridgend, Mid Glamorgan

Dr R. T. M. Edwards
Consultant Physician
Dewi Sant Hospital
Pontypridd
Mid Glamorgan

Dr A. C. Elias-Jones
Senior Registrar in Paediatrics
Nottingham City Hospital
Nottingham

Dr C. J. K. Ellis
Consultant Neurologist
Poole General Hospital
Poole,
Dorset

Dr R. Elwes
Research Registrar
King's College Hospital
London

Dr J. Fallowfield
Manchester

Dr P. R. W. Fawcett
Consultant Clinical Neurophysiologist
Newcastle General Hospital
Newcastle-upon-Tyne

Dr J. A. Finnegan
Consultant Clinical Neurophysiologist
Selly Oak Hospital
Birmingham

Dr E. Fischbacher
Associate Specialist in Mental Handicap
Gogarburn Hospital
Edinburgh

Dr H. M. Fleet
Consultant Paediatrician
High Wycombe Hospital
High Wycombe,
Bucks

Dr D. M. Flynn
Consultant Paediatrician
Royal Free Hospital
London

Dr H. Foley
Consultant Neuropaediatrician
St Luke's Hospital
Guildford,
Surrey

Mrs J. Forbes
Manchester

Dr W. I. Forsythe
Consultant Paediatrician
Leeds General Infirmary
Leeds

Dr T. J. Fowler
Consultant Neurologist
Brook Hospital
London

Dr J. E. Fox
Consultant Clinical Neurophysiologist
Midland Centre for Neurosurgery and
Neurology
Smethwick

Dr T. French
Consultant Paediatrician
Musgrove Park Hospital
Taunton, Somerset

Dr M. K. Ghosh
Consultant Physician in Geriatric Medicine
Rotherham District General Hospital
Rotherham

Dr J. D. Gibson
Consultant Neurologist
Derriford Hospital
Plymouth

Dr R. Godwin-Austen
Consultant Neurologist
University Hospital
Nottingham

Dr A. Goodwin
Consultant Paediatrician
West Wales Hospital
Carmarthen, Dyfed

Dr R. H. Gosling
Consultant in Pharmaceutical Medicine
Altrincham, Cheshire

Dr J. Gray
Consultant Physician
Quarriers Homes Epilepsy Centre
Bridge of Weir, Renfrewshire

Dr R. C. D. Greenhall
Consultant Neurologist
Radcliffe Infirmary
Oxford

Dr E. J. W. Gumpert
Consultant Neurologist
Royal Hallamshire Hospital
Sheffield

Dr A. K. Gupta
Consultant Neurophysiologist
Dudley Road Hospital
Birmingham

Dr D. Hall
Consultant Paediatrician
St George's Hospital
London

Dr Y. Hart
Clinical Research Fellow
Chalfont Centre for Epilepsy
Chalfont St Peter, Bucks

Dr O. Hensey
Consultant Paediatrician
Central Remedial Clinic
Dublin, Republic of Ireland

Dr E. M. Hicks
Consultant Paediatric Neurologist
Royal Belfast Hospital for Sick Children
Belfast, NI

Dr M. Hildick-Smith
Consultant in Geriatric Medicine
Nunnery Fields Hospital
Canterbury, Kent

Dr D. Hilton-Jones
Consultant Neurologist
Radcliffe Infirmary
Oxford

Dr P. Hoare
Senior Lecturer in Child Psychiatry
Royal Hospital for Sick Children
Edinburgh

Dr J. M. Hockaday
Consultant Paediatric Neurologist
John Radcliffe Hospital
Oxford

Dr S. Hollins
Senior Lecturer in Mental Handicap
St George's Hospital Medical School
London

Mr A. E. Holmes
Consultant Neurosurgeon
Addenbrooke's Hospital
Cambridge

Mr R. Holmes
Chief Executive
Irish Epilepsy Association
Dublin, Republic of Ireland

Dr H. Hood
Regional Director
British Epilepsy Association
Belfast, NI

Dr D. J. Howard
Consultant Geriatrician
St Margaret's Hospital
Swindon, Wilts

Dr F. M. Howard
Consultant Paediatrician
Frimley Park Hospital
Camberly, Surrey

Dr D. P. M. Howells
Consultant Physician
Burton General Hospital
Burton on Trent, Staffs

Dr J. Inglis
Consultant Paediatrician
Doncaster Royal Infirmary
Doncaster

Dr I. A. Ismail
Consultant Psychiatrist
Leicester Frith Hospital
Leicester

Professor P. M. Jeavons
Visiting Professor
Department of Vision Sciences
Aston University
Birmingham

Dr J. Jenkins
Consultant Paediatrician
Waveney Hospital
Ballymena, Co. Antrim, NI

Dr S. K. M. Jivani
Consultant Paediatrician
Queen's Park Hospital
Blackburn

Dr A. L. Johnson
Medical Statistician
MRC Biostatistics Unit
Cambridge

Dr M. Johnson
Consultant Neurologist
St James's University Hospital
Leeds

Dr R. Johnson
Director of Postgraduate Medical Education
John Radcliffe Hospital
Oxford

Mr F. G. Johnston
Lecturer in Neurosurgery
Atkinson Morley's Hospital
London

Dr R. H. T. Jones
Consultant Paediatrician
Princess of Wales Hospital
Bridgend, Mid Glamorgan

Mr R. M. Kalbag
Consultant Neurosurgeon
Newcastle General Hospital
Newcastle-upon-Tyne

Dr C. B. Karki
Senior Registrar
Stoke Park Hospital
Bristol

Dr D. A. J. Keegan
Consultant Physician
Altnagelvin Hospital
Londonderry, NI

Mr A. Kelleher
Manchester

Dr R. E. Kelly
Hon. Consultant Neurologist
National Hospital for Nervous Diseases
London

Dr C. Kennard
Consultant Neurologist
The London Hospital
London

Mr A. Keogh
Consultant Neurosurgeon
Royal Preston Hospital
Preston

Dr A. Khan
Consultant Physician
Royal Shrewsbury Hospital
Shrewsbury

Dr J. G. Kirker
Consultant Neurologist
St James's Hospital
Dublin, Republic of Ireland

Dr D. R. Knight
Consultant Psychiatrist
St Crispin Hospital
Northampton

Dr P. Lakhani
Consultant Paediatrician
Milton Keynes Hospital
Milton Keynes, Bucks

Dr M. J. Ledwith
Medical Director
Brothers of Charity
Limerick, Republic of Ireland

Dr M. M. Liberman
Consultant Paediatrician
Northwick Park Hospital
Harrow, Middlesex

Dr J. Lim
Consultant Paediatrician
Waveney Hospital
Ballymena, Co. Antrim, NI

Dr S. M. J. Linford
Consultant Psychiatrist
Royal Shrewsbury Hospital
Shrewsbury

Dr L. A. Loizou
Consultant Neurologist
Pinderfields General Hospital
Wakefield, W. Yorkshire

Dr M. Loizou
Consultant Psychiatrist
Norman House
Harrogate, W. Yorks

Dr M. F. Lowry
Consultant Paediatrician
Sunderland District General Hospital
Sunderland

Dr B. M. MacArdle
Consultant Paediatrician
Northwick Park Hospital
Harrow, Middlesex

Dr I. G. Mannall
Consultant Paediatrician
Halifax General Hospital
Halifax, W. Yorks

Dr D. Manning
Senior Registrar in Paediatrics
Ryegate Children's Centre
Sheffield

Dr B. Mason
Consultant Paediatrician
Worcester Royal Infirmary
Worcester

Dr R. F. Massey
Consultant Paediatrician
Hull Royal Infirmary
Hull

Mr J. W. McIntosh
Consultant Neurosurgeon
North Staffs Royal Infirmary
Stoke-on-Trent

Dr J. McKenna
Consultant Physician
Sligo General Hospital
Sligo, Republic of Ireland

Dr R. O. McKeran
Consultant Neurologist
Atkinson Morley's Hospital
London

Dr J. B. McMenamin
Consultant Paediatric Neurologist
Our Lady's Hospital for Sick Children
Dublin, Republic of Ireland

Dr G. P. McMullin
Consultant Paediatrician
Warrington District General Hospital
Warrington

Dr P. K. A. McWilliam
Hospital Practitioner in Paediatrics
The General Infirmary
Pontefract, W. Yorks

Dr H. G. H. Meierkord
Clinical Research Registrar
The National Hospital
London

D. W. Michael
Consultant Neurologist
Brook Hospital
London

Mr C. Middlefell
Manchester

Dr R. Miles
Consultant Paediatrician
Hinchingbrooke Hospital
Huntingdon, Cambs

Dr J. D. Mitchell
Consultant Neurologist
Royal Preston Hospital
Preston

Dr P. D. Mohr
Consultant Neurologist
Hope Hospital
Salford

Dr H. P. Monaghan
Consultant Neuropaediatrician
Our Lady's Hospital for Sick Children
Dublin, Republic of Ireland

Dr J. I. Morrow
Hon. Senior Registrar/Clinical Lecturer
University of Wales College of Medicine
Cardiff

Mr A. Muirhead
Manchester

Dr M. A. Nasar
Consultant Paediatrician
Bridlington & District Hospital
Bridlington

Dr C. G. H. Newman
Consultant Paediatrician
Queen Mary's Hospital
London

Dr E. A. Nieman
Consultant Neurologist
St Mary's Hospital
London

Mr D. Nodder
Manchester

Dr M. J. Noronha
Consultant Paediatric Neurologist
Royal Manchester Children's Hospital
Manchester

Dr G. O'Brien
Director of Mental Handicap
Brothers of Charity Services
Waterford, Republic of Ireland

Dr A. Palit
Consultant Paediatrician
Withybush Hospital
Haverford West, Dyfed

Dr D. M. Park
Consultant Neurologist
Southend Hospital
Westcliff on Sea, Essex

Dr J. L. W. Parker
Consultant Physician
St George's Hospital
Lincoln

Dr J. D. Parkes
Reader in Neurology
King's College Hospital
London

Dr H. R. Patel
Consultant Paediatrician
Joyce Green Hospital
Dartford, Kent

Dr J. M. S. Pearce
Consultant Neurologist
Hull Royal Infirmary
Hull

Dr E. W. Poole
Consultant in Clinical Neurophysiology
The Radcliffe Infirmary
Oxford

Dr D. J. Poulton
Hon. Senior Registrar in Paediatrics
John Radcliffe Hospital
Oxford

Dr M. Prendergast
Consultant Child Psychiatrist
Birmingham Children's Hospital
Birmingham

Dr R. W. G. Prescott
Consultant General Physician
Bishop Auckland General Hospital
Bishop Auckland, Co. Durham

Dr P. Price
Consultant Physician
Princess Margaret Hospital
Swindon, Wilts

Dr B. L. Priestley
Consultant Paediatrician
The Children's Hospital
Sheffield

Dr R. E. Pugh
Leighton Hospital
Crewe

Dr R. J. M. Quinn
Consultant Paediatrician
Altnagelvin Hospital
Londonderry, NI

Dr P. A. B. Raffle
Chairman
Medical Commission on Accident Prevention
London

Dr E. Ragi
Senior Registrar in Clinical Neurophysiology
Dudley Road Hospital
Birmingham

Dr C. Rajagopal
Consultant Paediatrician
Duchess of Kent's Military Hospital
Catterick, N. Yorks

Dr R. J. Regan
Consultant Physician
Amersham General Hospital
Amersham, Bucks

Dr B. Reynolds
Consultant Paediatrician
Grimsby District General Hospital
Grimsby

Dr I. F. Roberts
Consultant Paediatrician
Chesterfield & North Derbyshire
Royal Hospital
Chesterfield

Dr A. Robinson
Consultant Paediatrician
Wythenshawe Hospital
Manchester

Mr P. Rogan
Chairman
Mersey Epilepsy Association
Liverpool

Dr S. H. Roussounis
Consultant Paediatrician
St James' University Hospital
Leeds

Dr N. de M. Rudolf
Consultant Clinical Neurophysiologist
Charing Cross Hospital
London

Dr S. A. W. Salfield
Consultant Paediatrician
Rotherham District General Hospital
Rotherham

Dr J. W. Sander
Clinical Research Fellow
Chalfont Centre for Epilepsy
Chalfont St Peter, Bucks

Dr W. H. Schutt
Consultant Paediatric Neurologist
Tyndalls Park Children's Centre
Bristol

Dr M. S. Schwartz
Consultant Neurophysiologist
Atkinson Morley's Hospital
London

Dr O. E. P. Shanks
Consultant Psychiatrist
Muckamore Abbey Hospital
Muckamore, Co. Antrim

Dr D. I. Shepherd
Consultant Neurologist
North Manchester General Hospital
Manchester

Dr F. G. Simpson
Consultant Physician
Shotley Bridge General Hospital
Consett, Co. Durham

Mr W. Singarayer
Manchester

Dr D. Smith
Research Registrar
Walton Hospital
Liverpool

Dr D. P. L. Smythe
Consultant Paediatrician
St Mary's Hospital
London

Dr J. A. Spillane
Consultant Neurologist
Midland Centre for Neurosurgery & Neurology
Smethwick

Dr E. G. S. Spokes
Consultant Neurologist
Leeds General Infirmary
Leeds

Dr G. D. Stark
Consultant Paediatrician
Royal Hospital for Sick Children
Edinburgh

Mr I. Steward
Manchester

Dr R. J. Stocks
Consultant Paediatrician
James Paget Hospital
Gt Yarmouth, Norfolk

Dr D. W. Sumner
Hon. Lecturer in Neurology
University of Leeds
Leeds

Dr G. Supramanian
Consultant Paediatrician
Watford General Hospital
Watford

Dr N. J. Tangney
Consultant Paediatrician
Bon Secours Hospital
Cork, Republic of Ireland

Dr M. A. Tettenborn
Consultant Paediatrician
Eastbourne District General Hospital
Eastbourne, East Sussex

Dr P. J. B. Tilley
Consultant Neurologist
General Hospital
Middlesbrough, Cleveland

Dr P. C. Trevisol-Bittencourt
Research Fellow
Chalfont Centre for Epilepsy
Chalfont St Peter, Bucks

Dr M. R. Trimble
Consultant Physician
The National Hospital for Nervous Diseases
London

Dr A. M. Turner
Consultant Neurologist
Southampton General Hospital
Southampton

Dr R. M. Tyler
Consultant Paediatrician
Chesterfield & North Derbyshire Royal Hospital
Chesterfield

Mr D. Uttley
Consultant Neurosurgeon
Atkinson Morley's Hospital
London

Dr M. J. Vaizey
Consultant Paediatrician
Pilgrim Hospital
Boston, Lincs

Dr G. S. Venables
Consultant Neurologist
Royal Hallamshire Hospital
Sheffield

Dr H. Vaughan
Manchester

Dr C. M. Verity
Consultant Paediatric Neurologist
Addenbrooke's Hospital
Cambridge

Dr G. B. Wallace
Senior Registrar in Paediatric Neurology
Booth Hall Children's Hospital
Manchester

Mr A. Waters
Hon. Consultant Neurosurgeon
Addenbrooke's Hospital
Cambridge

Dr R. W. Watt
Consultant Paediatrician
Bolton General Hospital
Bolton

Mrs P. Watts
Manchester

Dr L. A. Wilson
Consultant Neurologist
Royal Free Hospital
London

Mr R. A. Wing CBE
Manchester

Mr G. Yaffé
Manchester

Dr J. A. Young
Consultant Paediatric Neurologist
Ninewells Hospital
Dundee

Dr Z. Zaiwalla
Clinical Lecturer
Park Hospital for Children
Oxford
Mrs P. Castree
Mrs S. Mangan
Sanofi UK Limited
Manchester

INTERNATIONAL DELEGATES

Belgium
Dr P. Boon
Mr P. Verschelde

Denmark
Dr Grethe Anderson
Dr Mogens Angelo-Nielsen
Dr Jette Boas
Dr Marit Dahl
Dr Mogens Laue Friis
Dr Flemming Juul Hansen
Dr Per Evald Hansen
Dr Vibeke Holsteen
Dr Hans Hogenhaven
Dr J. P. A. Jensen
Dr Bo Johansen
Dr Finn Ursin Knudsen
Dr Axel Lademann
Dr Inge-Merete Nielsen
Mr Hans Orum
Dr Soren Anker Pedersen
Dr Knud Kjaersgaard Pedersen
Dr Jorge Petrera
Dr Niels H. Rasmussen
Dr Anne Sabers
Dr Niels Simonsen
Dr Jogen Therkelsen
Dr Sven Vestermark
Dr Jorgen Wendelboe
Dr Mogens Worm
Dr Jorgen Worm-Petersen

Finland
Mr Juhani Hares
Dr Tapani Karanen
Dr Matti Livanainen
Dr Mauri Reunanen
Mr Kauka Ruppa
Dr Matti Sillanpaa
Dr Olli Waltimo

France
Professor Michel Baldy-Moulinier
Mlle Viviane Broustassoux
Professor J. P. Cano
Dr Patrick Chauvel
Dr Claudine Colas
Mr P. Douillet

Dr Paul Favel
Dr Joseph Feurstein
Dr Gerard Frangin
Dr Pierre Genton
Dr Pierre Jallon
Dr Andre Perret
Dr Joseph Roger
Dr Guy Venaud

Federal Republic of Germany
Professor H. H. von Albert
Dr H. E. Boenigk
Dr P. Bulau
Dr N. Diederich
Dr G. Gulla
Professor Korinthenberg
Professor R. Kruse
Dr M. C. Laub
Professor D. Palm
Dr S. Read
Mr H. E. Salzmann
Dr H. Schneble
Dr G. Schreiber
Dr Schulz
Dr S. Stodieck
Mr H. R. Thorbecke

Greece
Dr A. Kovanis
Dr E. Zografos

The Netherlands
Dr G. Akkerhuis
Dr H. Anten
Dr W. Arts
Dr P. Beneder
Ms H. de Boer
Dr M. Bomhof
Dr A. Boon
Mr J. Bot
Dr H. Bottger
Dr T. Breuer
Dr O. Brouwer
Dr F. Bussemaker
Dr J. Doelman
Dr C. van Donsellaar
Mr M. Duinspee
Dr H. Evenblij
Dr C. Franke
Dr J. Geelen
Dr R. de Graaf
Dr van der Graaf
Dr C. Gijsbers
Dr G. de Haan
Dr G. Hageman
Dr W. Hoefnagels
Dr R. ten Houten
Madam L'Huizer

Dr G. de Jong
Dr P. de Jong
Dr A. Koelemay
Dr E. Koppejan
Dr J. Kuster
Dr P. Lambregts
Dr G. Lassouw
Dr G. van Meer
Dr J. van de Meulen
Dr R. Meijer
Dr O. Mulder
Mr J. de Neef
Dr L. Oei
Dr C. van Oorschot
Dr R. Oosterkamp
Mr C. Peper
Dr A. Peters
Mr P. Pop
Dr P. Raedts
Dr W. Renier
Dr L. Rotteveel
Dr F. Scholtes
Dr T. Segeren
Dr H. Stroink
Dr P. Stuurman
Dr C. Tijssen
Dr J. Vanneste
Dr M. Veering
Dr P. Verlooy
Dr P. Vink
Dr J. Vles
Dr E. Vries
Dr P. Voskuil
Dr M. Wittebol

Hong Kong
Dr Virginia Wong

India
Dr Chakravarty
Dr U. P. Dave
Dr V. S. Saxena

Portugal
Dr Jose Pimental
Dr Margarida Santiago
Dr Antonio N. Da Silva

Spain
Professor Manuel Nieto Barrera
Mr Luis Oller Ferrer-Vidal
Professor Manuel Noya
Mr Ignacio Pascual-Castroviejo
Mm Ines Picornell
Professor Javier Salas Puig
Mlle Fabiola Rius Vesga

Mr Jose Prats Vinas
Professor Cesar Viteri

Sweden
Dr Gunnar Ahlsten
Dr Bo Andersson
Dr Jurgen Bensch
Dr Gosta Blennow
Mr Bo Creutzer
Dr Milada Duchek
Professor Orvar Eeg-Olofsson
Dr Rolf Ekberg
Mr Goran Ericson
Dr Hans Gylje
Dr Per Hilton-Brown
Dr Bengt Hindfeldt
Dr Eva Hoglund-Kumlien
Dr Bengt Holmberg
Dr Stig Kihlstrand
Dr Jorgen Kinnman
Dr Marten Kyllerman
Dr Bo Laestadius
Dr Hans Lindehammar
Dr Per Lindstrom
Dr Bjorn Lundberg
Dr Kikael Lundvall
Dr Bengt Nilsson
Dr Gunnar Nordin
Dr Lars Noren
Dr P-O. Osterman
Dr Sven Palhagen
Dr Ragnar Palm
Dr Lennart Persson
Dr Bo Stromberg
Dr Anders Sundqvist
Dr Bernt Tonnby
Dr Jan-Eric Wedlund

Switzerland
Dr A. Beaumoir
Dr B. Blajev
Professor G. Dumermuth
Mr M. Favrod
Dr B. Geudelin
Dr Ch. Haenggeli
Dr U. E. Honegger
Dr A. Kohler
Mr F. Leunenberger
Dr R. Markoff
Dr H. Matthis
Dr G. de Meuron
Dr Ch. Meyer
Dr J. Penzien
Dr P. V. Rai
Dr O. Staheli
Professor F. Vassella
Dr S. Zagury

Contents

Group Response Interactive Video System

During the Fourth International Symposium on Sodium Valproate and Epilepsy delegates had a chance to respond to speakers directly by using new technology in the shape of a Group Response Interactive Video System.

Each delegate was provided with an individual calculator style keypad, which was connected to all the other keypads in the main auditorium and to a microcomputer.

Each speaker was asked before the symposium whether they would like to pose multiple choice questions to the audience. A number of speakers accepted this invitation. These questions were posed, as were other spontaneous questions by both Chairmen and speakers.

The collective audience responses were displayed on a screen as histograms showing the percentage of the audience choosing each answer option.

Owing to lack of space in this publication it has not been possible to show the audience response in the form of histograms but only in the form of a printed question and response.

The Sanofi Epilepsy Essay Competition

This was a competition sponsored by Sanofi Pharma in which Registrars and Senior Registrars were invited to submit essays on a choice of topics associated with Epilepsy.

The titles were as follows:

1. 'The Financial and Social Costs of Epilepsy'.

   OR

2. 'Advances in Genetics and their Application to Epilepsy'.

The winner, Dr Jo Poulton, Honorary Senior Registrar in Paediatrics, John Radcliffe Hospital, Oxford, presented her paper at the Fourth International Symposium on Sodium Valproate and Epilepsy.

There were also two joint runners up:

Dr Hartmut Meierkord, Registrar, the National Hospital for Nervous Diseases, London.

AND

Dr James Morrow, Senior Registrar, University of Wales College of Medicine, Cardiff

The awards were presented by Professor Peter Jeavons, visiting Professor in the Department of Ophthalmic Optics, University of Aston, Birmingham.

Sodium Valproate (or Valproic Acid) is available in those countries from which delegates participated in the 4th International Symposium on Sodium Valproate and Epilepsy in Jersey as follows:

EPILIM   UK, Republic of Ireland and Hong Kong

DEPAKINE   Belgium, France, Greece, Portugal, Spain, Switzerland and the Netherlands

DEPRAKINE   Denmark and Finland

ERGENYL   Federal Republic of Germany and Sweden

EPILEX   India

DEPAKENE   USA

Introduction

It is a pleasure to welcome you to this Fourth International Symposium on Sodium Valproate and Epilepsy.

The first was held at Nottingham University in 1975 shortly after the introduction of sodium valproate to the United Kingdom market. The second Symposium was held in Birmingham in 1979 and a third in Guernsey in 1983. On each occasion there have been increasing numbers of participants from outside the United Kingdom and I would particularly like to welcome speakers and delegates from France, Republic of Ireland, Switzerland, Federal Republic of Germany, Belgium, The Netherlands, Sweden, Denmark, Finland, Spain, Portugal, Greece, Hong Kong, India and the United States of America.

The programme is extensive and varied and offers the opportunity to assess the place of sodium valproate as a mature antiepileptic drug in the management of epilepsy. The speakers all enjoy an international reputation and I am sure we can expect the scientific content of the programme to be of the highest standard. The subjects covered include the applications of sodium valproate in childhood and adult epilepsies and its adverse effects as well as broader questions of patient management and quality of life in epilepsy. The field of new indications for the use of valproate is also covered. As well as formal presentations we are using interactive video techniques to facilitate communications and your involvement in the Symposium. I hope that we shall have a lively and enjoyable Symposium and I greatly appreciate the honour of being asked by Sanofi to be the President of this Symposium.

David Chadwick
Consultant Neurologist
Walton Hospital, Liverpool

OPENING SESSION

The classification of epilepsy

S. D. Shorvon

Institute of Neurology, National Hospital, London, UK

INTRODUCTION

Throughout its history, epilepsy has been classified in many different ways, none of which have been either comprehensive or completely satisfactory. A major issue has been the distinction between an empirical and a scientific classification. This was recognized by Hughlings Jackson (1), over a century ago. Jackson realized that many classifications were groupings simply for convenience. Such an empirical classification would not necessarily follow a scientific principle, and although an empirical classification might well suit physicians for normal clinical purposes, it would fail to satisfy the needs of scientific enquiries. As Jackson elegantly wrote: 'Whilst it is convenient to consider a whale as a fish for legal purposes, it would never do to consider it so in zoology!' As usual, Jackson had put his finger on the crucial dilemma facing all those constructing modern epilepsy classifications, and this dilemma has yet to be fully resolved.

Epilepsy might be classified in any one of a number of ways (Table 1). A classification by aetiology, for instance, might seem appropriate as the aetiology of many neurological diseases is of paramount importance. However, the same aetiology may produce seizures of widely differing types in differing people, or indeed different types of seizures at different times in the same person. A cerebral glioma for instance, may cause apparently primary or secondarily generalized seizures, complex partial or simple partial seizures. This is a reflection of the fact that the phenomenon of epilepsy is largely dependent on electro-physiological and anatomical features, rather than the underlying causative pathology. A classification on an anatomical basis has attractions because the clinical phenomenology of the seizure is to a large extent a reflection of the part of the brain activated by the electrical disturbance. An anatomical classification is particularly useful in focal neocortical seizures, especially of frontal or occipital origin, but is less satisfactory for mesial temporal lobe attacks, or limbic seizures, perhaps due to the rapid and diffuse spread of the seizure activity. Anatomical classifications are also much less satisfactory in regard to generalized seizures, reflecting our ignorance of the underlying anatomical basis of most generalized seizure types. The demonstration that focal stimulation of certain cortical areas, especially mesial frontal cortices, can produce generalized seizures (absence or tonic-clonic), for instance, makes an anatomical classification difficult to apply or utilize coherently. In the recognition, perhaps, that epilepsy is a functional event, overriding anatomical or aetiological factors, a classification might be based on EEG findings. In some instances, for example in petit mal attacks, this approach is worthwhile, and a reasonably consistent entity can be defined in terms of its EEG. However, even here, this pattern is not specific and the three Hz spike-wave discharge, which is typical of petit mal, may also be seen rarely in some focal epilepsies and in other types of generalized epilepsies, which neither have the form of petit mal, nor are necessarily primarily generalized. In routine practice also, the EEG is often normal and the ictal and interictal EEGs may be contradictory or confusing. Furthermore, EEG findings may differ minute by minute and a classification on the basis of EEG would therefore not be easy to apply. Classification by age is

Fourth international symposium on sodium valproate and epilepsy, edited by David Chadwick, 1989; Royal Society of Medicine Services International Congress and Symposium Series No. 152, published by Royal Society of Medicine Services Limited.

Table 1 *Possible criteria for classifying the epilepsies*

Aetiology
Anatomical basis
EEG
    ictal
    interictal
Age
Clinical phenomenology (e.g. seizure type)

another possible way of differentiating epilepsy, particularly in young children where the forms of epilepsy may most reflect the stage of cerebral maturity, rather than the aetiology EEG or anatomy of the epilepsy. It is not uncommon, for instance, for a child with tuberous sclerosis to develop clonic seizures in infancy, which evolve to infantile spasms in the first year of life, and subsequently to complex partial or grand mal seizures in later childhood. In adult epilepsy, however, the classification by age has little attraction and age is a poor determinant of most features of the epilepsy.

ILAE CLASSIFICATION OF SEIZURE TYPE (2,3)

The commonest method of classifying epilepsy is by its clinical phenomenology—especially by seizure type. Before 1969, there were a number of classifications in common use, and the International League Against Epilepsy (ILAE) set up a Commission of Classification to review, simplify and rationalize these schemes. A new classification scheme was produced in 1969, which was a landmark in epilepsy history (2). In 1981, this classification was revised and the 1981 revision is shown in Table 2 (3). The principal changes between the 1969 and 1981 classification are shown in Table 3. This ILAE seizure type classification has proved enormously successful, and has been widely taken up. It should not be forgotten, however, that this is still an *empirical* classification and *non-scientific* in Jackson's terms; and as such has definite limitations. The classification is so well known that there is no need to describe it in detail, although it would be worth outlining some problems which limit its value.

There are several problems of definition. Simple and partial seizures are to be distinguished in this classification scheme by whether or not consciousness has been impaired. Consciousness is notoriously difficult to define (and indeed is not clearly defined

Table 2 *1981 Classification of epileptic seizures*

Partial seizures (seizures beginning locally)
(A) Simple partial seizures (consciousness not impaired)
    1. With motor signs
    2. With somatosensory or special sensory symptoms
    3. With autonomic symptoms
    4. With psychic symptoms
(B) Complex partial seizures (with impairment of consciousness)
    1. Beginning as simple partial seizures and progressing to impairment of consciousness
    2. With impairment of consciousness at onset
        (a) With impairment of consciousness only
        (b) With automatisms
(C) Partial seizures secondarily generalized

Generalized seizures (bilaterally symmetrical and without local onset)
(A) 1. Absence seizures
    2. Atypical absence
(B) Myoclonic seizures
(C) Clonic seizures
(D) Tonic seizures
(E) Tonic-clonic seizures
(F) Atonic seizures

Unclassified epileptic seizures (incomplete data)

Table 3 *Changes made to the 1981 classification from the 1969 scheme*

1. Anatomical basis, aetiology and age are ignored
2. The differentiation between simple and complex partial seizures is made on the basis of whether consciousness is impaired or maintained.
3. Unilateral seizures are classified under partial seizures
4. Compound forms, mixed forms and akinetic seizures are omitted
5. The classification allows progression from one seizure type to another

in the classification scheme), and its impairment is also notoriously difficult to detect. Furthermore, in some patients, the same seizure may cause loss of consciousness on one occasion and not on another. To base a primary division of epilepsy on such a distinction is therefore problematical. In practice, this distinction works well in most types of partial seizure (e.g. in the distinction between the Jacksonian motor seizure and the psychomotor temporal lobe seizure), but in a minority of cases difficulties arise. A second problem concerns the large number of seizures which may cross boundaries of the clinical classification. For instance, the commonly encountered attack in which a patient blanks out and falls to the ground and in which the EEG may show non-specific changes, may be classified by one physician as a complex partial seizure, by others as tonic, atonic, atypical absence or even atypical tonic-clonic seizures. A third problem concerns the concept of focality itself. The major categorization of this classification is into partial and generalized seizures. This distinction is based on whether a seizure begins locally or is bilaterally symmetrical without local onset. Again this differentiation works well with focal cortical seizures on the one hand and with the genetically determined generalized grand mal and absence seizures with three Hz spike-wave on the other. There are, however, many seizures in which it is unclear whether there is a focal or a generalized onset, and where this distinction is rather meaningless. This is further complicated by the well known clinical observation that stimulation of many cortical regions (e.g. mesial frontal regions), can produce apparently generalized absence and tonic-clonic seizures with EEG and clinical phenomenology which show no trace of a focal origin. It is also common clinical experience to find a cerebral tumour causing apparently generalized seizures. Indeed, it seems likely that many apparently generalized seizures may have a focal origin; and to base our classification on this distinction is often illusory. A final problem concerns the incorporation of the EEG. The 1981 classification is a classification of seizure type and EEG, yet the manner in which EEG data is to be incorporated is not clearly specified. In a complex partial seizure, for instance, the EEG can show a variety of forms or indeed be normal, even in the same patient, and yet the classification pays no cognizance of this. The fact that the interictal and ictal EEG may be so different is also a confounding feature. If one remembers that the

Table 4 *Anatomical and physiological classification of the epilepsies*

Frontal lobe epilepsies	—Rolandic epilepsy —Supplementary motor area epilepsy —Anterior frontal epilepsy —Mesial frontal —Frontal-polar —Orbital frontal
Temporal lobe epilepsy	—Mesial temporal sclerosis —Temporal neocortex —Limbic system epilepsy —Amygdala epilepsy
Parietal lobe epilepsy	
Occipital lobe epilepsy	
Cortico-reticular epilepsy	
Sub-cortical epilepsy	
Centrencephalic epilepsy	
Multifocal epilepsy	

classification of seizure type is essentially an empirical description, with limited anatomical, physiological or aetiological correlations, these anomalies should not surprise us.

COMPOUND CLASSIFICATIONS

It was in recognition of the limitations of the seizure type classification that other classifications have been proposed, based on aetiology, anatomical and physiological data and also clinical phenomenology. Such compound classifications are valuable in that they recognize the multitudinal influences in the production of epilepsy. One such classification is shown in Table 4 and is based on anatomical and physiological data. This is a useful approach, and one which is more closely tied to the essential basis of epilepsy, although such a classification poses a severe test to the physician or non-specialist neurologist. Furthermore, such a classification implies that we understand the anatomical and physiological basis of most epilepsy, which is patently not the case.

ILAE CLASSIFICATION OF EPILEPSIES AND EPILEPTIC SYNDROMES (4,5)

Because of the incomplete nature of other classifications, the ILAE commission on classification and terminology proposed a new classification scheme in 1985 (2). This was a classification of epilepsies and epileptic syndromes, rather than of seizure type. This classification is less well known, and yet is an important step towards reconciling the empirical and scientific approaches to epilepsy classification. The ILAE classification of epilepsies and epileptic syndromes is outlined in Table 5. The terminology is clumsy, and the classification complex, but this should not detract from its essential value.

As in the classification of epileptic seizures, the major groupings are according to whether the epilepsies have a focal or generalized nature. The focal epilepsies are called 'localization-related', and are divided into idiopathic and symptomatic categories. At present two idiopathic syndromes are established, which are the benign childhood epilepsies with centro-temporal spikes, and the childhood epilepsies with occipital paroxysms. Other syndromes may be established in the future, as these are recognized. It is noticeable that within this category are incorporated criteria of age, aetiology, EEG and clinical phenomenology. The anatomical and physiological basis of these epilepsies is currently unknown.

Amongst the symptomatic localizational epilepsies are all those syndromes which are the result of known or suspected cerebral pathology. Included here are the epilepsies associated with cerebral tumour, infection and so on. The individual seizure type will largely reflect the anatomical localization and the patterns of seizure spread, and the clinical features of these epilepsies will vary widely.

The generalized epilepsies are again defined as idiopathic or symptomatic. The idiopathic generalized epilepsies are divided into age-related syndromes, and no doubt this list will increase as the nosologists get to work. Currently there are seven categories, including benign neonatal familial convulsions, benign myoclonic epilepsy in infancy and juvenile absence and myoclonic epilepsies.

A second category of idiopathic and/or symptomatic epilepsies has been formed, which includes the West syndrome, Lennox-Gastaut syndrome and various forms of myoclonic epilepsy. These idiopathic generalized epilepsies pose a real difficulty in classification, and whether each is a specific syndrome is debatable. The Lennox-Gastaut syndrome for instance is felt by many to be a heterogeneous group of conditions, without internal coherence. The juvenile absence and myoclonic epilepsies and the awakening grand mal epilepsies may also be simply variations of the syndrome of primary generalized epilepsy. In such idiopathic cases, of course the underlying genetic or physiological basis is uncertain, and classification is therefore certain to be arbitrary.

The next category is that of the symptomatic generalized epilepsies. These are divided into those with a non-specific aetiology and those with a specific identifiable cause. The principle distinctions between the idiopathic generalized and the non-specific symptomatic

Table 5   *1985 International classification of epilepsies and epileptic syndromes*

1. Localization-related (focal, local, partial) epilepsies and syndromes
1.1 Idiopathic (with age-related onset)
   —benign childhood epilepsy with centro-temporal spike
   —childhood epilepsy with occipital paroxysms
1.2 Symptomatic
   This comprises various syndromes with identified aetiology.
   The phenomenology of the epilepsy will be based on anatomical localization, clinical features, and the patterns of speech.

2. Generalized epilepsies and syndromes
2.1 Idiopathic (with age related onset—listed in order of age)
   —benign neonatal familial convulsions
   —benign neonatal convulsions
   —benign myoclonal epilepsy in infancy
   —childhood absence epilepsy (pyknolepsy)
   —juvenile absence epilepsy
   —juvenile myoclonic epilepsy (impulsive petit mal)
   —epilepsy with grand mal seizures (GTCS) on awakening
   Other generalized idiopathic epilepsies, if they do not belong to one of the above syndromes, can still be classified as generalized idiopathic epilepsies.
2.2 Idiopathic and/or symptomatic (in order of age)
   —West syndrome (infantile spasms, Blitz-Nick-Salaam Krampfe)
   —Lennox-Gastaut syndrome
   —Epilepsy with myoclonic-astatic seizures
   —Epilepsy with myoclonic absences
2.3 Symptomatic
2.3.1 Non-specific aetiology
   —Early myoclonic encephalopathy
2.3.2 Specific syndromes
   —Epileptic seizures may complicate many disease states
   Under this heading are included those diseases in which seizures are a presenting or predominant feature.

3. Epilepsies and syndromes undetermined whether focal or generalized
3.1 With both generalized and focal seizures
   —Neonatal seizures
   —Severe myoclonic epilepsy in infancy
   Acquired epileptic aphasia (Landau-Kleffner syndrome)
3.2 Without unequivocal generalized or focal features
   All cases with generalized tonic-clonic seizures where clinical and EEG findings do not permit classification as early generalized or localization-related.

4. Special syndromes
4.1 Situation-related seizures
   —Febrile convulsions
   —Seizures related to other identifiable situations such as stress, hormonal, drugs, alcohol, sleep deprivation, etc.
4.2 Isolated apparently unprovoked epileptic events
4.3 Epilepsies characterized by specific modes of seizure precipitation
4.4 Chronic progressive epilepsia partialis continua of childhood

[*Based on (2) and (4)*].

generalized epilepsies is that the former are said to commence more often on a background of normal development and are not associated with abnormal neurological signs or interictal EEG disturbances. Such a distinction is difficult in such syndromes as the Lennox-Gastaut syndrome, and some syndromes are likely to change categorization as knowledge becomes more complete. In general, this classification of the generalized epilepsies is less satisfactory than other parts of this scheme.

The third major category in this classification scheme are 'epilepsies and syndromes undetermined whether focal or generalized'. These are sub-divided into those with generalized and focal seizures and those without unequivocal generalized or focal features.

This is a rather unsatisfactory rag-bag, which includes neonatal seizures and the acquired epileptic aphasia (Landau-Kleffner syndrome). Finally, the fourth category are the specific syndromes. These are divided into four sub-categories, the first being the 'situation-related' seizures, which include febrile convulsions and also seizures related to identifiable environmental precipitants such as alcohol, sleep deprivation and so on. The second category is isolated apparently unprovoked epileptic events. The third category is of the epilepsies characterized by specific modes of seizure precipitation and here are included the seizures precipitated by photic or auditory stimulation. The fourth subdivision is the chronic progressive epilepsia partialis continua of childhood.

The best thing about this new classification is that it is both flexible and expandable, and also not restricted to a classification by seizure type, with all the limitations that this implies. Rather it tries to incorporate aetiology, age, EEG, anatomical features and seizure type and precipitations. As new syndromes are identified, they may be easily slotted in. It also avoids the problem of defining consciousness and other seizure phenomenology.

There are, however, a number of difficulties, which should be outlined. Firstly, the classification is complex and clearly unusable in normal clinical circumstances. The terminology is clumsy, and at times obscure. The second problem is that the dichotomy between the generalized and focal epilepsies is still maintained. It is perhaps in recognition of this, and the fact that a proportion of epilepsies are not easily thus categorized, that the classification has a section of 'epilepsies and syndromes undetermined whether focal or generalized', and a final section of 'special syndromes'. A third point is that because this classification attempts to be all inclusive and comprehensive, it becomes extremely unwieldy. Mixed in with common syndromes are those which are extremely rare and also included are syndromes whose identity is contentious. In normal clinical practice, the majority of epilepsy seen will fall into categories 1.2, 3.2 and 4.1, and these categories are generally poorly defined. It might have been better not to attempt to be comprehensive, but to make a classification of well-defined syndromes only.

This classification nevertheless remains a useful framework on which to base our clinical and research experience. Eventually, such a classification of the epilepsies and epilepsy syndromes will replace the more limited seizure type classifications. In doing so, a step away from empiricism towards a more rational scientific approach will have been taken.

ACKNOWLEDGMENTS

I would like to acknowledge the support of the Sir Jules Thorn Charitable Trust, the Wellcome Trust and the National Fund for Crippling Diseases, for support for this work.

REFERENCES

(1) Taylor J, ed. *The selected writings of John Hughlings Jackson.*
(2) Gastaut H. Classification of the epilepsies. Proposal for an international classification. *Epilepsia* 1969; **10** (Suppl 3): 14–21.
(3) Commission on Classification and Terminology, International League Against Epilepsy. Proposed revision of clinical and electroencephalographic classification of epileptic seizures. *Epilepsia* 1981; **22**: 480–501.
(4) Commission on Classification and Terminology, International League Against Epilepsy. Proposal for classification of epilepsies and epileptic syndromes. *Epilepsia* 1985; **26**: 268–78.
(5) Dreifuss FE. The different types of epileptic seizures, and the international classification of epileptic seizures and of the epilepsies. In: A Hopkins, ed. *Epilepsy* London: Chapman & Hall, 1987: 83–113.

DISCUSSION

Dr Rajagopal *(Catterick, UK):* The problem with classification is that after a few years it becomes useless. Also there are children who have accommodation of more than one type, who do not fit any category at all.

Dr Shorvon *(Chalfont St Peter, UK):* I absolutely agree. The essential problem of classification is that our current classification schemes are based on empiric rather than rational data, because we do not fully understand the physiological basis of epilepsy. As our understanding increases, so perhaps, our classifications will improve. In the classification of seizure type and epileptic syndromes there is a space for unclassified attacks, and many children's epilepsies will fall into this category.

Professor Dreifuss *(Virginia, USA):* I would like to comment on the classification as it has been presented. One of the problems with people who interpret the classifications, is that they do not read the introduction, which clearly states how the classification has developed. It is inherent in this statement that the classification is expected to change with time and with the acquisition of new knowledge. In addition there are places in the classification which allow for evolution of individual seizures and syndromes, from the West syndrome to the Lennox-Gastaut syndrome. Finally one of the rationales for classification that is becoming increasingly evident is definition and identification of some of the syndromes on the human genome. For instance, juvenile myoclonic epilepsy, which is a disease and not just a syndrome, one can now supply a gene locus on the short arm of the sixth chromosome which in time will result in the unravelling of the genetic problem and the associated biochemical disturbance. For these reasons it is important to continue to try and refine the classification.

Dr Abraham *(London, UK):* It seems to me that a good classification survives because it is simple, particularly in a subject like epilepsy which is multi-disciplinary. The 1981 classification was simple and could be easily adapted by people who were not specialists in epilepsy whereas the 1985 classification that you advocate has the disadvantage that it cannot be rapidly incorporated by non-epileptologists.

Dr Shorvon *(Chalfont St Peter, UK):* I quite agree. This is a perennial problem. I am not sure that the 1981 classification was entirely understood by the majority of non-specialists, many of whom still talk about 'major' and 'minor' epilepsy. The problem with our attempts at classification is that if one attempts to refine it, it becomes intolerably complicated, but if one tries to simplify it, then errors and confusion arise.

Professor Tallis *(Salford, UK):* When you are defining a classification you have first to decide what you are doing. One aim is to help people distinguish, for instance, West syndrome or juvenile myoclonic epilepsy. The other apparent purpose of a classification system is to bring together in a single hierarchical tree the aetiology, neurophysiology, clinical phenomena etc. and that is where the problem arises. I think we have to distinguish between clearly differentiating separate conditions and the organization into a single hierarchical tree.

Dr Shorvon *(Chalfont St Peter, UK):* I fully agree. Some people, particularly non-specialists, assume the seizure type classification is the only classification of epilepsy. That is incorrect; and we should continually emphasize the difference between classification of seizure type and of the epilepsies. This problem, however, is compounded by the epilepsy specialists who continue to talk about seizure type classification as if it was the only possible scheme. That is why the classification of syndromes is so important.

SESSION I

ASPECTS OF PATIENT MANAGEMENT

Chairman: E. H. Reynolds

Cranial imaging in epilepsy

R. Duncan, I. Bone, D. Hadley and J. Patterson

Institute of Neurological Sciences, Southern General Hospital, Glasgow, UK

INTRODUCTION

The diagnosis of epilepsy is in most cases a clinical one. As yet no cranial imaging technique has any place in confirming that diagnosis, so that the indications for such investigation in epilepsy fall into two categories: imaging undertaken to establish a cause for seizures and imaging undertaken to locate the source of a seizure focus so that surgery can take place. The former is the indication for most examinations at present, but the latter will assume increasing importance as surgical treatment for epilepsy is more frequently considered. X-ray computed tomography (CT) and magnetic resonance imaging (MRI) image brain structure. Positron emission tomography (PET) and single photon emission tomography (SPECT) image brain function.

X-RAY COMPUTED TOMOGRAPHY (CT)

CT continues to be the most commonly used technique to detect or exclude a structural cause for seizures. It is not carried out in all patients with epilepsy, so can widely accepted guidelines for its use be established?

The incidence of focal causative lesions demonstrated on CT rises with age (1–3). Approximately 60% of patients over 70 years of age show a focal lesion on CT, most commonly stroke (1,4). While in the majority of cases the demonstrated cause requires no specific treatment (5), one series found five out of 80 epileptic patients presenting with epilepsy at over 40 years of age to have meningiomas (6). The incidence of focal structural lesions is higher in epilepsy of focal onset, particularly in focal motor epilepsy (1,5,7). When epilepsy presents with status epilepticus, a significant proportion of patients have a structural lesion, often of the frontal lobe (8). The demonstration of focal pathology does not necessarily alter management. Surgically accessible benign lesions such as arteriovenous malformation or meningioma may be partially or totally removed in order to influence the progression of the disease process, but in those circumstances the epilepsy may not be improved by such treatment, and indeed may worsen. There is no evidence that early detection and aggressive treatment of malignant lesions by surgery or radiotherapy will greatly improve the duration or quality of remaining life (9).

Clear guidance on the use of CT can therefore be given in some situations at least. Epilepsy presenting with status epilepticus, focal motor seizures (or generalized seizures with focal motor onset), and epilepsy with progressively deteriorating control are all indications for CT. Patients with indications of structural disease such as focal neurological signs or focal delta discharge on EEG should have CT. It should be remembered that a symptomatic tumour may present with epilepsy while still too small to show on CT (5), underlining the need for clinical review, and a readiness to repeat scanning if need be. There is, however, no clear indication in the literature whether epilepsy of onset after a given age is in itself an indication for CT. It would seem reasonable to recommend that patients presenting

Fourth international symposium on sodium valproate and epilepsy, edited by David Chadwick, 1989; Royal Society of Medicine Services International Congress and Symposium Series No. 152, published by Royal Society of Medicine Services Limited.

with their first seizure from the ages of 30 to 60 should be scanned. After the age of 60, the chances of a lesion responsible for seizures being in itself amenable to therapy become small, but there may be justification for CT even then. The detection of a structural lesion may well lead to earlier treatment of the epilepsy (1), and may be of value in determining long term prognosis. Moreover, the therapeutic value of the negative scan should not be underestimated (10).

MAGNETIC RESONANCE IMAGING (MRI)

Many of the considerations applying to CT also apply to MRI, but its increased sensitivity to small changes in tissue water content and binding (11) give it an overall advantage in detecting subtle lesions in epilepsy. Several studies have compared the two imaging modalities in temporal lobe epilepsy (12–16). Most have been of patients with intractable disease, and have shown abnormalities in 10–25% of patients with normal CT. In one study of CT-normal patients with well controlled disease (16) MRI detected abnormalities in 50%. This superiority applies even where low field MRI is compared with high resolution CT using cuts angled to image temporal lobe structures with minimum bone interference (17). Pathological correlation of MRI findings following temporal lobectomy showed that a variety of lesions such as low grade gliomas, haematomas, vascular malformations and mesial temporal sclerosis were responsible for the signal abnormalities (Fig. 1) (14,18). While CT

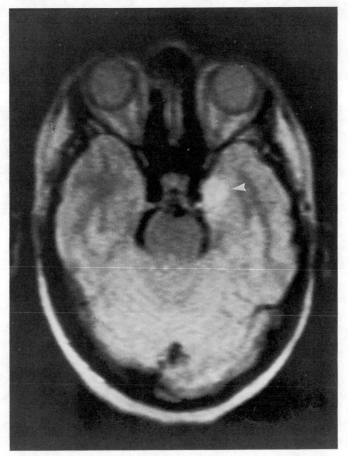

Figure 1 *Axial T2 weighted MRI image showing a high signal area in the mesial left temporal lobe (arrow) of a 31 year old woman with temporal lobe epilepsy. CT was normal.*

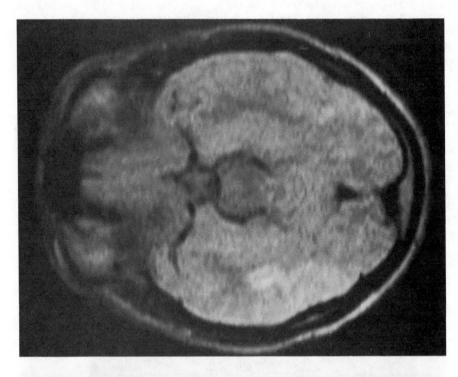

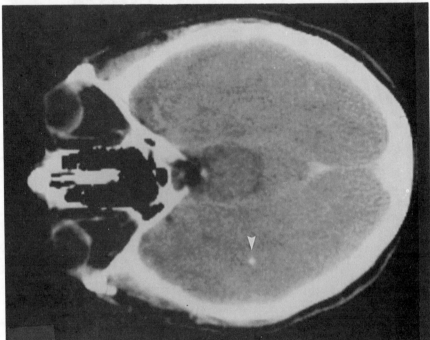

Figure 2   (a) Axial CT image showing a small calcified lesion in the right temporal lobe of a 29 year old man with temporal lobe epilepsy (arrow). (b) Axial T2 weighted MRI image of the same patient, showing the lesion as an area of high signal with low signal at its centre (arrow).

is more likely to detect calcium, areas of calcification are usually associated with abnormal tissue detectable using MRI (Fig. 2) (12,17). While most studies have been undertaken to evaluate MRI as a lateralizing investigation in the work-up for temporal lobectomy in intractable cases, the superiority of the technique is equally applicable to the detection of a cause for the epilepsy whatever its severity (16).

MRI mainly images brain structure, but can also image some aspects of function. The blood-brain barrier opens at the site of a focus during seizure activity (19) in animal models at least. MRI can show transient focal alterations in signal in epilepsy which are compatible with changes in water distribution occurring as a result of such opening of the blood-brain barrier (7,20).

POSITRON EMISSION TOMOGRAPHY (PET)

PET can image regional cerebral blood flow (rCBF) or metabolic parameters such as regional oxygen metabolism (rCMRO2) and regional glucose metablism (rCMRGlc). Simultaneous studies have shown that metabolism and blood flow are closely coupled in epilepsy, as in most other situations (21). In primary generalized epilepsy PET has shown a generalized increase in metabolism and blood flow ictally, with postictal depression and normal flow interictally (21). Few ictal studies have been done using PET, as its temporal

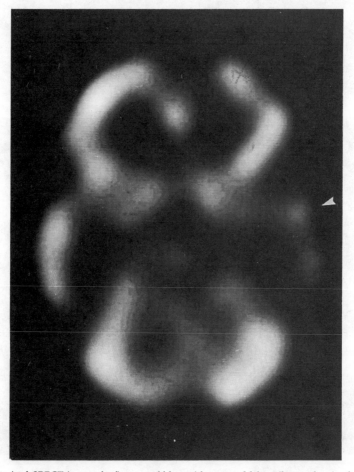

Figure 3 *Interictal SPECT image of a five year old boy with temporal lobe epilepsy, showing hypoperfusion of the left temporal lobe (arrow).*

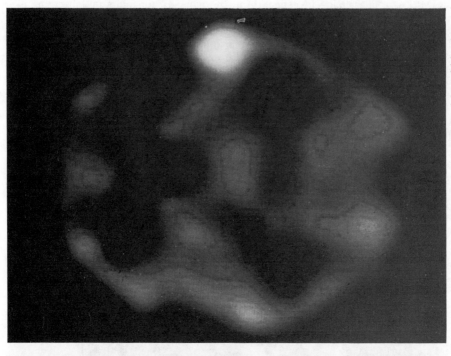

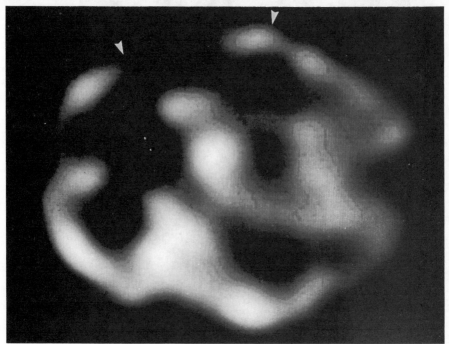

Figure 4 *(a) Interictal SPECT image of a 12 year old boy with temporal lobe epilepsy showing hypoperfusion of the left temporal and frontal lobes (arrows). (b) Ictal image of the same patient showing a hyperperfused focus in the originally hypoperfused area (the rest of the image appears dark because of the very high intensity of the hyperperfused area).*

resolution is of the order of minutes only, and ictal imaging presents practical difficulties. Most interest has centred on the abnormalities seen in focal epilepsy, particularly temporal lobe epilepsy.

Interictal studies in TLE have shown hypoperfusion and hypometabolism of the affected temporal lobe in around 70% of patients (21–28), with a minority of patients showing multiple or complex abnormalities. Ictally or postictally focal hyperperfusion and hypermetabolism have been seen in the affected temporal lobe (21,28), again with a minority of patients showing multiple abnormalities. While ictal hypermetabolism and hyperperfusion are thought to be due to increased metabolic demand from the mass of rapidly firing neurones around the site of the focus, the reasons for interictal hypometabolism and hypoperfusion are unknown.

The main clinical use for PET in epilepsy is to help lateralize a temporal lobe focus so that lobectomy can be carried out, and its usefulness in this respect is becoming established, as correlative studies with electrophysiological lateralization show good agreement (27). Already, the finding of unilateral hypoperfusion on PET is regarded in one centre at least as an indication that depth EEG studies need not be performed (29). Currently, despite its high spatial resolution and versatility, its high cost makes it essentially a research tool, available only at large centres.

SINGLE PHOTON EMISSION COMPUTED TOMOGRAPHY (SPECT)

Currently, SPECT can only be used to image regional cerebral blood flow, and is further disadvantaged *vis-à-vis* PET by having poorer spatial resolution, and by providing non-quantitative images. These disadvantages, however, mainly pertain to research applications. For clinical applications, SPECT has the enormous advantage that even 'state of the art' equipment is one-tenth of the cost of PET, and is able to produce images of resolution comparable to all but the most recent PET systems. Even rotating gamma camera systems, currently available in many hospitals in the UK, can provide images of regional cerebral blood flow which can be useful in the evaluation of patients for temporal lobectomy (30). The clinical application of SPECT has been further extended by the recent development of HM-PAO, a lipophilic compound to which the commonly used Technetium 99 m isotope can be attached. The compound crosses the blood brain barrier freely. On entering the cell, it then becomes hydrophilic, and cannot recross the blood brain barrier. Its distribution, and the tomographic image produced from it, remain constant for several hours. This allows a delay between the injection of isotope and scanning, making the technique ideal for studying paroxysmal events such as seizures (31).

The findings in epilepsy are similar to those using PET (30,32–37), with a similarly good correlation between rCBF abnormalities and electrophysiological findings (Fig. 3). The particular advantages of HM-PAO SPECT are likely to make it a powerful lateralizing tool in the preoperative assessment of patients for temporal lobectomy. The practice of admitting patients on reduced anticonvulsant treatment in order to record seizures by means of telemetry is established, and the same method has been used to produce ictal images of rCBF using SPECT (30,32) (Fig. 4). If these images are associated with a single or predominant seizure type, and are combined with an interictal image showing hypoperfusion on the same side, even current data suggest a high lateralizing reliability (30,32), and it seems likely that in the future ictal/interictal SPECT images will constitute the main lateralizing evidence in many patients.

CONCLUSION

The sensitivity of structural imaging techniques and the versatility and practicability of functional imaging techniques have considerably improved in recent years. MRI is established as the imaging modality of choice for detecting subtle structural lesions causing epilepsy, while SPECT shows imminent promise as a lateralizing investigation which will allow the expansion of the use of surgery in the treatment of temporal lobe epilepsy.

REFERENCES

(1) Ramirez-Lassepas M, Cipolle RJ, Morillo LR, Gumnit RJ. Value of computed tomographic scan in the evaluation of adult patients after their first seizure. *Ann Neurol* 1984; **15**: 536–43.

(2) Bauer G, Mayr U, Pallva A. Computerised axial tomography in chronic partial epilepsies. *Epilepsia* 1980; **21**: 227–33.

(3) Bogdanoff BM, Stafford CR, Green L, Gonzalez CF. Computerised transaxial tomography in evaluation of patients with focal epilepsy. *Neurology* 1975; **25**: 1013–17.

(4) Roberts MA, Godfrey JW, Caird FI. Epileptic seizures in the elderly: 1. Aetiology and type of seizure. *Age Ageing* 1982; **11**: 24–8.

(5) Young AC, Borg Constanzi J, Mohr PD, StClair Forbes W. Is routine axial tomography in epilepsy worthwhile? *Lancet* 1982; **ii**: 1446–7.

(6) Gillatt RW, Shorvon SD. Computerised tomography in epilepsy. *Lancet* 1983; **i**: 293.

(7) Theodore WH. Epilepsy. In: Theodore WH, ed. *Frontiers of clinical neuroscience Vol 4: Clinical neuroimaging*. New York: Liss, 1988.

(8) Oxbury JM, Whitty CWM. Causes and consequences of status epilepticus in adults. *Brain* 1971; **94**: 733–44.

(9) Wroe SJ, Fox PM, Williams IR, Chadwick DW, West C, Towns G. Differences between neurological and neurosurgical approaches in the management of malignant brain tumors. *Br Med J* 1986; **293**: 1015–18.

(10) Biehl JP. Computerised tomography in epilepsy. *Lancet* 1983; **i**: 293.

(11) Kucharczyk W, Brant-Zawadski M. Magnetic resonance imaging of cerebral ischemia and infarction. In: Kressel HY, ed. *Magnetic resonance annual*. New York: Raven Press, 1987: 49–69.

(12) Schorner W, Meenke HJ, Felix R. Temporal lobe epilepsy: comparison of CT and MR imaging. *Am J Neuroradiol* 1987; **8**: 773–81.

(13) Lesser RP, Modic MT, Weinstein MA, *et al*. Magnetic resonance imaging (1.5 Tesla) in patients with intractable focal seizures. *Arch Neurol* 1986; **43**: 367–71.

(14) Sperling MR, Wilson G, Engel J, Babb TL, Phelps M, Bradley M. Magnetic resonance imaging in intractable partial epilepsy: correlative studies. *Ann Neurol* 1986; **20**: 57–62.

(15) Theodore WH, Dorwart R, Holmes M, Porter RJ, DiChiro G. Neuroimaging in refractory partial seizures. Comparison of PET, CT and MRI. *Neurology* 1986; **36**: 750–9.

(16) Triulzi F, Franceschi M, Fazzio F, Del Maschio A. Nonrefractory temporal lobe epilepsy: 1.5T MR imaging. *Radiology* 1988; **166**: 181–5.

(17) Duncan R, Patterson J, Macpherson P, Hadley DM, Bone I. CT and MR imaging in temporal lobe epilepsy. Proceedings of the Association of British Neurologists. *J Neurol Neurosurg Psychiat* 1989; **52**: 1209.

(18) Kuzniecky R, DeLaSayette D, Ethier R, *et al*. Magnetic resonance imaging in temporal lobe epilepsy: pathological correlations. *Ann Neurol* 1987; **22**: 341–7.

(19) Cornford EM, Oldendorf WH. Epilepsy and the blood brain barrier. In: Delgado-Escueta AV, Ward AA, Woodbury DM, Porter RJ, eds. *Advances in neurology, Vol. 44*. New York: Raven Press, 1986.

(20) Stone JL, Hughes JR, Barr A, Tan W, Russel E, Crowell RM. Neuroradiological and electroencephalographic features in a case of temporal lobe status epilepticus. *Neurosurgery* 1986; **18**: 212–16.

(21) Kuhl DE, Engel J, Phelps ME, Selin C. Epileptic patterns of local cerebral metabolism and perfusion in humans determined by emission computed tomography of 18FDG and 13NH3. *Ann Neurol* 1980; **8**: 348–60.

(22) Kuhl DE, Fishbein D, Dubinsky R. Patterns of cerebral metabolism in patients with partial seizures. *Ann Neurol* 1988; **38**: 1201–6.

(23) Theodore WH, Newmark ME, Sato S, Brooks R, Patronas N, DeLaPaz R. 18F Fluorodeoxyglucose positron emission tomography in refractory complex partial seizures. *Ann Neurol* 1983; **14**: 429–37.

(24) Theodore WH, Dorwart R, Holmes M, Porter RJ, DiChiro G. Neuroimaging in refractory partial seizures. Comparison of PET, CT and MRI. *Neurology* 1986; **36**: 750–9.

(25) Theodore WH, Fishbein D, Dubinsky R. Patterns of cerebral glucose metabolism in patients with partial seizures. *Neurology* 1988; **38**: 1201–6.

(26) Abou Khalil BW, Siegel JG, Sackellares C, Gilman S, Hichwa R, Marshall R. Positron emission tomography studies of cerebral glucose metabolism in chronic partial epilepsy. *Ann Neurol* 1987; **22**: 480–6.

(27) Engel J, Kuhl DE, Phelps ME, Crandall PH. Comparative localisation of epileptic foci in partial epilepsy by PCT and EEG. *Ann Neurol* 1982; **12**: 529–37.

(28) Franck G, Sadzot B, Salmon E, *et al*. Regional cerebral blood flow and metabolic rates in human focal epilepsy and status epilepticus. In: Delgado-Escueta AV, Ward AA, Woodbury DM, Porter RJ, eds. *Advances in neurology*. New York: Raven Press, 1986; 935–44.

(29) Mazziotta JC, Engel J. The use and impact of positron computed tomographic scanning in epilepsy. *Epilepsia* 1984; **25**: S86–S104.

(30) Lee BI, Markand ON, Wellman HN, *et al.* HIDPM-SPECT in patients with medically intractable complex partial seizures. *Arch Neurol* 1988; **45**: 397–402.
(31) Neirinckx RD, Canning LR, Piper IM, *et al.* Technetium 99m d,l-HM-PAO: a new radiopharmaceutical for SPECT imaging of regional cerebral blood perfusion. *J Nucl Med* 1987; **28**: 191–202.
(32) Rowe CC, Berkovic SS, Austin M, McKay WJ, Bladin PF. Postictal SPECT in epilepsy. *Lancet* 1989; **i**: 389–90.
(33) Lee BI, Markand ON, Siddiqui AR, *et al.* Single photon emission computed tomography (SPECT) brain imaging using N,N,N′-trimethyl-N′-(2hydroxy-3-methyl-5-123I-iodobenzyl)-1,3-propanediamine 2 HCL (HIDPM): Intractable partial seizures. *Neurology* 1986; **36**: 1471–7.
(34) Lavy S, Melamed E, Portnoy Z, Carmon A. Interictal regional cerebral blood flow in patients with partial seizures. *Neurology* 1976; **26**: 418–22.
(35) Hougaard K, Oikawa T, Sveinsdottir E, *et al.* Regional cerebral blood flow in focal cortical epilepsy. *Arch Neurol* 1976; **33**: 527–35.
(36) Uren RF, Magistretti PL, Royal HD, *et al.* Single photon emission computed tomography. *Med J Aust 1983;* **1**: 411–13.
(37) Bonte FJ, Stokely EM, Devous MD, Homan RW. Single photon tomographic study of regional cerebral blood flow in epilepsy. *Arch Neurol* 1983; **40**: 267–70.

The diagnostic role of ambulatory cassette EEG

S. J. L. Howell and L. D. Blumhardt

Department of Neurological Science, University of Liverpool, Liverpool, UK

INTRODUCTION

Since its clinical introduction in the mid-1970s (1), ambulatory EEG recording on cassette tape (AEEG) has been applied for a variety of reasons, including the quantification of seizures, particularly petit mal absence attacks and the effects of medication (2–4,6–8), sleep studies (4,9), the characterization, localization and classification of the type of epilepsy (3,5,10–12), the timing of seizures and their precipitation (13) and the occurrence of new unexplained symptoms in known epileptics (3,8,14–16).

Table 1 *Relative advantages and disadvantages of AEEG*

	Advantages	Disadvantages
Versus REEG	Long duration recordings High quality ictal traces 100% sleep records Enhanced spikes/sharp waves Unrestricted patients	Fewer channels Patients unobserved Artefacts Analysis time Expense
Versus CEEG	Long duration recordings Natural environment Out-patient Unrestricted patient Fast playback analysis Economical	Fewer channels Patients unobserved/no video facility

The major practical clinical application, which is the subject of this brief review, is the investigation of patients with repeated, undiagnosed disturbances of consciousness which could be epileptic. Many reports have attested to the *diagnostic* usefulness of this technique (2,4,6,7,9–12,16–26). Its main advantage over routine EEG (REEG) is the facility to record for very long periods, commonly several days at a time, thus increasing the chances of recording both symptomatic attacks and clinically 'silent' abnormalities. Its main advantage over video-telemetry (CEEG) is that the recordings can be made at home, school, or work, thus avoiding an expensive hospital admission. The main disadvantages are that patients are unobserved during their attacks and special skills must be acquired to enable accurate high-speed review of the tape recordings. The most-quoted 'advantages and disadvantages' of AEEG, versus other tests, are listed in Table 1.

AEEG SENSITIVITY IN THE TARGET DISORDER—EPILEPSY

For AEEG to be of value to the clinician it must not only facilitate the *capture* of symptomatic events, but it must have a high sensitivity and specificity in patients with a firm clinical

Fourth international symposium on sodium valproate and epilepsy, edited by David Chadwick, 1989; Royal Society of Medicine Services International Congress and Symposium Series No. 152, published by Royal Society of Medicine Services Limited.

Table 2 *AEEG during symptomatic ictal attacks in clinically diagnosed epileptics*

Reference	n	AEEG seizure	AEEG equivocal	AEEG negative
Ives and Woods (1980) (27)	155 CPS	79%	5%	16%
	51 CP auras	10%	—	90%
Oxley and Roberts (1982) (15)	23 seizures	91%	—	9%
Oxley and Roberts (1985) (28)	31 seizures[a]	81%	—	19%
Blumhardt et al. (1986) (29)	74 CPS	89%	8%	3%
Smith et al. (1989) (30)	80 CPS	91%	9%	—

[a] Defined as 'severe' epileptic seizures.

diagnosis of epilepsy. Studies of clinically-diagnosed epileptics are still few, but the majority of attacks in these patients are confirmed to be associated with EEG seizure activity (Table 2). Unfortunately, a minority will not show recognizable EEG changes ('false negatives') during otherwise 'clinically-definite' seizures (Table 2), while in another group of patients, artefacts can confound interpretation of the traces leading to equivocal results.

The reasons for EEG negative-seizures are not unique to AEEG. The least likely explanation and the most frequently raised objection against AEEG, is that of 'insufficient spatial coverage through lack of recording electrodes'. This comment relates more to electroencephalographers pursuing focal theta 'abnormalities' of dubious clinical relevance, rather than to those experienced in the visual and auditory analysis of ictal recordings at sixty times real time.

Most published data has been obtained from 4-channel recorders generally using three channels for AEEG and one for an event marker and timer. The performance of these has been compared with the more recently introduced 8-channel machines and with 16-channel CEEG. In the only study of its type, there was a 100% detection rate by 3-channel AEEG of all seizures identified by CEEG (31). Although the differentiation from artefactual events was thought to be easier in 8-channel records (two such abnormalities were incorrectly interpreted as seizures in the 3-channel traces) the interpretations were made, rather unrealistically, without knowledge of the presence or timing of symptoms. Further, some epileptogenic abnormalities detected on 3-channel AEEG were missed in the 8-channel traces, as the large amount of data presented on the playback unit in this mode is difficult for observers to assimilate rapidly. A reduction in the inter-electrode distance with multi-channel montages may actually reduce the amplitude (and thus the ready recognition during fast playback analysis) of sharp waves and spikes. The numbers in this study were so small that the results cannot be regarded as justification for abandoning the use of 4-channel recorders. There is no other compelling evidence to suggest that increasing the number of channels significantly improves the *diagnostic* performance of AEEG (see below). It certainly increases the cost, the problem of analysing the records, the likelihood of errors of omission and the technician's time taken to fit the recorders.

What difference does the scalp position of AEEG electrodes make? It has been adequately demonstrated that limited spatial coverage is not a major limitation for *diagnostic* AEEG, provided appropriate recording sites are chosen. A 3-channel AEEG montage with a frontal transverse and two longitudinal channels is capable of detecting 74–100% of even the minor interictal epileptogenic abnormalities detected on simultaneous multi-channel CEEG (32). Almost any montage will pick up generalized seizure activity and, as the distribution of focal seizure activity across the scalp in epileptic populations is not random, but skewed with a fronto-temporal emphasis (32), appropriate montages can be designed to maximize the 'hit-rate', with four, three, or even two channels. A 3-channel fronto-temporal montage will reveal seizure activity in almost 80% of clinically symptomatic, focal, temporal lobe seizures (27). The 20% negative ictal recordings, in this and other studies, may be due in part to the presence of artefacts (chewing and movement) during seizures, electro-decremental seizure activity without spikes and rhythmic slow waves and, the failure of some seizures seen at depth electrodes to project to the scalp.

In one study, 90% of 'auras' and 20% of approximately 200 clinical CPS, had no definite AEEG accompaniments (27) (Table 1). As with all surface EEG recording, the possibility exists that seizures may occur deep in the brain without surface change (33).

Table 3 *Ictal AEEG/ECG in undiagnosed cases[a] with possible epilepsy*

	n	AEEG seizure	AECG arrhythmia	Equivocal AEEG	Negative AEEG/ECG
Wood & Ives (1977)[b] (24) (Capture rate 12/26, 46%)	12	2 (17%)	2 (17%)	2 (17%)	6 (50%)
Blumhardt (1985) (26) (Capture rate 48/145, 33%)	48	4[a] (8%)	3[a] (6%)	13 (27%)	29 (60%)

[a] From neurology clinics after neurological examination
[b] Selected by attack frequency

Diagnostic AEEG monitoring with depth electrodes (sphenoidal or foramen ovale) is currently under evaluation at several centres.

RESULTS IN PATIENTS WITH UNDIAGNOSED RECURRENT SYMPTOMS

A critical assessment of the diagnostic value of AEEG in this common clinical situation is difficult if not impossible to achieve from the current literature, as essential data on the patients and their symptoms is often lacking from reports. The populations studied clearly vary widely. For example, patients seen by a neurologist in a district general hospital or regional unit (18,26) will not be the same as the tertiary referrals to an epilepsy centre (31). AEEG may be worthwhile in some populations, but not in others: in one study, children referred by child psychiatrists with attacks of uncertain origin were much less likely to have seizure discharges on their AEEG than those referred by paediatricians (34), implying either different populations or different referral practice. The proportion of patients with major episodes of loss of consciousness versus minor disturbances of consciousness, will affect the proportion with ictal EEG seizure activity on AEEG (17,18,26) (Table 1).

The criteria for monitoring and the preliminary diagnostic work-up, is widely variable. In some studies pre-AEEG assessment by one or more neurologists (4,26), or by both a neurologist and a cardiologist (36) was reported. This improves the definition of the patient population, although explicit criteria for the diagnosis of 'unexplained symptoms', or of CPS, is generally not given. 'Capture rates' will vary if patients in some series are selected according to their symptom frequency. Some studies included cases only if they had had at least one attack per week (2,23), while others (26) attempting to answer different questions recorded patients regardless of attack frequency. Similarly, the proportion of patients in whom an ictal event is captured may obviously be increased simply by prolonging the duration of the recording. This varies greatly from study to study. Some patients have cyclical patterns to their attacks and rates of positive recordings will obviously be increased by careful timing of the recordings.

A further advantage of AEEG is the ability to obtain a simultaneous ECG record, although this is not mentioned in many series of 'undiagnosed' patients. Some authors monitored ECG in a minority of patients (4,25,37), although the criteria used to select cases is unclear. Neither the irregularities found, nor the outcome of cardiological treatments, are described in detail in any reports. Series which did obtain simultaneous EEG and ECG recordings in all cases, suggest that primary cardiac arrhythmias are the basis for the symptoms in a minority of neurological patients and these will not be detected by monitoring EEG alone (Table 3). In studies of undiagnosed populations taken from neurology clinics after full neurological investigations including REEG and ECG (i.e. a low prevalence population for serious dysrhythmias) one would expect the majority of recordings to be negative and only a few with atypical, non-specific, or unusually difficult clinical presentations to have demonstrated arrhythmias as a cause of their symptoms (Table 3).

VALIDATION OF RESULTS OF AEEG IN UNDIAGNOSED PATIENTS

The technical 'gold standard' against which AEEG must be evaluated is CEEG. In one study AEEG and CEEG were performed on 40 patients referred to an epilepsy centre,

Table 4 *Follow up diagnosis two years after AEEG ictal recordings in 48 patients according to AEEG result*

A/EEG result	n	Epilepsy	Follow-up diagnoses Cardiac	Other (ceased)
Seizure	4	4/4	—	—
Cardiac arrhythmia	3[a]	2/3[ab]	2/3[ab]	—
Equivocal EEG	13[a]	2/13[a]	—	11/13 (4)
EEG		(15%)		
Negative	29	2/29	2/29	25/29 (9)
		(7%)	(7%)	

[a,b] denote common patients

17 simultaneously and the rest sequentially with a 'blinded' tape review (38). Concurrence between AEEG and CEEG was 77% overall, 79% for focal and 100% for generalized interictal abnormalities. All seizures detected on CEEG were detected on AEEG.

An alternative approach, which is more realistic and appropriate to large numbers of patients with infrequent attacks, is the outcome of long-term follow up. This has seldom been attempted. One group reported a 12- to 60-month follow up of 12 treated patients (<21 yrs) whose ictal AEEG had been negative (21). On reassessment, six of these patients were no longer receiving anti-epileptic drugs and attacks had ceased in five. However, in four of the 12 a 'final diagnosis' of epilepsy had been made, although no details on how the diagnosis was reached were provided.

One other study has reported follow-up data on 145 patients with unexplained episodes of disturbed consciousness (26). One third of these (n=48) had had symptomatic attacks recorded. The results and the follow up data are shown in Table 4. Of nine patients who were eventually diagnosed as epileptic after two years, only four had been successfully predicted by AEEG. Two of the nine had had a negative ictal EEG and two an equivocal EEG. Furthermore, two patients with ictal cardiac arrhythmias had gone on to a diagnosis of epilepsy. Thus AEEG failed to detect at least 10% of patients who were later thought to have epilepsy.

INTERICTAL 'ABNORMALITY DETECTION'

If symptomatic attacks are too infrequent to be recorded even in long samples of AEEG recording, in a majority of undiagnosed patients unselected by symptom frequency, the question of AEEG versus REEG for detecting possibly helpful interictal 'epileptogenic' abnormalities must be addressed. In most reports, AEEG has been almost invariably superior to REEG in this respect (Table 5). However, since the type of AEEG and REEG 'abnormalities' are rarely detailed, it is difficult to be sure of their relationship, if any, to symptoms occurring at other times. While much effort has been expended to demonstrate the presence of these abnormalities, there have been remarkably few attempts to determine whether these observations have any prognostic significance. A two-year follow-up study of 97 patients in whom no attacks had been captured, suggested that an AEEG recording

Table 5 *Studies comparing AEEG with REEG for detection of interictal abnormalities*

Reference	REEG	AEEG	Comment
Clinically diagnosed epileptics			
Bridgers & Ebersole, (1985) (11)	6/25 (24%)	12/25 (48%)	Spike/sharp waves only
Sivenius et al. (1984) (12)	0/13	6/13 (46%)	'Irritative EEG'
Unexplained episodes (Suspected epilepsy)			
Green et al. (1980) (39)	33/74 (45%)	41/74 (55%)	Abnormalities not defined
Cull, (1985) (18)	16/62 (26%)	21/62 (34%)	Including slow waves

Table 6 *Sensitivity, specificity and predictive value of interictal AEEG[a] two years after recording in 97 patients with undiagnosed episodes of disturbed consciousness (26)*

A/EEG Result	Clinical diagnosis of epilepsy Present	'Absent'	AEEG prediction
+ve	6	5	6/11 PPV = 56%
−ve	8	78	78/86 NPV = 91%
Totals	14 (Sensitivity 43%)	83 (Specificity 94%)	97 PREV = 14%

[a] AEEG captured asymptomatic interictal abnormalities only (PPV and NPV = positive and negative predictive values, PREV = prevalence of epilepsy).

Table 7 *AEEG findings in patients with suspected 'pseudoseizures'*

Reference	Total patients n	Capture rate	AEEG seizure
Davidson et al. (1981) (6)	10	5 (50%)	1/5 (20%)
Ives et al. (1981) (23)	27	16 (59%)	2/16 (13%)
	13[a]	6 (46%)	3/6
Oxley & Roberts (1982) (15)	7	7 (100%)	0
Sivenius et al. (1984) (12)	25	15 (60%)	2/15 (13%)
	38[a]	15 (39%)	8/15 (53%)
Blumhardt (1985) (26)	14[a]	10 (71%)	4/10 (40%)
Totals	142	74 (52%)	20/74 (27%)
	65[a]	31 (48%)	15/31 (50%)

[a]Patients with epilepsy and suspected pseudoseizures.

of sharp waves or spikes in a patient with unexplained symptoms was far from infallible as an indicator of epilepsy, at least in the short term (26). Within two years of monitoring, 45% of patients with 'epileptogenic' features had not reached a diagnosis and, in many of these, symptoms had ceased altogether. Subclinical rhythmic slow activity appears to be a very poor indication that epileptic attacks will be confirmed in that individual in the future (hardly surprising in mobile, unobserved patients) (26). Furthermore, the completely negative recording appears to have a 'false-negative' predictive rate of *at least* 8% (Table 6) (further cases may occur on long term follow-up). As a result of poor sensitivity in this low prevalence population, the *interictal* AEEG result hardly affected the probability of epilepsy (Table 6), suggesting that the cost-effectiveness of AEEG could be improved by concentrating on symptomatic event analysis (26).

'PSEUDOSEIZURES' OR NON-EPILEPTIC (HYSTERICAL) ATTACKS

The non-epileptic attack, often referred to as a 'pseudoseizure', is a special type of undiagnosed episode which has been addressed in a number of AEEG studies. Some authors appear to conclude that a negative AEEG during a symptomatic attack excludes epilepsy and indicates a non-epileptic seizure. For the reasons above, this conclusion is incorrect. In the author's opinion, unless there eventually proves to be a characteristic AEEG pattern of a 'pseudoseizure', which would seem rather unlikely, the technique is best used in a positive manner to *exclude* the label of 'pseudoseizure' for a particular attack or symptom, by demonstrating the coincidence of EEG seizure activity. Thus in several studies of patients suspected to have 'pseudoseizures', AEEG recordings have demonstrated the epileptic nature of the attacks in almost one-third of cases, or in almost one-half of those with a previous diagnosis of epilepsy (Table 7).

CONCLUSION

There seems little doubt that the technique of out-patient EEG recording in mobile patients, particularly as the methodology for data acquisition and analysis improves, will find a place as a major diagnostic test in future years. However, no matter how sophisticated the future technical developments, clinicians will still require careful clinical correlations validated by follow-up analyses, to clarify the type of patient and the circumstances in which AEEG is indicated. The currently available data, although encouraging, is still deficient in a number of important areas.

REFERENCES

(1) Ives JR, Woods JF. 4-channel 24 hour cassette recorder for long term EEG monitoring of ambulatory patients. *Electroenceph Clin Neurophysiol* 1975; **39**: 88–92.
(2) Stores G. Differential diagnosis of seizures: psychiatric aspects. In: Dam M, Gram L, Penry JK, eds. *Advances in epileptology; XIIth international symposium*. New York: Raven Press, 1981: 259–63.
(3) Oxley J, Roberts M. Clinical evaluation of 4-channel ambulatory EEG monitoring in the management of patients with epilepsy. *J Neurol Neurosurg Psychiat* 1985; **48**: 930–2.
(4) Docherty TB. Ambulatory encephalogram: monitoring in routine clinical practice. *Electrophysiol Technol* 1981; **7**: 141–58.
(5) Declerck AC, Martens WLJ, Schiltz AM. Evaluation of ambulatory EEG cassette recording. In: Stefan H, Burr W, eds. *Mobile long term EEG monitoring*. Stuttgart: Fischer, 1982: 29–36.
(6) Davidson DLW, Fleming AMM, Kettles A. Use of ambulatory EEG monitoring in a neurological service. In: Dam M, Gram L, Penry JK, eds. *Advances in epileptology: XIIth international symposium*. New York: Raven Press, 1981: 319–21.
(7) Bruens JH, Kniff W. Ambulatory EEG monitoring with a 24 hour cassette recorder in epileptic patients. Chapter In: *Epilepsy: clinical and experimental research*, Basle: Karger, 1980: 295–7. (Monograph Neurol Sci; vol. 5.).
(8) Stores G. Ambulatory EEG monitoring in neuropsychiatric patients using the Oxford Medilog 4-24 recorder with visual playback display. In: Stott FD, Raftery EB, Goulding L, eds. *Proc third international symposium on ambulatory monitoring*. London: Academic Press, 1980: 399–406.
(9) Powell TE, Harding GFA. Twenty-four hour ambulatory EEG monitoring: development and applications. *J Med Eng Technol* 1986; **10**: 229–38.
(10) Jerret SA. Ambulatory EEG: a community hospital prospective study with analysis of patient outcome. *Clin Electroenceph* 1985; **16**: 161–6.
(11) Bridgers SL, Ebersole JS. The clinical utility of ambulatory cassette EEG. *Neurology* 1985; **35**: 166–73.
(12) Sivenius J, Keranen T, Reinikainen K, Yletyinen I, Partanen J, Riekkinen P. Diagnostic evaluation of ambulatory, cassette EEG monitoring in 100 epileptic patients. *Acta Neurol Scand Suppl* 1984; **68**: 99–100.
(13) Stores G, Lwin R. A study of the factors associated with the occurrence of generalized seizure discharge in children with epilepsy. In: Dam M, Gram L, Penry JK, eds. *Advances in epileptology: XIIth epilepsy international symposium*. New York: Raven Press, 1981: 421–2.
(14) Oxley J, Roberts M, Dana-Haeri J, Trimble M. Evaluation of prolonged 4 channel EEG taped recordings and serum prolactin levels in the diagnosis of epileptic and non epileptic seizures. In: Dam M, Gram L, Penry JK, eds. *Advances in epileptology: XIIth epilepsy international symposium*. New York: Raven Press, 1981: 343–55.
(15) Oxley J, Robert M. The role of prolonged ambulatory monitoring in the diagnosis of non-epileptic fits in a population of patients with epilepsy. In: Stott FD, Raftery EB, Goulding L, eds. *Proc fourth international symposium on ambulatory monitoring*. London: Academic Press, 1983: 195–202.
(16) Bachman DS. 24 hour ambulatory electroencephalographic monitoring in paediatrics. *Clin Electroenceph* 1984; **15**: 164–6.
(17) Callaghan N, McCarthy N. Twenty-four-hour EEG monitoring in patients with normal routine EEG findings. In: Dam M, Gram L, Penry JK, eds. *Advances in epileptology: XIIth international symposium* New York: Raven Press, 1981: 357–9.
(18) Cull RE. An assessment of 24 hour ambulatory EEG/ECG monitoring in a neurology clinic. *J Neurol Neurosurg Psychiat* 1985; **48**: 107–10.
(19) Blumhardt LD, Oozeer R. Simultaneous ambulatory monitoring of the EEG and ECG in patients with unexplained transient disturbances of consciousness. In: Stott FD, Raftery EB, Goulding L, eds. *Proc fourth international symposium on ambulatory monitoring* London: Academic Press, 1983: 171–82.
(20) Berkovic SF, Bladin PF, Conneely MD, Gossat LA, Symington GR, Vajda FJE. Experience with continuous ambulatory EEG monitoring. *Clin Exp Neurol* 1984; **20**: 37–46.
(21) Powell TE, Harding GFA, Jeavons PM. Ambulatory EEG monitoring: a preliminary follow-up study. In: Ross E, Chadwick D, Crawford R, eds. *Epilepsy in young people*. Chichester: Wiley, 1987: 131–9.
(22) Powell TE, Jeavons PM, Harding GFA. An evaluation of 3 and 8 channel ambulatory EEG monitoring. In: Dal Palu C, Pessina AC, eds. *Proc fifth international symposium on ambulatory monitoring*. Padova: Cleup, 1986: 625–32.

(23) Ives JR, Hausser C, Woods JF, Andermann F. Contribution of 4 channel monitoring to differential diagnosis of paroxysmal attacks. In: Dam M, Gram L, Penry JK, eds. *Advances in epileptology: XIIth epilepsy international symposium*. New York: Raven Press, 1981: 326–36.

(24) Woods JF, Ives JR. Prolonged monitoring of the EEG in ambulatory patients. In: Penry JK, ed. *Epilepsy, the eighth international symposium*. New York: Raven Press, 1977: 109–13.

(25) Ramsay RE. Clinical usefulness of ambulatory EEG monitoring of the neurological patient. In: Stott FD, Raftery EB, Goulding L, eds. *Proc fourth international symposium on ambulatory monitoring*. London: Academic Press, 1983: 151–6.

(26) Blumhardt LD. The diagnostic value of ambulatory ECG/EEG recording: a follow-up study of 145 patients with unexplained transient non-focal neurological symptoms. In: Dal Palu C, Pessina AC, eds. *Proc fifth international symposium on ambulatory monitoring*. Padova: Cleup, 1986: 675–83.

(27) Ives JR, Woods JF. A study of 100 patients with focal epilepsy using a 4-channel ambulatory cassette recorder. In: Stott FD, Raftery EB, Goulding L, eds. *Proc third international symposium on ambulatory monitoring*. London: Academic Press, 1980: 383–92.

(28) Oxley J, Roberts M. Clinical evaluation of 4-channel ambulatory EEG monitoring in the management of patients with epilepsy. *J Neurol Neurosurg Psychiat* 1985; **48**: 930–2.

(29) Blumhardt LD, Smith PEM, Owen L. Electrocardiographic accompaniments of temporal lobe epileptic seizures. *Lancet* 1986; **i**: 1051–6.

(30) Smith PEM, Howell SJL, Owen L, Blumhardt LD. Instant heart rate profiles during partial seizures. *Electroenceph Clin Neurophysiol* 1989; **72**: 207–17.

(31) Ebersole JS, Bridgers SL. Direct comparison of 3 and 8 channel ambulatory cassette EEG with intensive inpatient monitoring. *Neurology* 1985; **35**: 846–54.

(32) Leroy RF, Ebersole JS. An evaluation of ambulatory cassette EEG monitoring: I. Montage design. *Neurology* 1983; **33**: 1–7.

(33) Lieb JP, Walsh GO, Babb TL, Walter RD, Crandall PH. A comparison of EEG seizure patterns recorded with surface and depth electrodes in patients with temporal lobe epilepsy. *Epilepsia* 1976; **17**: 137–60.

(34) Stores G. Comparison of video and ambulatory (cassette) monitoring in the investigation of attacks in children. In: Dal Palu C, Pessina AC, eds. *Proc fifth international symposium on ambulatory monitoring*. Padova: Cleup, 1986: 633–8.

(35) Callaghan N, McCarthy N. Ambulatory EEG monitoring in fainting attacks with normal routine and sleep EEG records. In: Stefan H, Burr W, eds. *Mobile long-term EEG monitoring*. Stuttgart: Fischer, 1982: 61–5.

(36) Graf M, Brunner G, Weber H, Auinger C, Joskowicz, G. Simultaneous long-term recording of EEG and ECG in 'syncope' patients. In: Stefan H, Burr W, eds. *Mobile long-term EEG monitoring*. Stuttgart: Fischer, 1982: 67–75.

(37) Jeffreys DE. The clinical usefulness of the ambulatory 24 hour EEG monitor. *Am J EEG Technol* 1981; **21**: 129–40.

(38) Ebersole JS, Leroy RF. Evaluation of ambulatory cassette EEG monitoring: III Diagnostic accuracy compared to intensive inpatient EEG monitoring. *Neurology* 1983; **33**: 853–60.

(39) Green J, Scales D, Nealis J, Schott G, Driber T. Clinical utility of ambulatory EEG monitoring. *Clin Enceph* 1980; **11**: 173–9.

SPECT-scanning and magnetic resonance imaging in epilepsy

A. R. Andersen[1] M. Herning[2] and M. Dam[3]

[1]University Clinic of Neurology, Rigshopitalet, [2]University Clinic of Magnetic Resonance and [3]Neurology, Hvidovre Hospital, Copenhagen, Denmark

---

INTRODUCTION

Single photon emission computed tomography (SPECT) of regional cerebral blood flow (rCBF) changes measures a functional parameter, while magnetic resonance imaging (MRI) yields structural (anatomical) information. SPECT of rCBF has been valuable in the description of major cerebral disorders, such as stroke (1), dementia (2) and classical migraine (3). MRI has been used in the evaluation of a number of neurological disorders, such as multiple sclerosis, cerebrovascular lesions and neoplasms. In the last decade the SPECT studies of rCBF changes in patients suffering from epilepsy have also been of increasing importance.

It has been known for many years, that both generalized and focal epileptic seizures are associated with an increase of blood flow and of oxidative metabolism (4,5,6). Using the intra-arterial xenon-133 clearance technique with stationary gamma-detectors (not SPECT) Ingvar clearly showed the ictal flow increased in patients with partial epilepsy and he reported that in the interictal state the focal area had a decrease in flow to below the normal level (7).

Several studies using positron emission tomography (PET) and tracers for imaging metabolism or blood flow extended these early observations to larger series of patients (8,9,10,11). Engel and associates (9) used PET imaging as an aid in localizing the affected side in drug-resistant cases of temporal lobe epilepsy (DRTLE), that due to the severity of the disease were candidates for temporal lobectomy (8,9).

Similar studies based on SPECT have now been published from several groups reporting both ictal and interictal changes of CBF distribution (12–17).

Magnetic resonance imaging (MRI) has advanced the non-invasive visualization of human tissue begun by cranial computerized tomography. The advantages of MRI are readily apparent. MRI does not require ionizing radiation; medial temporal lobe and posterior fossa structures are readily seen, unencumbered by bone artifact, and the potential for using physiological variables in delineating human anatomy may be possible by altering the techniques used in the imaging process.

METHODOLOGY

SPECT

The basic instrumentation is a SPECT, a rotating gamma camera. Essential in such an instrument is the perforated lead shield, *the collimator*, positioned between the head of the patient and the detectors. It determines the direction of the photons (gamma-rays) seen

---

Fourth international symposium on sodium valproate and epilepsy, edited by David Chadwick, 1989; Royal Society of Medicine Services International Congress and Symposium Series No. 152, published by Royal Society of Medicine Services Limited.

by the camera. The camera records a series of evenly spaced views ('projections') of the head. This is accomplished by having the whole camera rotate around the head, or by merely having the collimator rotating. The data sampling lasts typically 20–30 min when using tracers that are well retained in the brain (see below) and 4–5 min with freely diffusible tracers such as xenon-133. The projection data are reconstructed transaxially so that a set of transverse images, basically of the same type as with CT scanning is obtained. By stacking these images coronal and sagittal planes can also be reconstructed.

Conventional single-headed low speed SPECT yields a resolution of about 15–20 mm (FWHM). Brain dedicated SPECT systems have a spatial resolution of 9–10 mm using Tc99m. Some SPECT devices also allow rapid (dynamic) tomograms, albeit with lesser resolution. It should be noted, that the spatial resolution now routinely obtainable for CBF with SPECT is comparable to that obtained for CBF by PET.

Xenon-133 is a rather weak photon emitter (0.81 keV). As it arrives in the brain and washes out quite rapidly (18,19) a fast, highly sensitive SPECT system is needed for the scanning. Tracers for CBF labelled with Tc99m or Iodine-123, are also available. These isotopes have physical properties more suitable for SPECT. The labelled molecules have been designed to be retained in the initial flow-dominated distribution pattern for at least 60 min. The Iodine-123 isotope has been complexed with amines of the amphetamine type (20), while the Tc99m isotope has formed a lipophilic molecule with d,l-hexamethylene-propyleneamine oxime (HMPAO) (21). The pharmacokinetics of this compound have recently been published (22). Tc99m is cheaper and much easier to handle in the laboratory than is Iodine-123. The physical half-life is 6.1 h. It decays to Tc99 with the emission of a single gamma ray (140 KeV), which is optimal for tomographic imaging by SPECT. The isotope is available every day.

MRI

MRI relies on the fact that a sample of matter placed in a magnetic field is magnetized, that the magnetization is acted upon by electromagnetic waves of the proper wavelength whereby energy is stored in the system, and that this energy is given off during the relaxation of the system towards equilibrium in the form of radiation (electromagnetic waves in the radiofrequency range) which can be monitored by a receiver.

When a small sample is placed in a homogeneous magnetic field the sample is magnetized with the magnetization (vector) in the direction of the field. This macroscopic magnetization is made up of contributions from the small magnetic dipoles of the individual spinning nuclei, e.g. protons, which are aligned with the external field. These dipoles are precessing (rotating like a top) around the direction of the field with a frequency which for a given nucleus is dependent upon the strength of the magnetic field (Larmor frequency). If the sample is irradiated with electromagnetic waves with a frequency equal to the Larmor frequency (resonance), then the magnetization vector is turned into the plane perpendicular to the external field direction. The magnetization vector will precess (rotate) in the plane with the Larmor frequency thereby inducing an electrical signal of the same frequency in a receiver coil with an amplitude proportional to the number of nuclei from which it stems.

By applying weak, linearly varying magnetic fields (gradients) on top of the strong external field the Larmor frequency of the nuclei of the different parts, that make up an extended body, also varies in a linear way: the frequency is coding for location. After application of an electromagnetic pulse, whose frequency range spans the range of Larmor frequencies of the body a complicated signal, which is a superposition (sum) of the signals stemming from the small parts, that make up the body, is induced in the receiver coil.

Subsequently the signal is operated upon by the Fourier transformation which sorts out the different amplitudes according to their frequencies thereby synthesizing an image of the original body.

The timing scheme describing the sequence of field gradients, electromagnetic pulses, and data acquisition periods is called a pulse sequence, e.g. inversion recovery or spin echo sequences. After excitation the spin system is relaxing towards its equilibrium according to two processes with two characteristic time constants, the longitudinal and the transverse relaxation times, T1 and T2. These relaxation processes influence the signals

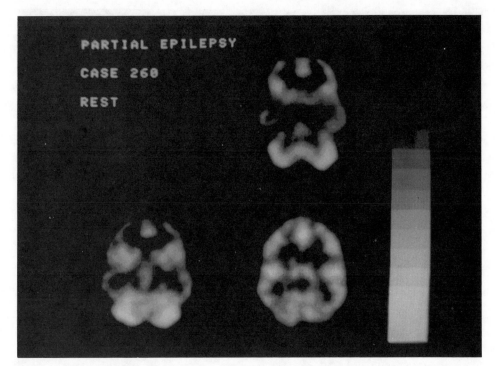

Figure 1 *Interictal SPECT images of rCBF. Case 260 studied by Tc99m-HMPAO injection. Left is situated to the left and the nose of the patient is pointing up. The blood flow distribution in the horizontal plane situated 2.3 cm, 3.6 cm, and 5 cm above the orbito meatal plane are given. A low flow region is evident in the left temporal lobe, but the side to side asymmetry is not very impressing.*

from the different tissues modifying the amplitudes of the signals and consequently the contrast of the images.

CLINICAL STUDIES

We have at present studied rCBF in 28 patients with complex, partial epilepsy using SPECT; the majority of the patients have DRTLE characterized by frequent seizures, despite optimal antiepileptic treatment. They exhibit simple or complex partial seizures with or without secondary generalization. Most of the patients have been studied by SPECT as a part of a presurgical evaluation programme*.

Regional CBF was measured by a brain dedicated SPECT-scanner, TOMOMATIC 64 (Medimatic Inc., Copenhagen) using xenon-133 inhalation and Tc99m-HMPAO injection. Using xenon-133 mean rCBF and the standard error is calculated in any region of interest, based on the clearance and the bolus distribution principle.

Tc99m-HMPAO was injected intravenously 1 h later. Usually the patients are positioned so that a series of nine parallel slices at a 1.3 cm distance are obtained, situated at OM + 1 cm, OM + 2.3 cm etc. up to OM + 11.6 cm. The HMPAO images are evaluated visually without knowledge of the case history or other patient data and compared to the 200 other patient studies performed by our group during the same period. CT and MR scanning was also performed using a Siemens CT scanner (Somatom DRG), and Magnetom® (1.5 Tesla) respectively.

---

* The study group comprises Dam M, Gram L, Andersen AR, Kjær L, Fuglsang-Frederiksen A, Herning M, Lassen NA, Friberg L., Kruse Larsen C, Waldemar G.

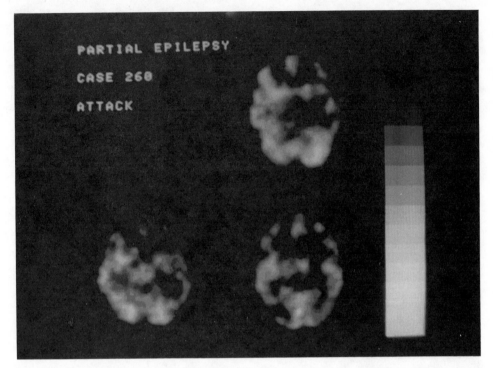

Figure 2 *Case 260 studied during a complex partial attack. The distribution of CBF at the orbito-meatal plane + 2.3 cm, + 3.6 cm and + 5 cm are given. The very high blood flow values in the left frontotemporal region are evident. They corresponded to a spike focus measured by EEG at the time of injection. MRI and CT-scan did not detect significant focal changes*

Sixteen-channel EEG-recordings (Siemens-Elema) were obtained, using a standard 10/20 electrode placement including zygomatic or sphenoidal electrodes. Sleep-recordings, and thiopental activation, were performed in all patients.

RESULTS

In 24 of our 28 patients we observed an obvious low flow region in one temporal lobe using Tc99m-d, l-HMPAO. In the remaining four patients unilateral lesions were present as borderline cases. The low flow regions were demarcated from normal tissue and in many cases also involved higher (parietal and frontal) homolateral regions of the brain. In 13 patients a smaller region of low flow was observed in the contralateral (mirror) temporal lobe. The perfusion asymmetry of the temporal lobes was obvious in 16 of the 27 patients studied by xenon-133 inhalation SPECT. SPECT was superior to CT as well as MR for visualizing the focal epileptogenic region suggested by the EEG.

MR has so far been performed in 21 patients. A result congruent with the functional tools (SPECT and EEG) was found in 12 cases. In seven of the MR and CT negative cases a consistent diagnosis was made by combining the results of the functional tools.

DISCUSSION

The results correspond closely to those presented by Mazziotta and Engel (8) using PET. Our results are also in accordance with previous comparative investigations of EEG and SPECT in patients with partial epilepsy (Stefan *et al.* (15)). In our series the long-term success can not be assessed yet, but the short term success is evident:

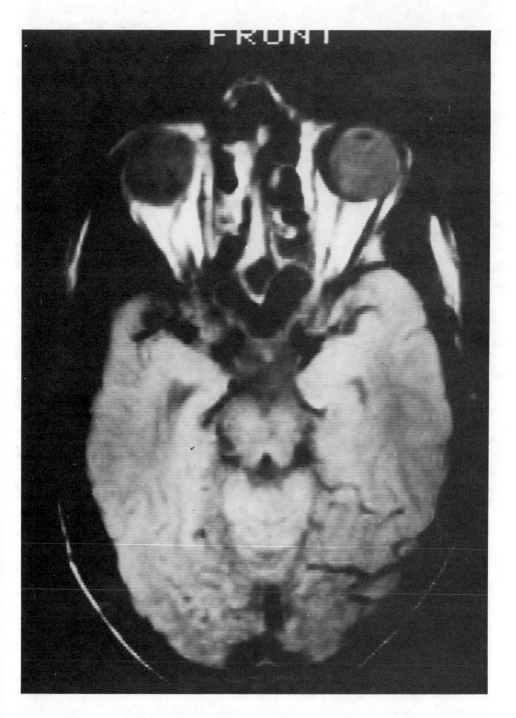

Figure 3 *Axial MR image (Magnetom 1.5 T Siemens, TR 1.8 s, TE 28 ms) shows no focal change in signal intensity but a clear asymmetry of the temporal horns with size reduction of the right hippocampus.*

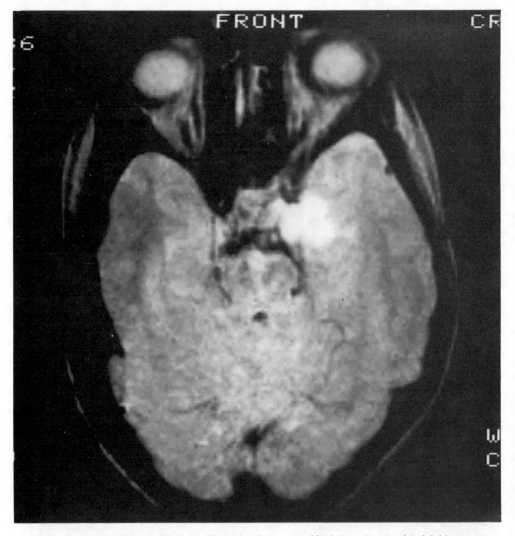

Figure 4 *Axial MR image (TR 1.8 s, TE 90 ms) shows area of high-intensity signal in left hippocampus.*

all 10 operated patients have been relieved from their very frequent and otherwise intractable attacks.

Using the I-123 HIPDM and SPECT Lee *et al.* studied 16 patients with DRTLE (12). Ictal HIPDM localized epileptic foci in 13 of 14 patients with a unilateral temporal focus and provided confirmative evidence of an epileptic focus in 11 patients by demonstrating maximally increased rCBF in epileptic foci that had shown decreased activity in a previous interictal study. Correlation with simultaneously recorded ictal EEG provided further clues for localizing the epileptic focus.

The overall results from SPECT studies of CBF in temporal lobe epilepsy show an average detection rate of significant focal rCBF changes in about 75% of the patients (12–17).

The idiopathic epileptic syndromes that often are genetic in nature are most reasonably caused by some unknown generalized biochemical nervous system abnormality. The use of SPECT in generalized epilepsy is controversial and still doubtful. MRI has not been helpful in delineating abnormalities in these patients. This finding is consistent with the results of CT-scan, which is normal in 90% of the patients (23,24). In symptomatic generalized epilepsies MRI has been shown to be superior to the CT-scan in the childhood leukodystrophies (25). White matter lesions are more easily seen with MRI especially with the spin-echo technique.

In mesial temporal sclerosis there seems to be correlations between the frequency of abnormal MRI and the degree of gliosis in the abnormal temporal lobe tissue (26). It is important to realize that transient MRI abnormalities may be seen during focal status epilepticus (27). Such lesions may be due to oedema in a site of high metabolic activity.

Partial epilepsy is the area for neuroimaging. In 100 consecutive patients with partial seizures, the EEG was most sensitive in diagnosing epilepsy (28). Thirty-six patients had an abnormal CT-scan, 45 had an abnormal MRI. Seven of the nine patients with abnormal MRI and normal CT-scan had lesions of possible surgical significance.

MRI seems to be able to reveal differences in temporal lobe size as well as more focal lesions compared to CT-scan (29). Calcific lesions are missed by MRI, but few focal findings seen on CT-scan are missed by MRI. MRI uncovers low grade gliomas better but may miss small thrombosed arteriovenous malformations seen on CT-scan (30).

Overall, there is approximately a 10% higher yield for abnormalities with MRI on patients with epilepsy, predominantly partial epilepsy. The typical findings not seen by CT-scan include low grade gliomas, small vascular lesions and severe gliosis. MRI will not identify calcific lesions and possibly some cases of atrophy or mild gliosis (31).

Most studies have utilized MRI scanners of less than one Tesla strength. Increased strength of 1.5 Tesla may result in an increased sensitivity in the evaluation of epilepsy (31).

MRI has proved advantageous in the post-operative management of patients with epilepsy. Callosotomy is used to ameliorate seizures in patients suffering from intractable generalized epilepsy. The determination of the exact surgical lesion made with the operation can be evaluated.

CONCLUSION

Our preliminary experience shows that in many patients with DRTLE in whom there is doubt with regard to localization of the seizure-eliciting area of the brain, the site of the epileptogenic focus can be identified by SPECT. As a consequence, surgical therapy may be offered to more of these patients, if they fulfil the clinical criteria for this therapy. SPECT or PET scanning would to us seem indispensable for optimal presurgical work-up of patients with partial epilepsy.

MRI is the imaging modality of choice in the evaluation of anatomical lesions in patients with partial epilepsy. A variety of disease processes associated with epilepsy are imaged better with MRI, e.g. low grade gliomas and higher grades of gliosis.

Stronger magnets and contrast agents may be of benefit in increasing sensitivity as well as specificity.

ACKNOWLEDGMENTS

This study was supported by the Danish Medical Research Council and by the Danish Hospital Foundation for Medical Research and the Lundbeck Foundation.

REFERENCES

(1) Vorstrup S. Tomographic cerebral blood flow measurements in patients with ischemic cerebrovascular disease and evaluation of the vasodilatory capacity by the acetazolamide test. *Acta Neurol Scand* 1988; **77** (Suppl 114): 1–48.
(2) Smith FW, Gemmel HG, Sharp PF. The use of Tc99m-d, l-HMPAO for the diagnosis of dementia. *Nucl Med Commun* 1987; **8**: 525–33.
(3) Andersen AR, Friberg L, Olsen TS, Olesen J. SPECT demonstration of delayed hyperemia following hypoperfusion in classic migraine. *Arch Neurol* 1988; **45**: 154–9.

(4) Penfield W, Von Santha K, Cipriani A. Cerebral blood flow during induced epileptiform seizures in animal and man. *J Neurophysiol* 1939; **2**: 257–67.
(5) Plum F, Posner JB, Troy B. Cerebral metabolic and circulatory responses to induced convulsions in animals. *Arch Neurol* 1968; **18**: 1–13.
(6) Brodersen P, Paulson OB, Bolwig TG, *et al*. Cerebral hyperemia in electrically induced epileptic seizures. *Arch Neurol* 1973; **28**: 334–8.
(7) Ingvar DH. Regional cerebral blood flow in focal cortical epilepsy. *Stroke* 1973; **4**: 359–60.
(8) Mazziotta JC, Engel J. The use and impact of positron computer tomography scanning in epilepsy. *Epilepsia* 1984; **25** (Suppl 2): S86–S104.
(9) Engel J. The role of neuroimaging in the surgical treatment of epilepsy. *Acta Neurol Scand* 1988; **45** (Suppl 117): 84–9.
(10) Latack JT, Abou-Khalil BW, Siegel GJ, Sackellares JC, Gabrielsen TO, Aisen AM. Patients with partial seizures: Evaluation by MR, CT, and PET imaging. *Neuroradiology* 1986; **159**: 159–63.
(11) Theodore WH, Newmark ME, Sato S, *et al*. F-18-fluorodeoxyglucose positron emission tomography in refractory complex partial seizures. *Ann Neurol* 1983; **14**: 429–37.
(12) Lee BI, Markand ON, Wellman HN, *et al*. HIPDM-SPECT in patients with medically intractable complex partial seizures. Ictal study. *Arch Neurol* 1988; **45**: 397–402.
(13) Ryding E, Rosen I, Ingvar DH. SPECT measurements with Tc99m-HMPAO in focal epilepsy. *J Cerebr Blood Flow Metab* 1988; **8**: S95–S100.
(14) Sanabria E, Chauvel P, Askienazy S, *et al*. Single photon emission computed tomography (SPECT) using I-123-isopropyl-iodo-amphetamine (IAMP) in partial epilepsy. In: Baldy-Moulinier *et al.*, eds. *Current problems in epilepsy: Cerebral blood flow, metabolism and epilepsy*. London: John Libbey, 1983: 82–7.
(15) Stefan H, Kuhnen C, Biersack HJ, Riechmann K. Initial experience with 99m Tc-hexamethyl-propylene amine oxime (HMPAO) single photon emission computer tomography (SPECT) in patients with focal epilepsy. *Epilepsy Res* 1987; **1**: 134–8.
(16) Gjerstad L, Nyberg-Hansen R, Taubøll E, Rootwelt K, Russell D. Some aspects of regional cerebral blood flow (rCBF) in epilepsy, using single photon emission computer tomography (SPECT). In: Dam M, Johannessen SI, Nilsson B, Sillanpää M, eds. *Epilepsy: Progress in treatment*. Chichester: John Wiley, 1987; 69–80.
(17) Andersen AR, Gram L, Kjær L, *et al*. SPECT in partial epilepsy: Identifying side of the focus. *Acta Neurol Scand* 1988; **45** (Suppl 117): 90–4.
(18) Celsis P, Goldman T, Henriksen L, Lassen NA. A method for calculating regional cerebral blood flow from emission computed tomography of inert gas concentrations. *J Comput Assist Tomogr* 1981; **5**: 641–5.
(19) Lassen NA, Sveinsdottir E, Kanno I, Stokely EM, Rommer P. A fast moving single photon emission tomograph for regional cerebral blood flow studies in man. *J Comput Assist Tomogr* 1978; **2**: 661–2.
(20) Kuhl DE, Barrio JR, Huang SC, *et al*. Quantifying local cerebral blood flow by N-isopropyl-p(I-123) iodo amphetamine tomography. *J Nucl Med* 1982; **23**: 196–203.
(21) Neirinckx RD, Canning LR, Piper IM, *et al*. Technetium-99m-d, l-HMPAO: A new radiopharmaceutical for SPECT imaging of regional cerebral blood perfusion. *J Nucl Med* 1987; **28**: 191–202.
(22) Lassen NA, Andersen AR, Friberg L, Paulson OB. The retention of Tc99m-d, l-HMPAO in the human brain after intra-carotid bolus injection; a kinetic analysis. *J Cerebr Blood Flow Metab* 1988; **8** (Suppl 1): S13–S22.
(23) Gastaut H, Gastaut JL. Computerized transverse axial tomography in epilepsy. *Epilepsia* 1976; **17**: 325–36.
(24) Yang PJ, Berger PE, Cohen ME, Duffner PK. Computerized tomography and childhood seizure disorders. *Neurology* 1979; **29**: 1084–8.
(25) Young RSK, Osbakken MD, Alger PM, Ramer JC, Weidner WA, Daigh JD. Magnetic resonance imaging in leukodystrophies of childhood. *Pediat Neurol* 1985; **1**: 15–9.
(26) Kuzniecky R, De La Sayette V, Ethier R, *et al*. Magnetic resonance imaging in temporal lobe epilepsy: pathologic correlations. *Ann Neurol* 1987; **22**: 341–7.
(27) Kramer RE, Lüders H, Lesser RP, *et al*. Transient focal abnormalities of neuroimaging studies during focal status epilepticus. *Epilepsia* 1987; **28**: 528–32.
(28) Riela AR, Penry JK, Laster DW, Schwartze GM. Magnetic resonance imaging and complex partial seizures. In: Ellington RJ, Murray NMF, Halliday AM, eds. *The London Symposium (EEG Suppl 39)*. Elsevier, 1987: 161–73.
(29) Schörner W, Meencke HJ, Felix R. Temporal-lobe epilepsy: comparison of CT and MR imaging. *Am J Radiol* 1987; **149**: 1231–9.
(30) Ormson MJ, Kispert DB, Sharbrough FW, Houser OW, Earnest F, Scheithauser BW, Laws ER. Cryptic structural lesions in refractory epilepsy: MR imaging and CT studies. *Radiology* 1986; **160**: 215–9.
(31) Riela A, Penry JK. Magnetic resonance imaging and epilepsy. In: Dam M, Gram L, eds. *Epileptology—An international perspective*. New York: Raven Press, 1989: in press.

Discussion after Drs Bone and Blumhardt and Professor Dam

Dr Kennard *(London, UK):* I was not clear when you were talking about SPECT, whether or not there were patients who had abnormalities on the SPECT scans but did not have any abnormalities on the EEG.

Dr Bone *(Glasgow, UK):* Patients whose CT and MRI scans were normal had SPECT scans. An EEG was carried out at the time of injection of Ceretec, but there was no correlation between the surface EEG and the finding of hypoperfusion.

Dr Genton *(France):* Dr Blumhardt, in a patient in whom you are considering withdrawal of medication, is there a place for ambulatory monitoring of the EEG before withdrawal of the drug when the patient has no seizure?

Dr Blumhardt *(Liverpool, UK):* I know of no study that has actually looked at this. You might expect the very long temporal samples to be a better predictor of outcome than routine EEG.

Dr Reynolds *(Chairman):* Is this something you do Dr Genton?

Dr Genton *(France):* No, I have no experience of that.

Dr Binnie *(London, UK):* One series on antiepileptic drug withdrawal included a period of telemetric monitoring, which demonstrated that 10% of the patients who believed themselves, and who were believed by others, to be seizure free, were not.

Dr Verity *(Cambridge, UK):* I was interested to hear your comments on the number of channels available and surprised that an increased number of channels did not necessarily improve the quality of recording. Would you comment on that?

Dr Blumhardt: If epileptiform abnormalities were randomly distributed across the scalp then three channels would obviously not be as good as eight channels. Because studies of routine EEGs have shown that there is a frontotemporal emphasis, then the montage can be tailored to pick up those predominantly frontotemporal abnormalities. Electrodes can be placed in such a way with 3 channels to produce satisfactory results. With more channels there is a slight improvement in terms of ictal diagnosis, but the majority of interictal abnormalities can be picked up with two or three channels.

Dr Besag *(Surrey, UK):* We found ambulatory monitoring tremendously helpful for children who appear rather 'switched off' in the mornings, and we have discovered that a lot of them have silent nocturnal seizures which are missed. Similarly, for nocturnal wetting in some youngsters who are not showing overt seizures, the ambulatory monitoring is absolutely invaluable. The quantitative analysis of ambulatory monitoring is extremely tedious and we have overcome that difficulty for children who are showing frank spike and wave by devising a new device which automatically monitors and logs the spike and wave and also allows a playback of the events, the duration of all spikes and waves, the number of events where they occurred and at what time. So instead of taking three days to analyse the record it can be done in a matter of minutes.

Dr Blumhardt: The detection of silent seizures is a point well made. But to look through all the tapes in order to detect silent seizures in that sort of child is expensive and time consuming. Only 2% of our series of adult patients with 'turns' of uncertain aetiology had silent seizures which they did not report in their diaries. The situation is of course very different in severely epileptic populations where there are large numbers of silent seizures.

Dr Nasar *(Bridlington, UK):* In what age group did you look at the ambulatory monitoring?

Dr Blumhardt: 15–90.

Dr Nasar: Did you find any difference between the elderly and the adult in the rate of pickup?

Dr Blumhardt: No, but we only have 145 cases. We are currently analysing nearly 500 cases that have been followed-up for five years, so we might get some break down by age group eventually.

Professor Dam *(Copenhagen, Denmark):* Would you recommend us now to drop the number of electrodes during ambulatory EEG and use only three in our normal recordings?

Dr Blumhardt: If you have got eight channels then you should use them.

Professor Dam: But for the normal routine EEG, if we go back from 24 or 16 to only three it would save a lot of time.

Dr Blumhardt: It depends on the reasons for doing an EEG. Most commonly I believe you do it for localization and lateralization and the identification of focal (i.e. phase-reversals) abnormalities, the detection of which is notoriously poor with ambulatory EEG monitoring.

Professor Dam: Would it not be useful to have the focus on the ambulatory monitoring and be able to see focal changes?

Dr Blumhardt: It would, but you would need many more channels to do that, and the problem is that you get an enormous number of artefactual slow wave abnormalities which can mimic focal abnormalities on ambulatory monitoring. It is a very different situation recording 16 or 24 channels in a patient lying in an EEG room, to recording a patient at home. If you did a blind analysis of that, the results would be quite hopeless.

I would be interested to know what the audience feels about the routine use of ambulatory EEG in their clinics. What proportion actually uses ambulatory EEG as a routine diagnostic test in patients seen in the clinic, when you are not sure about the diagnosis?

Interactive questions from Dr Blumhardt

		Response
1. Do you have access to ambulatory monitoring?		
	1 Yes	64%
	2 No	33%
	3 Don't know	3%
2. Those of you who have access to ambulatory monitoring, do you use it on a regular daily basis?		Response
	1 Yes	30%
	2 No	68%
	3 Don't know	2%

Dr Reynolds: Most people who have access to it do not actually use it on a regular basis.

Dr Blumhardt: This is what I suspected.

Interactive question from Professor Dam	
Is it possible to demonstrate hippocampal sclerosis by MR scan?	**Response**
1 Yes	65%
2 No	8%
3 Don't know	27%

Dr Reynolds: A lot of don't knows there, would you like to comment on this Dr Dam?

Professor Dam: I think that not many people have an MRI and have tried to see whether they can see hippocampal sclerosis. You need to have a neuropathological investigation afterwards to see if there was a hippocampal sclerosis, but you can often see it with MI while you can never see it with a CT scan.

Dr Zagury *(Switzerland):* Does Dr Dam routinely use gadolinium injection with magnetic resonance in epileptic patients?

Professor Dam: No, we have just started using this contrast medium.

Dr Reynolds: Dr Bone said that MRI picked up everything that his CT picked up and more, whereas in your talk Dr Dam you implied that there were things picked up on CT that were not picked up on MRI. This is a very important issue for those of us who have not got access to MRI. What is the relative role of these two imaging techniques, could you expand on that?

Professor Dam: I think in patients with epilepsy MRI is clearly much better, but if you study infarctions and arterial venous malformations, CT scan can be better.

Dr Reynolds: Does everyone agree with that?

Dr Peters *(Netherlands):* I do not agree that a CT is better in picking up arterial/venous malformation than MRI. On the contrary, in the literature there are many examples of patients who have a negative CT whereas a clear flow phenomenon can be seen with the MRI.

Depth electrodes in seizure mapping— selection of patients

C. D. Binnie

The Maudsley Hospital, London, UK

INTRODUCTION

The main difficulties and complexities of epilepsy surgery lie in preoperative assessment rather than in the surgical procedures themselves. The preoperative programme which may be required in any given patient is rarely obvious at the point of referral. As the flow chart in Fig. 1 indicates, patients undergo a phased assessment and at various points a decision is made to operate, to give up, or to proceed to further investigations.

Phase Ia comprises the basic clinical assessment, interictal EEG investigations (including studies in sleep and possibly with sphenoidal or other special electrodes), neuroradiological imaging, and initial neuropsychological evaluation. These will suffice to identify some patients who are clearly unsuitable for surgery, others who have gross radiologically demonstrable lesions requiring removal, and those whose seizures can best be relieved by hemispherectomy or callosotomy. Phase Ib involves ictal EEG recording with scalp and/or sphenoidal or foramen ovale electrodes, possibly further radiological imaging (MRI and PET), if not done before, and often a carotid amytal test to lateralize cognitive functions and determine the possible intellectual deficits which might result from surgery. At this point it may be discovered during telemetry that some patients have pseudoseizures or that, having seen the inside of a neurosurgical unit, they no longer want operative treatment. Patients with an unequivocally localized, unilateral, temporal origin of their seizures may be identified at this point and offered surgery ('simple temporal lobe epilepsy' in the flow chart). The remainder will proceed to Phase II, involving more invasive methods of electrophysiological investigation with intracranial electrodes. The figures in the flow chart indicate the courses typically followed by 100 patients referred to the Maudsley epilepsy surgery programme. Approximately one-quarter reach Phase II. These comprise mainly patients with complex partial seizures which cannot be confidently localized to one temporal lobe (' "difficult" C.P.S.' in Fig. 1), and those with a presumed seizure origin over the convexity, whether frontal, central or parietal ('lateral focus' in the figure).

The extent to which use is made of intracranial recording varies greatly between centres. To some extent this reflects different philosophies, but also the facilities that are available and the referral patterns. A centre without sophisticated neurophysiological support may only carry out Phase Ia of the programme, removing radiologically demonstrable lesions and performing hemispherectomy and callosotomy where appropriate, and rejecting as inoperable (or referring elsewhere) those patients who require more complex assessment. Some centres receive large numbers of patients with classical clinical radiological and electrophysiological features of mesial temporal sclerosis and these patients can generally be identified and successfully treated on the basis of Phases Ia and b. At the Maudsley Hospital such patients make up nearly a third of our referrals and, before facilities were available for sub-acute intracranial recording, represented the majority of those undergoing operation. Conversely, in some countries there is reluctance to refer patients for surgery

Fourth international symposium on sodium valproate and epilepsy, edited by David Chadwick, 1989: Royal Society of Medicine Services International Congress and Symposium No. 152, published by Royal Society of Medicine Services Limited.

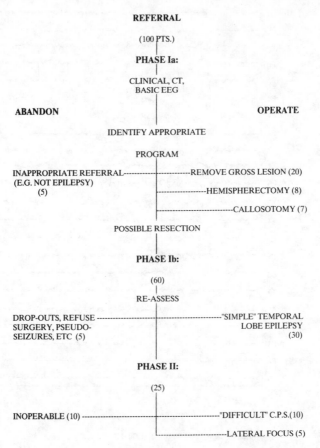

REFERRAL

(100 PTS.)

PHASE Ia:

CLINICAL, CT,
BASIC EEG

ABANDON   **OPERATE**

IDENTIFY APPROPRIATE

PROGRAM

INAPPROPRIATE REFERRAL--------------------REMOVE GROSS LESION (20)
(E.G. NOT EPILEPSY)
(5)   --------------------HEMISPHERECTOMY (8)

                                           --------------------------CALLOSOTOMY (7)

POSSIBLE RESECTION

PHASE Ib:

(60)

RE-ASSESS

DROP-OUTS, REFUSE --------------------------"SIMPLE" TEMPORAL
SURGERY, PSEUDO-   LOBE EPILEPSY
SEIZURES, ETC (5)   (30)

PHASE II:

(25)

INOPERABLE (10) --------------------------"DIFFICULT" C.P.S.(10)

                              --------------------------LATERAL FOCUS (5)

Figure 1 *Investigation and decision-making in 100 patients referred for preoperative assessment, see text.*

and only those with the most complex problems are seen, with a variety of lesions, traumatic, infective etc., often located outside the temporal lobes. Such patients usually require Phase II assessment.

FORAMEN OVALE ELECTRODES

The need for insertion of extensive arrays of intracranial electrodes has been significantly reduced by development of foramen ovale electrodes (1). In contrast to sphenoidal electrodes placed outside the foramen ovale and recording little which cannot be detected with suitably positioned surface contacts, foramen ovale electrodes are inserted into the subdural space and come to lie alongside mesial temporal structures, providing a true intracranial recording.

As shown in Figs 2 and 3 they pick up both interictal and ictal discharges which may be unrecognizable on the surface. Where a temporal origin for a patient's seizures is probable but not certain, or where there is doubt concerning the lateralization of seizure onset, ictal recordings with foramen ovale electrodes may suffice to identify the causative focus. They also have a more specialized use in distinguishing mesial from lateral temporal foci, a discrimination which may determine the choice between treating temporal lobe epilepsy by *en bloc* resection or selective amygdalo-hippocampectomy. No less importantly, foramen ovale recording may establish that the seizures are not of temporal origin, reinforcing a decision to embark on Phase II investigations (Fig. 4).

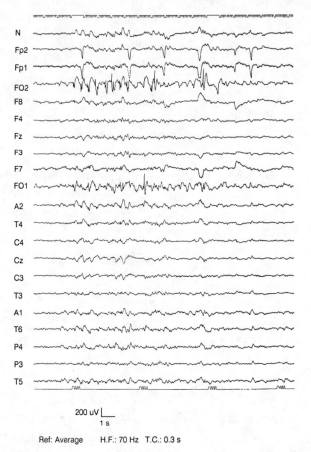

N

Fp2

Fp1

FO2

F8

F4

Fz

F3

F7

FO1

A2

T4

C4

Cz

C3

T3

A1

T6

P4

P3

T5

200 uV
1 s

Ref: Average   H.F.: 70 Hz   T.C.: 0.3 s

Figure 2 *Interictal recording of spike-wave discharges at foramen ovale electrodes. Electrode designations: FO2 and FO1—right and left foramen ovale, others according to usual international 10/20 convention.*

DEPTH AND SUBDURAL ELECTRODES

Apart from foramen ovale electrodes three different technologies are generally used for chronic intracranial recording:

Mats, or rectilinear arrays of multiple contacts mounted on plastic sheets, may be placed over the cerebral convexity. They provide excellent recordings and are eminently suitable for functional mapping by electrical stimulation or by evoked response studies. They are subject to the obvious drawback that a craniotomy is required for their insertion, indeed a bilateral craniotomy if the side of seizure origin is in doubt, and that they provide no coverage of less accessible areas such as mesial temporal and orbital frontal regions.

Subdural strips are constructed by essentially the same technologies as mats but being narrower can be inserted through burr holes and slipped down the mesial aspect of the hemispheres and under the inferior surfaces of the frontal and temporal lobes. Obviously this technology too will fail to detect seizure onset in deep structures such as the amygdalo-hippocampal complex.

Depth electrodes are multicontact electrode bundles inserted stereotactically into targets considered most likely to be the source of ictal activity. Most often they are inserted

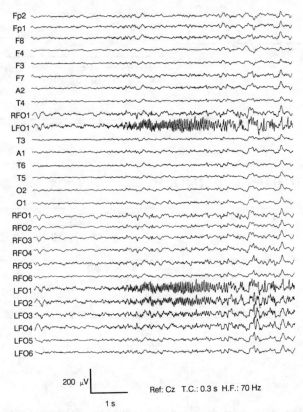

Figure 3 *Onset of complex partial seizure in left mesial temporal structures. Multipolar foramen ovale contacts right (RFO) and left (LFO) numbered 6 to 1 from region of foramen ovale to depth of 4 cm. Note that discharges are maximal at deepest contact (LFO1) and are virtually undetectable either in surface EEG or in region of foramen ovale (LFO6), i.e. close to conventional sphenoidal electrode site.*

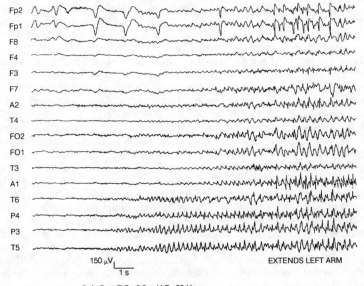

Figure 4 *Ictal recording of complex seizure not arising at foramen ovale electrodes, origin was subsequently shown to be right parieto-temporal. (Same patient as Fig. 12).*

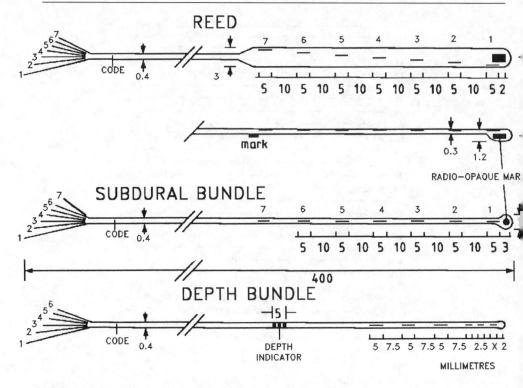

Figure 5 *Subdural and depth electrodes described by Van Veelen et al. (in press).*

horizontally using a technique described by Bancaud and Talairach (2). Whilst the contacts closest to the tip of each bundle record from mesial temporal structures or the mesial aspects of the hemispheres, the more laterally placed contacts record from the cortical convexity at the point of penetration. Each contact samples the electrical activity of only a very small volume of brain. Consequently, it may be necessary to employ a large number of bundles and to have a clear hypothesis concerning the probable site of seizure onset before embarking on their use. The incidence of significant morbidity is about 1 per 1000 electrodes inserted and many centres will use upwards of a dozen bundles (3,4).

At the Maudsley Hospital we do in fact use mats and strips for patients with seizures thought to arise from the cerebral convexity (e.g. simple partial seizures with exclusively motor symptoms). However, for other purposes and particularly in patients with complex partial seizures we employ a somewhat innovative technology developed by Storm van Leeuwen and colleagues in Utrecht (5) using combined depth and subdural electrodes. It would obviously be difficult to combine mats or strips with horizontally inserted depth electrodes and our technique depends upon inserting both depth electrodes and slender flexible subdural 'reeds' and bundles radially from two central trephine holes. The subdural electrodes, being flexible, can be manipulated through the subdural space under fluoroscopy, reaching sites as inaccessible as the orbital surface of the frontal lobe. Generally, seven contact bundles are used but if difficulty is experienced in passing these in the required direction 'reeds' are substituted. These are flattened, and being therefore compliant in only one dimension, are easier to guide to the target (Fig. 5). Having obtained an extensive coverage of all regions of the convexity and undersurface of the hemispheres likely to be relevant we place depth electrodes only in a few selected targets, typically the amygdala, anterior and mid-hippocampus on one or both sides and possibly through the cingulum into the infero-medial frontal region in patients whose seizures appear to be of possible frontal origin. This allows the use of a minimum number of depth electrodes to study the suspected site of seizure origin, whilst providing extensive coverage or other regions to guard against the working hypothesis being incorrect.

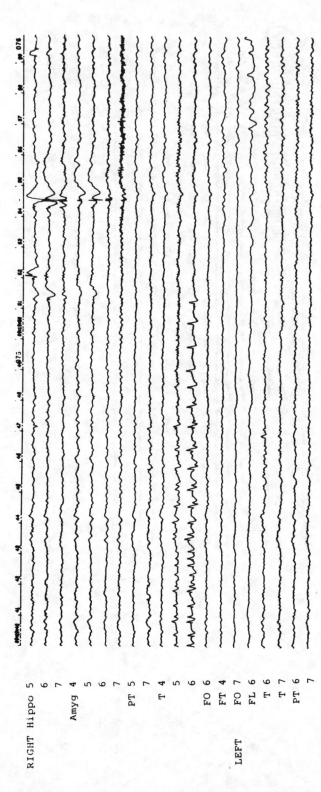

Figure 6a,b,c *Recording with depth and subdural electrodes of seizure arising in right amygdala (see text). Key: Depth contacts: hippo—hippocampus, amyg—amygdala; Subdural: PT—posterior temporal, T—mid-temporal, FO—orbital frontal, FT—fronto-temporal, FL—lateral frontal. Reprinted with permission from Binnie CD. Electroencephalography. In: Laidlaw J, Richens A, Oxley J, eds. A textbook of epilepsy. London: Churchill Livingstone, 1988: 236–306.*

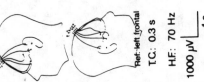

Figure 6b

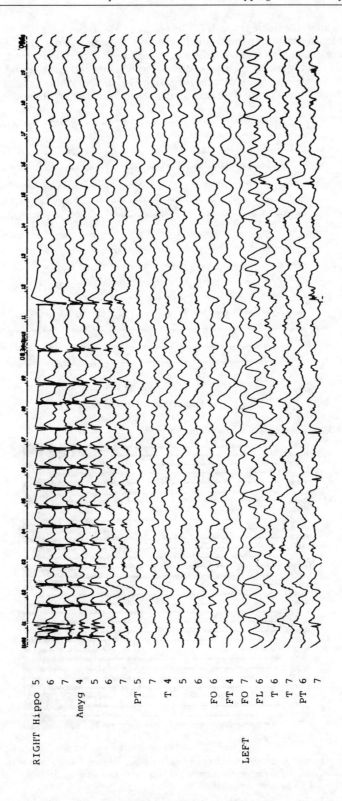

Figure 6c

The justification for this approach is illustrated in Fig. 6, which makes several points of general interest concerning intracranial recording. This shows an ictal record of a patient with right mesial temporal sclerosis who is now seizure-free following temporal lobectomy. Both amygdali and hippocampi have been implanted and subdural electrodes are located over both hemispheres. The interictal recording is characterized by spikes which were present almost continually at a right mid-temporal subdural contact (channel 12). At seizure

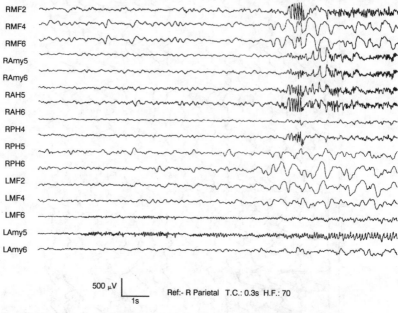

Figure 7a   *Onset of complex partial seizure in left amygdala.*

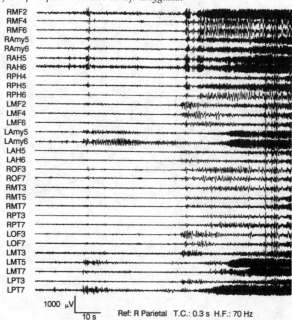

Figure 7b   *Same seizure, 31 channel recording on greatly reduced time scale. Key: Depth contacts: MF—mesial frontal, Amy—amygdala, AH—anterior hippocampus, PH—posterior hippocampus; Subdural: OF—orbital frontal, MT—mid-temporal, PT—posterior temporal.*

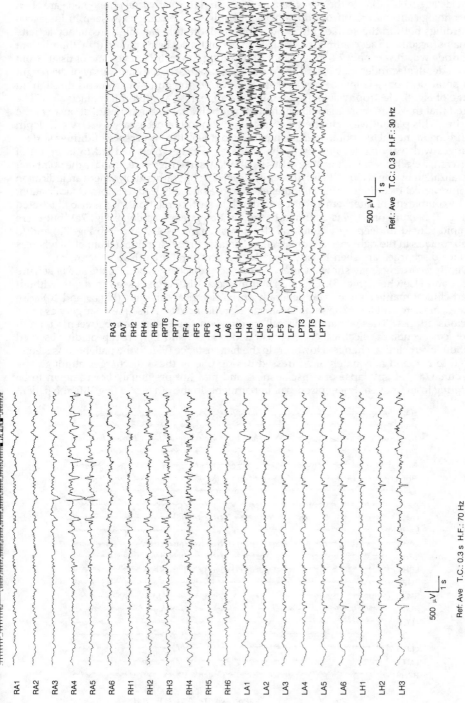

Figure 8a *Interictal recording with depth electrodes, note right and left-sided independent discharges in amygdala (RA and LA) and anterior hippocampus (RH and LH).*

Figure 8b *Diffuse left-sided onset of seizure in hippocampus and lateral frontal contact (LF7) in same patient—see text.*

onset these cease and instead high frequency multiunit activity appears at a contact in the right amygdala (channel 7). This illustrates both that inter-ictal discharges do not necessarily provide a reliable guide to the site of seizure onset, and that early ictal phenomena are often morphologically different from the spikes and spike-wave complexes seen in inter-ictal recordings both in the surface EEG and in depth. Note that this high frequency activity remains for some 15 sec confined to a single contact and is not being picked up at the adjacent electrode which was only 2.5 mm distant, illustrating the restricted volume of tissue from which depth electrodes may record. As the seizure progresses the entire array of deep right temporal electrodes is invaded by spikes (Fig. 6b). At the end of Part a and throughout Part b of Fig. 6, electrophysiological changes are appearing at subdural contacts. It will be noted that these are more marked on the left, contralateral to the true site of onset of the seizure. This patient was admittedly atypical: it is not often necessary to carry out depth recording in mesial temporal sclerosis and indeed it was the occurrence of diffuse surface changes with varying asymmetry in the ictal scalp EEGs which had led to insertion of intracranial electrodes. The purpose of this illustration is not, therefore, to make the point that lateralization by the scalp EEG is necessarily unreliable but rather that, where an indication for intracranial recording exists, subdural electrodes alone may lead to incorrect localization.

The complexity of interhemispheric and depth to surface relationships is also illustrated in Fig. 7. Seizure onset was confined to the left amygdala (see detail Fig. 7a), but there is rapid spread to deep right temporal structures (channels 4–7 and 9 in Fig. 7b) and to deep contacts in the right mesial frontal region, notably in the cingulum (channel 1), whereas surface discharges are seen mostly over the left temporal area (last 4 channels).

Depth recordings may show a variety of inter-ictal discharges both at the site of seizure onset and elsewhere (Fig. 8). Often a rhythmic ictal discharge is seen in depth without overt clinical manifestations and generally such 'electrical seizures' (Figs 9 and 10) arise at the same site and have the same localizing significance for subsequent surgery as more obvious attacks. These phenomena call in question the distinction between ictal and inter-ictal events: the electrical events illustrated in Figs 9 and 10 were repeatedly observed without overt clinical change. However, in the first instance (Fig. 9) the patient consistently failed to respond adequately if addressed during one of these discharges although she was unaware of any lapse of consciousness and had not previously been known to be suffering from frequent brief episodes of impairment. In the other case (Fig. 10), the patient

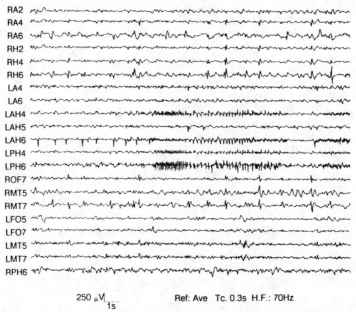

250 μV / 1s   Ref: Ave   Tc. 0.3s   H.F.: 70Hz

Figure 9   *Apparently subclinical 'electrical seizure' in left anterior and posterior hippocampus (LAH, LPH). Patient showed transitory cognitive impairment. (See also overt seizure, Fig. 11).*

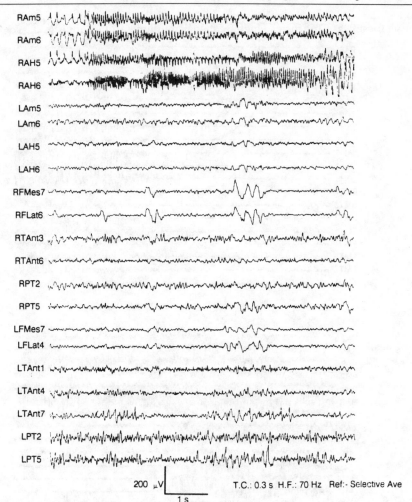

Figure 10 *Apparently subclinical seizure in right amygdala and anterior hippocampus (RAm, RAH). Patient was taught to recognize clinical symptoms accompanying discharge.*

responded adequately during the discharges and initially denied any clinical symptoms. However, after being repeatedly challenged during several similar discharges, she began to recognize that they were accompanied by a characteristic abdominal sensation and thereafter was able reliably to signal their occurrence by the pressing of an event marker button.

The complexity of ictal spread was noted above and this on occasions gives rise to the difficulties in confidently identifying seizure onset. Figure 11 shows a typical sequence of events in the overt seizures of a patient whose 'subclinical' discharges were illustrated in Fig. 9. After a left hippocampal onset the discharges spread to the deep structures on the right, and those on the left abruptly ceased. All clinical features of the patient's seizures except the initial event (tingling in the right side of the face), could be replicated by electrical stimulation of the right hippocampus. The picture was further complicated by the fact that, when antiepileptic drugs were withdrawn in order to increase the rate of seizure capture, attacks were seen starting in the right hippocampus without the initial left-sided events. This pattern was reversed when the drugs were reinstituted. The patient is now seizure-free following removal of a sclerotic left hippocampus and amygdala, the clinical response and pathology confirming the accuracy of the eventualy localization. In this context it may be added that antiepileptic drug withdrawal is in general held to be a suitable method of increasing seizure frequency during monitoring with depth electrodes (6), but Engel and Crandall (7) have also reported one similar incidence of AED withdrawal altering the electrographic seizure pattern.

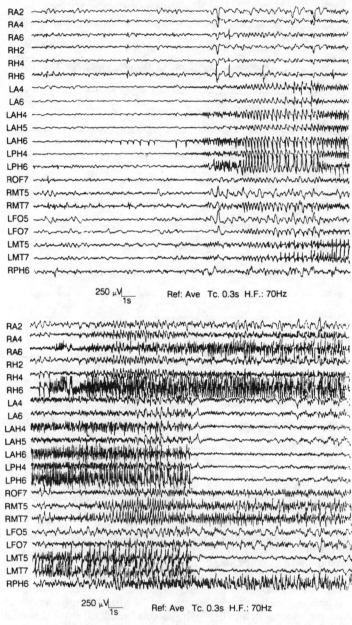

Figure 11a,b *Consecutive sections of ictal recording from same patient as Fig. 9. Onset in left anterior hippocampus (LAH6) with rapid spread to right hemisphere.*

It is far from the case that depth recording invariably provides clear evidence of the site of seizure onset and a basis for a surgical resection. Where the majority of the inter-ictal discharges, the subclinical electrical seizures and the overt attacks all clearly start at a single anatomically restricted site, and precede the appearance of clinical events, one may be reasonably confident of localization, particularly so when the initial events consist of high frequency multiunit activity as in Figs 6 and 12. Where multiple foci of seizure onset or initially generalized discharges are seen, one may conclude that the patient is inoperable (8). Greater difficulty arises where initial ictal changes are seen at several ipsilateral but not closely related electrodes suggesting spread from another, unidentified site. Similarly, the

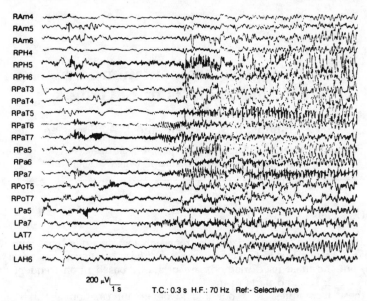

RAm4
RAm5
RAm6
RPH4
RPH5
RPH6
RPaT3
RPaT4
RPaT5
RPaT6
RPaT7
RPa5
RPa6
RPa7
RPoT5
RPoT7
LPa5
LPa7
LAT7
LAH5
LAH6

200 μV|
1 s   T.C.: 0.3 s H.F.: 70 Hz Ref:- Selective Ave

Figure 12 *Seizure onset with high frequency multiunit activity chiefly in right parieto-temporal region (RPaT7) and posterior hippocampus (RPH5). Same patient as Fig. 4.*

appearance of relatively low frequency wave forms, sharp and slow wave complexes or an electrodecremental event accompanied by a DC shift, suggests again that these changes may be secondary to seizure onset at an undetected site. The ictal record in Fig. 8b has all these features. In making a decision one may need to take account of other factors such as changes in threshold for producing after-discharges by electrical stimulation, replication of clinical seizure patterns by stimulation at a suspected site of onset, and the effects of sleep and intravenous barbiturates on inter-ictal discharges; where there are multiple foci, that from which the seizures arise is most likely to be activated and resistant to suppression by intravenous barbiturates and is less likely to show marked changes in discharge rate with waking and sleep. These criteria were met by the left-sided focus in the patient illustrated in Fig. 8, who is now seizure-free after left temporal lobectomy.

In conclusion, depth recording is not necessary in all patients undergoing epilepsy surgery and does not invariably provide the evidence required to justify operative treatment. It is a major undertaking in terms of technical resources and the risks and stress to which the patient is exposed, and should only be undertaken after careful patient selection in the context of an integrated pre-operative assessment programme.

REFERENCES

(1) Wieser HG, Elger CE, Stodieck SRG. The 'Foramen Ovale Electrode': a new recording method for the preoperative evaluation of patients suffering from mesio-basal temporal lobe epilepsy. *Electroenceph Clin Neurophysiol* 1985; **61**: 314–22.

(2) Bancaud J, Talairach J, Bonis A, *et al. La stereoencephalographie dans l'epilepsie.* Paris: Masson, 1965.

(3) Ajmone Marsan C. Depth electrography and electrocorticography. In: Aminoff MJ, ed. *Electrodiagnosis in temporal lobe epilepsy.* Springfield: Thomas, 1980: 78–108.

(4) Spencer SS. Depth electroencephalography in selection of refractory epilepsy for surgery. *Ann Neurol* 1981; **9**: 207–14.

(5) Van Veelen CWM, Debets RMC, Van Huffelen AC, *et al.* Combined use of subdural and intracerebral electrodes in preoperative evaluation of epilepsy, submitted to *J Neurosurg.*

(6) Spencer SS, Spencer DD, Williamson PD, Mattson RH. Ictal effects of anticonvulsant medication withdrawal in epileptic patients. *Epilepsia* 1981; **22**: 297–307.

(7) Engel J, Crandall P. Falsely localizing ictal events with depth EEG telemetry during anticonvulsant withdrawal. *Epilepsia* 1983; **24**: 344–55.

(8) Lieb JP, Engel J, Gevins A, Crandall PH. Surface and deep EEG correlates of surgical outcome in temporal lobe epilepsy. *Epilepsia* 1981; **22**: 515–38.

Adaptive segmentation and clustering analysis of EEG-signals

P. Jennum[1], J. S. Hansen[2] and J. A. Sørensen[2]

[1]Department of Neurology, University Hospital, Copenhagen; [2]Electronics Institute, Technical University of Denmark, Lyngby, Denmark

INTRODUCTION

The use of quantitative (computerized) electroencephalography (EEG) has improved during recent years. Quantitative EEG includes various different statistical analytical techniques (Table 1), but the most used methods are primarily based upon frequency-amplitude detection of user-selected parts of the EEG (1).

Using these techniques, it is possible to obtain information about frequency and amplitudes of selected parts of the EEG-signals. However, an automatic classification of the EEG—either in the background or in transients of the EEG—is not obtained using these methods. For example, sleep stages or spike detection is not possible solely using amplitude and frequency analysis.

Because long-term recordings have found increasing use during recent years in clinical and experimental use and research, an increasing demand for automatic EEG-analysis technique has risen in order to avoid time-consuming visual analysis. Obvious applications of automated techniques of long-term recording include sleep research, long-term recordings in patients suffering from epilepsy, intensive care, anaesthesia and operative monitoring, and pharmaco-EEG, among others.

Table 1 *Examples of different methods used in the analysis of quantitative EEG*

Frequency domain
  Power spectrum
    Amplitude spectrum
Spatial domain
Coherence
Significant scores
Period-amplitude analysis
Zero-crossing analysis
Fast Fourier Transform
Autoregressive analysis
Digital filtration

In order to evaluate different algorithms to allow classification of the EEG, different linear models were compared. A review of linear models is given by Jansen (2). The techniques used in this presentation are a part of a larger methodological study to improve and select statistical algorithms to subdivide and classify EEG-signals by automatic techniques. The algorithm is implemented into a larger software system running on IBM-compatible computers.

Fourth international symposium on sodium valproate and epilepsy, edited by David Chadwick, 1989: Royal Society of Medicine Services International Congress and Symposium No. 152, published by Royal Society of Medicine Services Limited.

THE AR-MODEL

The autoregressive (AR) model can be viewed as a process-generator or as a process-analyser.

AR-process-generator

The input-signal to the AR-process-generator is a white noise discrete time series e(n) with a zero mean. The generated output is a discrete time series x(n), n=1,2,..N. For the AR-model of order p the present output sample x(n) is given from the p previous output samples $x(n-1)\cdots x(n-p)$ and the white noise signal as

$$x(n) = a_1 x(n-1) + a_2 x(n-2) + \cdots + a_p x(n-p) + e(n),$$

where a_i, $i=1,2,\cdots$, p is the weighting coefficient or the parameters of the auto-regressive-model.

AR-process-analyser

The AR-process-analyser is the inverse of the AR-process-generator. The discrete time series x(n), $n=1,2,\cdots,N$, is now the input signal. The output e(n) is a time series of residual values (prediction errors), which indicates how well the input signal matches the AR-model. The AR-model of order p for the AR-process-analyser is given by

$$e(n) = x(n) - a_1 x(n-1) - a_2 x(n-1) - \cdots - a_p x(n-p).$$

Given the parameters a_i, $i=1,\ldots,p$, the time series analysed by the AR-process-analyser will be equal to the time series generated by an AR-process-generator with the same parameters, if the prediction error is white noise.

AR-spectral estimate

The spectrum of the signal generated or analysed with the AR-model can be estimated as

$$S(f) = \frac{S_e(f)}{(1 - \sum\limits_{n=1}^{p} a_n \exp(-j2\pi nf/f_s))^2}$$

in which $S_e(f)$ is the power spectrum of e(n), f_s is the sampling frequency. If e(n) is a white noise signal then $S_e(f)$ can be replaced by σ_e^2/f_s, where σ_e^2 is the variance of e(n).

Segmentation

To be able to analyse long-term recordings, the EEG has to be subdivided (segmented) into smaller pieces (segments) which can then be analysed. This can be done either by using a fixed-interval or a variable-interval segmentation (adaptive segmentation).

Fixed interval segmentation

In fixed interval segmentation, the EEG is divided into segments of equal intervals (example: 1 second). If long segments are used then a larger part of the EEG is covered, but discrete and transient activity is overlooked. Moreover, more than one stage of the EEG is often included (example: both theta-activity and K-complexes). If the segments are very short, then part of the activity may be cut into small meaningless pieces. The most commonly used segment length is 1–2.5 s (2).

Adaptive segmentation

In order to overcome the problems using fixed-intervals for the division of the EEG, Bodenstein et al. (3) suggested subdividing the EEG based upon the changes in it.

The primary principle using these methods is to view a part of the EEG through a window, the fixed window. Another window, the moving window, is placed over the fixed window, and from there slid along the EEG. As the moving window is moved through the EEG the parts of the EEG seen through the two windows are continuously compared, and the similarity expressed as a difference measure. When the difference measure exceeds a preset threshold, a segment is identified, and the procedure is repeated for identifying the next segment. Using these methods the EEG is subdivided primarily upon the changes in rhythmicity (either in background activity or in transients). The main problem using this method is the definition of the point at which the changes in the background activity or in the transient patterns actually occur.

Methods for adaptive segmentation

Different methods have been suggested (3–7). In order to characterize the ability to separate changes in (a) background activity, and (b) transient patterns, four models have been compared.

Adaptive segmentation based on the AR-model

The AR-model has been used for adaptive segmentation (3,4). The AF-coefficients are found on a part of the EEG, and the EEG is used as input-signal to the AR-process-analyser (inverse filtering). The prediction error of the output signal will be white noise while the EEG is as it was generated by the AR-model. Changes in the EEG can now be identified by checking when the prediction error changes from white noise.

Adaptive segmentation based on the autocorrelation-function

The autocorrelation-function, contains information about the spectral properties of the EEG, and can be used to estimate the spectrum of the EEG. The autocorrelation-function has been used for adaptive segmentation (5–6), by comparing the autocorrelation-functions of the EEG seen through the two windows. In this way changes in the EEG are detected by identifying spectral changes.

Clustering

All segments are analysed, and the EEG in each segment is described by a number of measures giving a feature-vector. We have used an 11-dimensional feature-vector containing the mean power and 10 AR-coefficients of the segment. The similarity of the EEG in different segments can thereby be analysed by comparing the feature vectors as points in an 11-dimensional space; similar segments will group in the same area in the 11-dimensional space.

Application on artificial signals

The models have been tested on artificial signals, characterized by changes in (a) amplitude, (b) frequency.

The old methods of Bodenstein *et al.* (3) clearly show asymmetry, and cannot be used for adaptive segmentation. The other three methods (4–6) track the shift in both amplitude and in frequency. However, short transient shifts in the background activity are not invariably or precisely detected.

Applications on EEG-signals

The adaptive segmentation was applied on EEG-signals from normal waking and sleeping subjects. The recordings were performed from central and occipital recordings (C3, C4, 01 and 02). Sampling rate was 100 Hz and the resolution was 12 bit. Filter settings were 0.2 and 40 Hz, 70 dB/octave. All data were analysed on an 80386 computer system (HP Vectra 20/100).

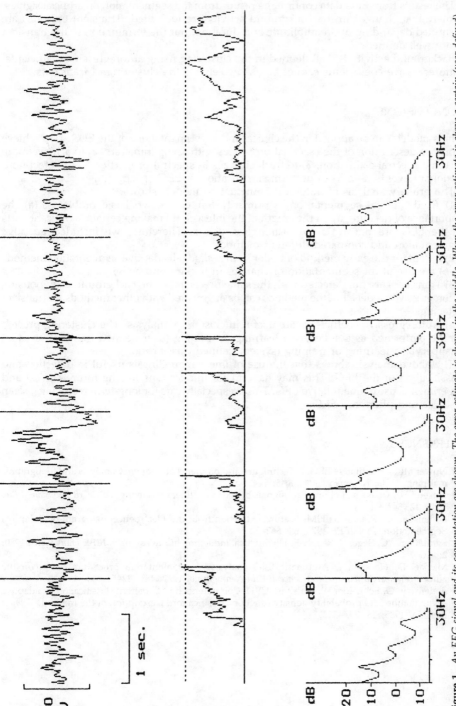

Figure 1 *An EEG signal and its segmentation are shown. The error estimate is shown in the middle. When the error estimate is above a certain (user defined) limit a segmentation is performed and a new feature extraction is defined. The spectral templates of the different segments are shown in the lower part.*

An example of the segmentation is shown in Fig. 1.

The results from EEG data confirm the results from the segmentation on artificial signals, namely that changes in the background activity are identified. Transient episodes are identified depending upon amplitude and duration, but the termination of the transient is not well defined.

Background activity is well defined in the clustering using autoregressive coefficients. Autoregressive coefficients cannot be used solely for the clustering of transients.

CONCLUSIONS

Linear models can be applied in the clinical and experimental use of the EEG: 1) to achieve a precise description of the essential properties with few parameters, 2) to achieve more accurate spectral estimation, 3) to track changes in spectral properties, 4) to detect non-stationary events, and 5) to perform classification of EEG spectra (2).

The primary analysis of different segmentation models shows:

1) fixed interval segmentation is primarily limited to two basic problems: (a) the importance of deciding upon the length of the interval, (b) making certain significant parts of the EEG are not cut into meaningless pieces. Therefore, we included adaptive segmentation and compared different methods.

2) Except for the early method of Bodenstein *et al.* (3) all adaptive segmentation methods (4–6) are useful for segmentation of changes in background activity.

3) Transients are not detected with the same precision as the background activity using autoregressive models, but the methods can be augmented with other methods for transient detection.

4) Autoregressive coefficients are useful in clustering analysis. The clustering process can be performed as a supervised learning or training (user-defined training) or as an unsupervised learning or training (system defined classification).

The above analysis shows that the use of linear modelling is useful in detection and classification of the EEG. This may have major implications for the future clinical and experimental use of quantitative EEG. This is especially true for long-term recordings, sleep research and pharmaco-EEG.

REFERENCES

(1) Nuwer MR. Quantitative EEG: I. Techniques and problems of frequency analysis and topographic mapping. *J Clin Neurophysiol* 1988; **5**: 1–43.
(2) Jansen BH. Analysis of biomedical signals by means of linear modeling. *CRC Crit Rev Biomed Eng* 1988; **12**: 343–92.
(3) Bodenstein G, Praetorius HM. Feature Extraction from the Electroencephalogram by Adaptive Segmentation. *Proc IEEE* 1977; **65**: 642–52.
(4) Sanderson AC, Segen J, Richey E. Hierarchical modelling of EEG signals. *IEEE Trans PAMI* 1980; **2**: 405–15.
(5) Michael D, Houchin J. Automatic EEG analysis: A segmentation procedure based on the autocorrelation function. *Electroenceph Clin Neurophysiol* 1979; **46**: 232–5.
(6) Bodenstein G, Schneider W, Malsburg CVD. Computerized EEG pattern classification by adaptive segmentation and probability density function classification. Description of the method. *Comput Biol Med* 1985; **15**: 297–313.

Discussion after Drs Binnie and Jennum

Interactive question from Dr Binnie

Should resective surgery be considered in:	Response
1 Only the most severely disabled patients	8%
2 Patients who have been intractable for 10 years	38%
3 Therapy resistant patients with partial seizures for 3 years	52%
4 Don't know	2%

Dr Binnie *(London, UK):* Perhaps I succeeded in persuading you that one should not be too reluctant to consider epilepsy surgery. There is good evidence that people with partial seizures who remain refractory for three years are most unlikely to get better, and particularly with a younger patient, the outcome of surgery both in terms of seizure control, and more importantly in terms of social development, is far better the sooner they are treated. It is tragic to see people successfully treated by surgery at the age of 30 remaining socially disabled, who could have been referred when they were 12.

Dr Price *(Swindon, UK):* One of the implications of what Dr Binnie has said is that patients who were rejected, say five years ago, as being unsuitable for surgery because it was thought that they did not have a well localized focus, should now be re-referred and reinvestigated with this more precise technology. Could you comment on that?

Dr Binnie: This is precisely the situation in our own practice. Since the introduction of depth recording and improved surgical procedures patients who have been previously rejected for surgery are being recalled, reassessed and operated on successfully.

Professor Mattson *(Connecticut, USA):* We have been doing intercranial recording for about 15 years and have studied around 200 patients, mostly with depth rather than sub-dural recording. However, the past 50 cases we have done by lateral depth as well as sub-dural recordings and we find that the sub-dural recordings do lateralize quite well. But overwhelmingly the more precise localization comes from the intercranial depth recording, partly because our depth electrode runs the length of the hippocampus and the majority of these intractable patients have their seizures arising from the hippocampus.

Dr Binnie: We share this view and it is worrying to see people rely solely on sub-dural recording. The advantage of combining sub-dural with depth is that you may be able to get away with fewer depth electrodes to cover the regions where you need to ensure that seizures are not starting. The morbidity of depth recording is dependent on the number of electrodes put in.

Dr Cumming *(Manchester, UK):* How long does this technique take and how many patients can be dealt with in a given period of time? When we start sending large numbers of patients, therapy resistant for three years, are there sufficient places available to deal with them?

Dr Binnie: The answer in Britain is 'no'. In continental Europe and the USA the number of centres providing these facilities is expanding rapidly. Each patient who requires depth recording has to go to the operating theatre three times—once to have the electrodes put in, once to have them taken out, and once for the definitive procedure. Telemetry may last from one to four weeks, and apart from the telemetric recording and the enormous amount of labour involved in assessing this, we usually take the opportunity to carry out stimulation studies and possibly evoked response studies as well. It is a very expensive process. The cost from beginning to end in North America is something of the order of \$50–70 000.

Dr Eames *(Bristol, UK):* There was a very dramatic demonstration of how one might get the site wrong with depth recordings, but might you not have avoided that with SPECT? Is there not some order of procedures which will produce the most efficient result? The ambulatory recording was claimed to be equivalent in efficiency in pickup and this might be a way of saving money. It might also make it more easy to do these kind of assessments in more centres in this country.

Dr Binnie: I was a little worried about being asked to give a presentation which dealt with one small aspect of pre-operative assessment out of context, because the whole point of pre-operative assessment is that it is a complicated, constantly changing, multi-disciplinary process involving many pieces of evidence. Before one ventures to put in depth electrodes one should develop a hypothesis about the origin and spread of the patient's seizures, and this will include all the available imaging techniques, neuropsychology, and conventional clinical assessment. Only when you have gone as far as you can with other sources should you resort to the ultimate invasive technique.

Dr Besag *(Surrey, UK):* The problem about referral is that we do not have the services to cope with them in Great Britain. Another brief point—you quoted an IQ cut-off at 70 points, but some patients have been operated on and investigated by your service whose IQ have been less than 70 but who have done remarkably well. I would not want that to be assumed as an absolute criterion.

Dr Fenwick *(London, UK):* What is the youngest age group that you feel that you can operate on?

Dr Binnie: In desperate circumstances I suppose, neonates.

Dr Fenwick: The question is, what is the youngest age of those people who have temporal lobe sizures who are going to get a good result from operation?

Dr Binnie: If you are talking of conventional complex partial seizures, then one has to have long enough to establish therapy resistance, which is going to be by age three or four. My remark about neonates was not a joke; sometimes in desperate situations one does operate on babies.

Dr Fenwick: And are you going to argue that three and four year olds should now come forward for temporal lobectomy on a routine basis?

Dr Binnie: If one is confident that therapy resistance has been established, then, yes. In practice, of course, the children with febrile convulsions typically start having fits when they are aged about four, so by the time therapy resistance is established they will be age seven.

Interactive question from Dr Jennum

Is it possible to perform spatial segmentation in order to visualize brain maps?	**Response**
1 Yes	5%
2 No	3%
3 Don't know	92%

Dr Jennum *(Vedback, Denmark):* That is a disappointing result. There has been a publication on this subject; it is possible.

Professor Baldy-Moulinier *(France):* Do you have any experience or any information on the effect of sodium valproate on EEG mapping in normal or in epileptic patients?

Dr Reynolds *(Chairman):* Why did you ask only about sodium valproate?

Professor Baldy-Moulinier: Because we know that it works, but we do not know what happens on EEG mapping.

Dr Jennum: No, we have not looked at that.

Dr Fenwick: I just want to encourage you with your work because I feel that techniques such as yours will produce a considerable amount of data on the times when seizures occur and the precursors of seizures, and I look forward to your next series of papers.

The Epicare system

W. J. K. Cumming

Withington Hospital, West Didsbury, Manchester, UK

The Epicare system has been devised to facilitate the management of patients with epilepsy.

The need for some sort of computerized record that can be easily and rapidly accessed, to provide information pertaining to the patient in question, is obvious. The patient, with notes running to three volumes, who arrives in a clinic asking the doctor to compare the events of the last three months with the time he lost his job five years ago, fills all of us with dread. Did we not promise the last time he was in the clinic that we would tidy-up the notes so that it could not happen again? But then another patient arrived, the clinic was overbooked, and so the good intention was lost; until the next time.

However, any computerized record system, to be of any value to the neurologist, has to be easy to use, has to provide information quickly and reliably and the initial (and subsequent) entry of data must be simply completed. Such a system (the Epicare system) is described below.

The system will run on any IBM-compatible PC with a hard disk including portables and requires little or no previous knowledge of computers or computing to be able to use it. The system is run from a menu whose options may be accessed by single key strokes (Fig. 1).

```
                           MENU
              A:   Base patient Data
              B:   Initial Examination
              C:   Patient History
              D:   Epilepsy & Seizure Type
              E:   Treatment Review
              F:   Consultation Notes
              G:   Seizure Record
              H:   Drugs, Concomitants, ADRs
              I:   Investigations
              J:   Checklist
              K:   Management of Status
              L:   Outcome of Pregnancy
              M:   Print GP Letters
              N:   System Facilities
```

Figure 1.

By simply typing 'A', the basic demographic details of the patient are displayed. The details of the examination done when the patient was first seen and the history, not only of epilepsy but also other medical conditions, are found in 'B' and 'C'. Information may be added and amended in each of these sub-sections by easily-identified key strokes. Information relating specifically to the patient's epilepsy is contained in sections 'D-H'. It is in these sections that most of the data regarding the patient's epilepsy history is contained.

'Treatment Review' (Fig. 2) provides a graphic display, covering 12 months at a time, of the patient's seizure frequency and drug dosage. This is a useful snapshot of events which may be interrogated further using options D,F,G and H.

Fourth international symposium on sodium valproate and epilepsy, edited by David Chadwick, 1989; Royal Society of Medicine Services International Congress and Symposium Series No. 152, published by Royal Society of Medicine Services Limited.

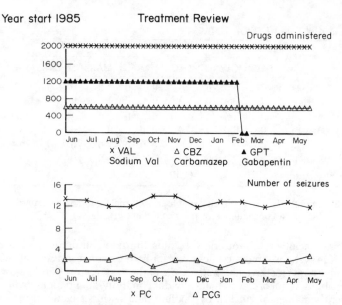

Figure 2 *Upper graph shows individual drugs and dosage. Lower graph shows seizure frequency of partial complex seizures and partial complex seizures with secondary generalizations.*

The Epilepsy and Seizure Type option (D), allows for the delineation of up to three seizure types, the particular seizure type being defined by an hierarchical system. This allows the doctor to define the seizure type in as much or as little detail as he wishes. There is also the ability to describe the seizure in free text. The seizure type(s) thus defined are carried forward throughout the rest of the system.

The Consultation Notes option (F), in addition to providing a date record of the patient's visits, allows the recording of information in a free text mode. This information may subsequently be incorporated into the GP letters (vide infra).

The Seizure Record option (G) (Fig. 3), provides a monthly record of seizure frequency for each seizure type as defined under 'D'. Where appropriate the reasons for any given set of seizures (e.g. alcohol, catamenial, poor compliance, etc.) may be recorded, and as a consequence, patterns not easily obtained from the notes may become apparent.

The Drugs, Concomitants, ADRs option (H), basically provides information regarding drugs, dosage and blood levels. These are recorded as and when the patient is seen. Any changes in the drug dosage, (e.g., no change, increased—blood level too low, stopped—ineffective, stopped—side effects etc.) are recorded. The module also allows for the recording of other drugs the patient may be taking for allied or independent conditions, thus making easier the recognition of actual or potential interactions. A separate subdivision of this module deals with adverse drug reactions (ADRs). These may be recorded in a systematic fashion and any which require onward transmission to the CSM are formatted accordingly.

The Investigation option (I), contains information regarding the EEG (standard, sleep, 24-h, etc.), radiological investigation (X-Ray, CT, MRI), haematological and biochemical investigations. These results are stored sequentially and any results which deviate from the normal range are highlighted.

The Checklist (J) provides a quick reminder of when important topics were last discussed with the patient (e.g. driving, contraception etc.).

The next two sections, K & L, (Management of Status, Outcome of Pregnancy) deal with special situations which are less common in routine practice. The ability to record such events according to a fixed format and to pool such data (*vide infra*) will provide important information which should be helpful in further patient management.

The ability to generate up to four letters (M—Print GP Letters) containing a combination of demographic details (A, B) and seizure and treatment information (D–H), permits rapid communication between the clinic and the general practitioner.

Livingston   SANOFI EPICARE   Fri, 18 Aug 1989
Current Patient:KL456/2—ALTERA, UNA   Seizure Record

No. of Seizures		1988				1989							
		SEP	OCT	NOV	DEC	JAN	FEB	MAR	APR	MAY	JUN	JUL	AUG
GTC	Awake	0	0	0	0	0	0	0	0	0	0	0	0
Generalis	Asleep	0	0	0	4	0	0	0	0	2	0	0	0
	Awake	0	0	0	0	0	0	0	0	0	0	0	0
	Asleep	0	0	0	0	0	0	0	0	0	0	0	0
	Awake	0	0	0	0	0	0	0	0	0	0	0	0
	Asleep	0	0	0	0	0	0	0	0	0	0	0	0
Reasons for seizure					CMP					CMP			

Figure 3 Twelve-month seizure record showing four nocturnal tonic-clonic seizures during December and two during May as a consequence of poor compliance (CMP).

The Systems Facilities sub-routine (N), aids the non-computer literate individual to manage disk file systems, an option designed for both personal and central analysis of data.

The description given above illustrates some of the basic features of the powerful Epicare system. The ability to record systematically data on individual patients will not only help in that patient's management, but by pooling data within a clinic, trends may become apparent which may help in overall patient management.

By pooling data between cooperating centres, (such data being stripped of any details that would identify the individual patient), a large database can be assembled to which referring centres would have access for specific research projects.

DISCUSSION

Interactive question from Dr Cumming

Would you find the Epicare System helpful?	**Response**
1 Yes	90%
2 No	5%
3 Don't know	5%

Dr Finnegan *(Birmingham, UK)*: Obviously the Epicare system outlined by Dr Cumming has a lot of appeal. It is clearly useful to be able to look at something comprehensively over a period of time. But in practice, how well does the system work in those patients in whom control is very erratic and difficult over a period of time? If you have a registrar or a senior registrar in your clinic, would each need a terminal to input data? Finally, another everyday practical problem, how easy is it to adapt that system to those common and troublesome patients who have a lot of pseudoseizures and partial seizures that are quite difficult to distinguish, however experienced one is?

Dr Cumming *(Manchester, UK)*: If I can answer in reverse order—I classify the pseudoseizures as 'other' at the moment, and I find it exceedingly difficult in any circumstance to distinguish them. One of the benefits of this system is in having a spread of so-called pseudoseizures or genuine seizures versus their drug therapy available to help make some decision as to whether or not you are doing any good.

When there is more than one person in the clinic, although it is possible to run multiple terminals off a single machine, not everyone would want to use a machine in the clinic. They would probably prefer to print out the information of those patients attending the clinic that day and have that with them. I opted for a portable system as I work on multiple sites and it is easier to carry it round with me than to use a modem back at the hospital. I have found it of most use in the problem patient and it gives me a chance to look for trends that I might not have seen previously.

Third World experiences of epilepsy

G. Hosking

The Ryegate Children's Centre, Sheffield, UK

Visitors to a developing country, whether it is for a short or a long period, may experience a variety of emotions. These may range from marvelling at the beauty of what is to be seen and experienced, to the feeling of anger that things do not happen that could or should. If one views the problems presented by persons with epilepsy, comparable emotions may arise. These can extend from feeling that the whole 'problem' could be cracked if wealthy pharmaceutical companies could be a little more charitable and provide low cost or free drugs, to the feeling that the 'problem' has little to do with drugs, but rather that health workers have more urgent things to attend to than treating a few patients with epilepsy. Obviously the 'problem' is complex, as it is in any society, and there is no single solution to providing an appropriate management to all persons that may have epilepsy.

What is the size of the 'problem'? There is no reason to suspect that epilepsy is less common in developing countries. Indeed a number of studies have demonstrated a very high incidence of epilepsy in a number of communities (1). If epilepsy is grouped together with other major non-communicable disorders in Africa—rheumatic heart disease, diabetes, and hypertension, it is at least as common and in most settings, more common, than these three, and the four together are more common than many of the communicable disorders that tend to receive significant attention in African and other developing countries. Most physicians and health workers that I have had contact with in developing countries recognize epilepsy as being a major clinical (and social) problem, with probably more than 80% of patients with epilepsy receiving no treatment whatsoever—except from traditional healers.

While my experience has been that clinicians are aware of the problems of persons with epilepsy, the same cannot be said of government health ministries. There is, therefore, in my opinion, a problem with awareness.

At the clinical level, there is, I feel, the problem in developing countries, as in the developed, of accurate clinical diagnosis. Peter Jeavons (2) has reminded us that maybe more than 20% of persons with a diagnosis of a seizure disorder do not have epilepsy. I have, on numerous occasions, encountered children in developing countries (as I have in my own developed country) being treated for epilepsy who do not have this disorder. Where a great reliance is placed upon non-medical health workers not only for diagnosis but for the provision of treatment, inevitably diagnosis has, I believe, to be of greater concern. EEG facilities seldom exist.

When the problems presented by persons with epilepsy are examined or discussed in developing countries, the problem of medication emerges rather rapidly.

When I administered a questionnaire to a group of 70 Nigerian doctors who were predominantly general practitioners, 43 (60%) thought that a greater availability of appropriate medication was the most important need that they had to improve their services to persons with epilepsy. This was more important than improving their own knowledge of epilepsy or receiving more help from specialist colleagues—the other two alternatives that they were given. But this study involved doctors predominantly in urban practice and their views do not necessarily represent those of the remainder of the country's doctors.

Fourth international symposium on sodium valproate and epilepsy, edited by David Chadwick, 1989; Royal Society of Medicine Services International Congress and Symposium Series No. 152, published by Royal Society of Medicine Services Limited.

Nevertheless, these views may reflect the needs that exist for all doctors.

While colleagues in India would probably not disagree with that belief, it has been pointed out to me that problems exist in terms of the quality of preparations. Some government hospitals, I have been told by many, are often supplied with very poor quality preparations of phenobarbitone and phenytoin, often with minimal active ingredient. Meanwhile retail outlets have higher quality preparations. Added to this, in the case of phenytoin, the differing bioavailability between different brands produces significant management problems in a number of patients.

The question of cost of medication cannot be avoided. A Tanzanian colleague calculated the relative cost of drugs for one day's treatment of a patient with epilepsy with phenobarbitone being unity. With this he ascertained that phenytoin would be 1.05, carbamazepine would be 29, ethosuximide—33, sodium valproate—40 and diazepam for oral administration—5. He had no figures for clonazepam. It is on this question of cost that emotions can run particularly high. In some countries the problem has been tackled by introducing differing tiers in terms of drugs that are allowed to be prescribed. With this the cheapest drugs can be prescribed by non-medical health workers and general medical officers, while the more expensive drugs can only be prescribed by certain more specialized and designated doctors.

In spite of this, there continues to be a demand for the pharmaceutical companies to cut their costs of the more expensive drugs. Superficially this would seem to be a straightforward question, but is it?

I cannot pretend to have detailed knowledge of how international pharmaceutical companies determine the prices of either the drugs that they export, or the 'transfer price' that is fixed for the raw materials necessary for drugs to be made up into the final products within a country. But simply having a very low transfer price for a poor country and a high one for a rich country is not necessarily the answer. The first outcome from that could be re-exporting of drugs from poor to rich countries in exchange for much needed foreign exchange. The desperate shortage of foreign exchange in very poor countries itself makes it virtually impossible to import drugs into the country. While India and some other countries have established their own pharmaceutical industries, in a number of other countries industrial activity is so run down that the prospects of creating an indigenous pharmaceutical industry are bleak. There are many more issues that bear in on the problem of availability of drugs for persons with epilepsy in developing countries, and amongst these is the question of distribution throughout a country. To reach people in remote rural areas can pose a major problem. I was impressed in rural Tanzania, by the health assistants who would carry huge cartons of drugs for miles to ensure that these reached remoter areas. But even with this commitment, a great number of people have no access to medication of any sort.

The problems do not end, however, with simply the question of access to drugs. I regret that too often I have seen needless polypharmacy instituted by doctors usually in urban private practice. The message of the importance of monotherapy has either not got through or it has been ignored as the 'good' doctor is the one that prescribes many different preparations rather than just one. This inevitably begs an important question of the need for further professional education.

Many doctors have complained to me about failure of follow-up in their patients. At the same time, however, the same doctors have noted that traditional healers have far better follow-up in spite of their useless and, at times, harmful treatment. The reasons for this may, of course, be as varied and complex as the problems of the availability of drugs—do they take time to explain the nature of the disorder that has been diagnosed and the need for continuous medication?

Epilepsy is, as we would all agree, a potentially socially disabling disorder. With this, the social aspects of the disorder cannot be ignored, whether one is talking about recognition, recognition that many can benefit from medication, and at ministerial level, the problem is important—much more important in most countries than leprosy.

Public education and information is, in my opinion, vital, if the needs of persons with epilepsy are to be recognized. Jilek (3) summarized the conceptualizations of epilepsy in a study in Tanzania under the following three headings:

Epilepsy as a punishment for sins
Epilepsy as bewitchment or possession
Epilepsy as a contagious disease.

While I do not feel that these conceptualizations differ greatly from conceptualizations in other cultures, including European cultures, it is my feeling that they are much more entrenched and stigmatizing than in our cultures in Europe. Certainly they indicate the issues that have to be addressed if progress is to be made in meeting needs. Added to these issues has to be a recognition that long-term medication, as it has been found in the treatment of hypertension, is alien to many.

In the same group of Nigerian doctors, to whom I have already made reference, when asked which of four persons or bodies may be the most supportive to persons with epilepsy, around 60% suggested that societies for persons with epilepsy would be the most helpful, while 30% suggested social workers, and the remainder suggested community leaders or religious leaders.

In concluding, I would like to do so on a note that contains optimism. My own feelings over meeting the needs of persons with epilepsy in rural Africa were considerably lifted by a recent article by Watts. Dr Watts published in the *British Medical Journal* her experience of providing a service for persons with epilepsy in rural Malawi. From humble beginnings, Dr Watts evolved a service with over 3000 persons receiving regular treatment at 45 health units throughout Malawi (4). Her article is, I feel, compulsory reading.

My own feelings over meeting the needs of persons with epilepsy are that three areas need to be considered. These are, that there should be a greater availability of appropriate drugs, there should be an improvement in the clinical knowledge of epilepsy—its diagnosis and its management, and there should be an increase in public awareness of epilepsy and what can be done to help persons that suffer from this disorder.

The challenge of doing this is one that clinicians in developed and developing countries and colleagues from the pharmaceutical industry can (and should) share together.

REFERENCES

(1) Jilek-Aall L. Epilepsy in the Wapogoro tribe in Tanganyika. *Acta Psychiatrica Scand* 1965; **41**: 57–86.
(2) Jeavons P. The practical management of epilepsy. *Hospital Update* 1975: 11–22.
(3) Jilek WG. The epileptic's outcast role and its background: a contribution to the social psychiatry of seizure disorders. *J Operat Psych* 1979; **10**: 127–33.
(4) Watts R. A model for managing epilepsy in a rural community in Africa. *Br Med J* 1989; **298**: 805–7.

DISCUSSION

Dr Bennett-Britton *(Sutton Coldfield, UK):* I have many patients who do not come from European countries, and I share your concern about compliance. How do we improve compliance in a nation which is not used to taking medication day in day out, year in year out? Can you help?

Dr Hosking *(Sheffield, UK):* I think it is important first to recognize and then to give greater prominence to the problems of compliance. Some doctors simply complain that their patients are uncooperative and they must be helped to understand that they are introducing something that is very new to people. On the other hand, we need the support of link workers who can explain to patients the importance of the therapy and the need for continuity. Simply to assume that it is accepted by somebody from a culture significantly different from a European one is inevitably going to end in non-compliance. I think you are helping yourself by recognizing that the problem exists. We need to approach it on a multi-cultural multi-professional front.

Dr Shanks *(Belfast, Northern Ireland):* I was lucky enough to hear Anne Watts describe her work. She addressed the issue of compliance and there were two factors that she mentioned as being particularly important. One of them was that all the medication was free, it was donated through churches, and she did not rely on the local supply at all. This was one of the factors that enabled her to have an 80% plus follow-up, with very good compliance.

Dr Chakravarty *(Calcutta, India):* We did some work on the problem of non-compliance and interestingly the majority of patients, when we asked them why they did not take the drugs, put the blame on the doctors. They said 'we are not told properly that we have to take the drugs'. Another factor was that they did not want to accept that they had epilepsy. Most of them understand what epilepsy is and what the implications are, but they did not want to face the fact. There are also those who believe that it is something like a 'demon' or something which would pass off on its own. And finally they alternate western medications with more traditional medicines.

Dr Hosking *(Sheffield, UK):* A newspaper article sent to me recently from Tanzania, which is written by someone anxious to exploit traditional remedies and who has asked the WHO to help them do so, said that they had stopped producing phenobarbitone because it was too expensive.

Dr Meinardi *(Heeze, Holland):* I am glad that you raised this problem even though you have no solution, because we still have time before October when we meet in India, at the International Epilepsy Meeting, to think about solutions. Cost is always given as the reason why the developing countries can not buy drugs, but on the other hand, a lot of money is spent on the traditional doctors and very little money spent on drugs. Finally, it is not only the drugs but also the health service which is not continuous; primary health workers tend to be there for a year or two, and then leave and new people have to take up the problems. Do you have any solution for that?

Dr Hosking: The question of availability is not necessarily one of cost, or one of distribution. There are also problems of importing, which can be bureaucratic as much as a lack of the necessary foreign exchange. So it is an immensely complicated problem.

SESSION II

CHILDHOOD EPILEPSY

Chairman: F. E. Dreifuss

INTRODUCTION

In 1770 Tissot with great prescience talked about epilepsy as consisting of two factors, a predisposition and a precipitating factor which it takes to produce a seizure. He recognized that there was an underlying condition and that the precipitating factor was necessary in order to trigger the seizure. The seizure is the phenomenon by which epilepsy expresses itself. Epilepsy is the disease of which the seizure is the symptom. And this is the crux of what was discussed earlier under 'classification', the difference between an epilepsy and a seizure. The seizure type is determined by the patient's behaviour and EEG pattern during the actual event. The epileptic syndrome on the other hand is defined not only by the seizure type but by the natural history of the disease, the EEG, the response to anti epileptic drugs, a family history, an aetiology and the pathology. I want to emphasize that there are epileptic syndromes because these are what the childhood epilepsies are, and they will be discussed in this session. The epileptic syndrome may be divided into those with focal and generalized seizures, but there is also the question of whether we are dealing with a primary or idiopathic condition or a secondary or symptomatic one. Some of the focal seizures may be seen in idiopathic form, such as the benign childhood epilepsies, or they might be seen in symptomatic form for example, lesional epilepsies. Similarly, the generalized seizures may be primary or idiopathic or secondary or symptomatic. This then is the framework for the following papers on the various diseases which go to make up the childhood epilepsies.

Epilepsies of childhood and adolescence: an update

J. Aicardi

Hôpital Necker Enfants Malades, Paris, France

INTRODUCTION

Considerable new knowledge on the epilepsies of children and adolescents has accumulated during the past few years. New aetiological factors have been uncovered. Epilepsy can be a manifestation of newly recognized conditions such as the mitochondrial encephalomyopathies (1) or of partial epilepsy with bilateral occipital calcifications without cutaneous angioma (2). Brain tumours have been found more commonly in children with seizures since the advent of modern imaging techniques (3,4). Hypothalamic hamartomas give rise to a syndrome of gelastic epilepsy of early onset, often associated with precocious puberty (5). However, this paper is mainly concerned with the clinical presentation of seizure disorders in childhood and adolescence, especially with the delineation of epileptic syndromes and a critical assessment of their significance.

MAIN EPILEPTIC SYNDROMES IN CHILDREN AND ADOLESCENTS

A syndrome is a cluster of signs and symptoms associated in a non-fortuitous manner. Epileptic syndromes are therefore characterized not only by the types of seizure that occur, but also by other neurological manifestations such as interictal electroencephalographic (EEG) abnormalities, and occasionally by other non-neurological disturbances (6). A list of the main epileptic syndromes in the age range considered appears in Table 1. The heterogeneous nature of the syndromes is evident. Some are well-defined from both clinical and EEG points of view, e.g. absence epilepsy, whereas others, in particular the grand mal epilepsies of childhood and adolescence, are rather loosely characterized, with both seizure types and EEG features that may also be observed in several other epileptic syndromes. Even well-defined syndromes can be subdivided into more specific types. The example is again typical absence epilepsy that includes the childhood and adolescence subtypes, as well as rarer forms such as myoclonic or clonic absences (6,15) and eyelid myoclonia with absence (16).

The syndromes that feature *myoclonic seizures in early childhood*, often in association with other brief seizures of tonic or atonic types or both, deserve more detailed discussion.

The *Lennox-Gastaut syndrome* is characterized clinically by the occurrence of tonic seizures and of atonic attacks and atypical absences. However, true myoclonic attacks may occur in 11 to 25% of cases and may be particularly prominent in some patients (17). The EEG is characterized by diffuse slow spike-wave activity (at a rate of less than 2.5 Hz) and often by runs of high amplitude 10 Hz rhythms during slow sleep, corresponding to subclinical tonic attacks. In many patients, faster ($\geqslant 2.5$ Hz) spike-wave activity is also present.

In *'true' myoclonic epilepsy of early childhood*, myoclonias are the sole or clearly predominant type of attack. They are characterized clinically by sudden shock-like jerks, usually bilateral, and electrophysiologically by bursts of fast ($\geqslant 2.5$ Hz) spike-wave activity, usually irregular in rhythm and with several spikes preceding a single slow wave (polyspike-wave

Fourth international symposium on sodium valproate and epilepsy, edited by David Chadwick, 1989; Royal Society of Medicine Services International Congress and Symposium Series No. 152, published by Royal Society of Medicine Services Limited.

Table 1   *Main epileptic syndromes in childhood and adolescence*

Early childhood	West syndrome
	Lennox-Gastaut syndrome[a]
	Myoclonic epilepsy (7)
	  severe type (8)
	  'benign' type (9)
	Febrile convulsions
	Grand mal epilepsy of early childhood (10)
	Partial epilepsy with brain damage[a]

Later childhood	Typical absence epilepsy Myoclonic epilepsies of late childhood (10) Grand mal epilepsy of late childhood (10) Partial epilepsy with rolandic spikes Partial epilepsy with occipital spikes Other partial benign epilepsies (10,11) Landau-Kleffner syndrome
Adolescence	Juvenile myoclonic epilepsy (Janz syndrome) (12) Grand Mal on awakening (13) Typical absence epilepsy of adolescence (14)

[a]*May begin also in late childhood and adolescence.*

complexes). However, tonic seizures can be observed in some patients and typical myoclonic jerks can be associated with slow spike-wave complexes (18).

It appears therefore that the Lennox-Gastaut syndrome and the myoclonic epilepsies of early childhood may be regarded as the two well-defined extremities of a spectrum of conditions that include multiple brief seizures of several types and may be impossible to precisely attribute to a specific syndrome (7).

The syndrome of *severe myoclonic epilepsy* as defined by Dravet *et al.* has distinctive features. Onset is in the first year of life, with generalized or more often unilateral clonic seizures. These are often of long duration and precipitated by viral infections with mild fever (8). Myoclonic jerks usually appear during the second year of life and arrest of neuromental development invariably sets in at the same time. Myoclonic jerks may be prominent or they may occur only briefly and infrequently. Indeed, many patients have a similar onset and course without ever displaying myoclonic attacks. The term 'polymorphic epilepsy of childhood' may thus be more appropriate than that of myoclonic epilepsy (7).

The *syndromes that feature partial epileptic seizures without evidence of brain damage* currently attract considerable attention. Their main interest is related to their outcome which appears to be favourable in most cases: the seizures tend to disappear before adulthood and neurological and mental development are unaffected.

The best known of these 'benign partial' epilepsies is *benign epilepsy of childhood with rolandic (or centrotemporal) spikes* or BECRS (19). Gastaut (20) has described another relatively well defined form characterized by partial seizures often with visual manifestations and, on the EEG, by the presence of a continuous, often rhythmic, spike-wave activity over one or both posterior regions of the scalp. This activity is partially or totally suppressed by opening the eyes. '*Benign occipital epilepsy*' is much less common than BECRS. The term benign may not be applicable in all cases as brain damage can produce a similar picture with a guarded prognosis (21).

Other 'partial benign epilepsies' may exist although there is not enough evidence to guarantee a favourable course from outset in most cases. 'Atypical partial benign epilepsy' was the term proposed for a small group of patients with features reminiscent of both partial rolandic epilepsy and the Lennox-Gastaut syndrome (22). The outcome for these patients was not as good as that of BECRS but it was vastly better than that of the Lennox-Gastaut syndrome, a diagnosis with which all these children were referred.

The term *Landau-Kleffner syndrome* is often applied to designate a group of children between 3 and 10 years of age who demonstrate a more or less complete loss of previously acquired language in association with paroxysmal EEG activity and, in 80% of cases, with seizures (23). The syndrome is probably heterogeneous with some children having mainly receptive aphasia whilst others have expressive difficulties. The course is variable, about two-thirds of the patients being left with significant difficulties of communication even at adult age. The mechanism of aphasia and its relationship with the abnormal EEG activity are poorly understood.

Among the epileptic syndromes of adolescence, *juvenile myoclonic epilepsy* has been particularly well described (24). It is characterized by conscious myoclonic attacks that affect mainly the upper limbs and occur, in isolation or in series, after awakening or when resting at the end of the day. Sleep deprivation is a major precipitating factor. Clinical attacks are associated with polyspike-wave discharges on a normal EEG background. In about 90% of patients, generalized seizures (*awakening grand mal*) are associated with the myoclonic jerks. They also occur on awakening and often follow a series of jerks, thus producing a clonic-tonic-clonic type of seizure (25). Such attacks are usually infrequent. In about 25% of patients with awakening grand mal or Janz syndrome or both, typical absence seizures are observed. These *typical absence seizures of adolescence* are generally much less frequently repeated than typical absences of childhood and tend to occur predominantly after awakening. The loss of consciousness is also less profound than in childhood absences and the patients are often aware of their having had an attack. The EEG may show rhythmical discharges of spike-wave complexes at 3 Hz or faster spike-wave activity at 4 or even 5 Hz which is almost specific of the generalized epilepsies of adolescence.

The three syndromes of juvenile myoclonic epilepsy, absence seizures of adolescence and grand mal on awakening constitute the *primary generalized epilepsies of adolescence*. This condition is usually well-controlled by drug treatment but the seizures tend to recur for very long periods and therefore require prolonged therapy. Status epilepticus, other than myoclonic status is exceptional and mentality is unaffected.

The usefulness and limitations of the concept of epileptic syndromes

The concept of epileptic syndrome is fundamentally of pragmatic significance. Recognizing a specific syndrome helps the physician select appropriate investigations, decide on optimal treatment and predict the outcome (6). The concept of epileptic syndromes dispenses with most of the assumptions about localization and mechanisms which are required when using other systems of classification. It is not necessary, in order to classify a case into an epileptic syndrome, to decide whether the seizures are 'generalized' or focal (localization-related), cryptogenic or symptomatic. Because such decisions are always largely arbitrary for want of sufficient neurophysiological knowledge, using a classification by syndromes avoids such arbitrary decisions and therefore facilitates classification. For this reason, the concept of epileptic syndromes has been incorporated in the International Classification of Epilepsies and Epileptic Syndromes, provisionally adopted in 1984 by the International League Against Epilepsy (26). Such classification is logically incompatible with the other criteria used in the same classification, which include the dichotomies generalized *vs* localized and cryptogenic *vs* symptomatic, the value of which remains uncertain.

Epileptic syndromes should not be misinterpreted as representing disease entities. Several different epileptic syndromes might well be determined by similar genetic factors: families are on record in which different syndromes are present in different members. Conversely, the same syndrome may be due to different unrelated causes. The West syndrome (so-called infantile or salaam spasms) is observed in several different diseases such as tuberous sclerosis or may be unassociated with any detectable brain abnormality. Typical absence seizures are usually 'cryptogenic' but may also occur with brain damage, especially involving the frontal lobes. As a consequence the concept of epileptic syndrome will probably be only temporarily useful. A classification based on disease entities or on systems involved in the genesis of various types of epilepsy is likely to replace eventually that founded on purely clinical and EEG features.

From a practical viewpoint the concept of epileptic syndromes has two major limitations. Only part of the cases fit in with the currently described syndromes. Although new syndromes will undoubtedly be delineated, excessive subdivision should be avoided, and only those syndromes that are generally recognized and accepted should be used for the purposes of classification. Conversely, physicians should resist the temptation of 'squeezing' atypical cases into recognized syndromes thus defeating the whole aim of delineating syndromes. In our experience many cases currently cannot be accommodated within syndromes that are sufficiently distinctive to be of general practical use. Delineation of disease entities based on mechanisms and aetiology remains the ultimate goal.

REFERENCES

(1) Chevrie JJ, Aicardi J, Goutières F. Epilepsy in childhood mitochondrial encephalomyopathies. In: Wolf P, Dam M, Janz D, Dreifuss FE, eds. *Advances in epileptology*, vol. 16, New York: Raven Press, 1987: 181–4.
(2) Gobbi G, Sorrenti G, Santucci M, Giovanardi Rossi P, Ambrosetto P, Michelucci R, Tassinari CA. Epilepsy with bilateral occipital calcifications: a benign onset with progressive severity. *Neurology* 1988; **38**: 913–20.
(3) Harbord MG, Manson JI. Temporal lobe epilepsy in childhood: reappraisal of etiology and outcome. *Pediatr Neurol* 1987; **3**: 263–8.
(4) Rutledge SL, Snead OC III, Morawetz R, Chanda-Sekar B. Brain tumors presenting as a seizure disorder in infants. *J Child Neurol* 1987; **2**: 214–9.
(5) Berkovic SF, Andermann F, Melanson D, Ethier RE, Feindel W, Gloor P. Hypothalamic hamartomas and ictal laughter: evolution of a characteristic epileptic syndrome and diagnostic value of magnetic resonance imaging. *Ann Neurol* 1988; **23**: 429–39.
(6) Aicardi J. Epileptic syndromes in childhood. *Epilepsia* 1988; **29** (Suppl 3): S1–S5.
(7) Aicardi J, Gomes AL. The myoclonic epilepsies of childhood. *Cleveland Clin J Med* 1989; **59**: S34–S39.
(8) Dravet C, Roger J, Bureau M. Severe myoclonic epilepsy of infants. In: Roger J, Dravet C, Bureau M, Dreifuss FE, Wolf P, eds. *Epileptic syndromes of infancy, childhood and adolescence*. London: John Libbey, 1985: 58–67.
(9) Dravet C, Bureau M, Roger J. Benign myoclonic epilepsy of infants. In: Roger J, Dravet C, Bureau M, Dreifuss FE, Wolf P, eds. *Epileptic syndromes in infancy, childhood and adolescence*. London: John Libbey, 1985: 51–7.
(10) Aicardi J. *Epilepsy in children*. New York: Raven Press, 1986.
(11) Deonna T, Ziegler AL, Despland PA, Van Melle G. Partial epilepsy in neurologically normal children: clinical syndromes and prognosis. *Epilepsia* 1986; **27**: 241–7.
(12) Delgado-Escueta AV, Enrile-Bacsal F. Juvenile myoclonic epilepsy of Janz. *Neurology* 1984; **34**: 285–94.
(13) Wolf P. Epilepsies with Grand Mal on awakening. In: Roger J, Dravet C, Bureau M, Dreifuss FE, Wolf P, eds. *Epileptic syndromes in infancy, childhood and adolescence*. London: John Libbey, 1985: 259–70.
(14) Wolf P. Juvenile absence epilepsy. In: Roger J, Dravet C, Bureau M, Dreifuss FE, Wolf P, eds. *Epileptic syndromes in infancy, childhood and adolescence*. London: John Libbey, 1985: 242–6.
(15) Tassinari CA, Bureau M. Epilepsy with myoclonic absences. In: Roger J, Dravet C, Bureau M, Dreifuss FE, Wolf P, eds. *Epileptic syndromes in infancy, childhood and adolescence*. London: John Libbey, 1985: 121–9.
(16) Jeavons PM, Harding GFA. *Photosensitive epilepsy: a review of the literature and a study of 460 patients*. London: Heinemann, 1975.
(17) Aicardi J, Levy Gomes A. The Lennox-Gastaut syndrome: clinical and electroencephalographic features. In: Niedermeyer E, Degen D, eds. *The Lennox-Gastaut syndrome*. New York: Allan Liss 1988; 25–46.
(18) Aicardi J. Course and prognosis of certain childhood epilepsies with predominantly myoclonic seizures. In: Wada JA, Penry JK, eds. *Advances in epileptology, the Xth epilepsy international symposium*. New York: Raven Press, 1980; 159–63.
(19) Lerman P, Kivity S. The benign focal epilepsies of childhood. In: Pedley TA, Meldrum BS, eds. *Recent advances in epilepsy*, vol. 3. Edinburgh: Churchill Livingstone, 1986; 137–56.
(20) Gastaut H, Zifkin BG. Benign epilepsy of childhood with occipital spike and wave complexes. In: Andermann F, Lugaresi E, eds. *Migraine and epilepsy*. London: Butterworths. 1987; 47–81.
(21) Newton R, Aicardi J. Clinical findings in children with occipital spike-wave complexes suppressed by eye-opening. *Neurology* 1983; **33**: 1526–9.
(22) Aicardi J, Chevrie JJ. Atypical benign epilepsy of childhood. *Dev Med Child Neurol* 1982; **24**: 281–92.
(23) Beaumanoir A. The Landau-Kleffner syndrome. In: Roger J, Dravet C, Bureau M, Dreifuss FE, Wolf P, eds. *Epileptic syndromes in infancy, childhood and adolescence*. London: John Libbey 1985; 181–91.
(24) Janz D. Juvenile myoclonic epilepsy—epilepsy with impulsive petit mal. *Cleveland Clin J Med* 1989; **56**: S23–S33.
(25) Asconapé J, Penry JK. Some clinical and EEG aspects of benign juvenile myoclonic epilepsy. *Epilepsia* 1984; **25**: 108–14.
(26) Commission on Classification and Terminology of the International League against Epilepsy. Proposal for revised clinical and electroencephalographic classification of epileptic seizures. *Epilepsia* 1981; **22**: 489–501.

DISCUSSION

Dr Vestermark *(Denmark):* According to one of Dr Aicardi's slides, febrile convulsions are included in the epileptic syndromes, I wonder if that can be correct?

Dr Aicardi *(Paris, France):* No, by definition epilepsy is supposed to be unprovoked seizures, but I included febrile convulsions for convenience because I think it is very difficult to leave aside such an important problem.

Professor Dreifuss *(Chairman):* In fact, probably all epileptic seizures are provoked. It is the underlying tendency which is unprovoked; ultimately there is a provocation to every seizure, even though we might not know it.

Dr Poole *(Oxford, UK):* Could someone clarify whether provocation is an important aspect in the classification? It seems to me that for seizures you require a tendency, and something which will provoke an occurrence. The febrile convulsion in childhood does not seem very different from the photosensitive adolescent in whom one can only find photosensitivity.

Dr Aicardi: I agree that primary seizures in adolescents are quite often provoked by a night without sleep or something similar. Most seizures are probably provoked by something, otherwise patients with epilepsy would be fitting all the time. There must be some sort of provocation, even if we do not know what it is.

Professor Dreifuss: I agree, because that is what sets apart those people who are epileptic by EEG and who never have a seizure, but they have relatives that have seizures. The EEG is important more as a confirmatory element in the diagnosis, while the condition, of course, is paramount in making a diagnosis of epilepsy.

The Paediatric EPITEG trial: A comparative multicentre clinical trial of sodium valproate and carbamazepine in newly-diagnosed childhood epilepsy.

A preliminary communication

Presented by
G. Hosking
on behalf of the Trial Participants

Ryegate Children's Centre, Sheffield, UK

INTRODUCTION

Jeavons *et al.* (1) reviewed their experience in the treatment of the generalized epilepsies of childhood and adolescence, and suggested that for this group sodium valproate was the drug of choice. No placebo was used in their studies, but the improvement in their patients was such as to leave no doubt as to the efficacy of the drug.

Shakir (2) when comparing the efficacy of carbamazepine and sodium valproate found that either drug was equally effective in controlling seizures of various types in an outpatient population (ages 7–56, mean 21 years).

Callaghan *et al.* (3) in a study of 181 patients of widely varying ages found no difference between the efficacy of carbamazepine, phenytoin and sodium valproate, but with all three drugs found them to be less effective in the partial seizures than in the generalized seizures.

Loiseau (4), while acknowledging the existence of previous reports that sodium valproate was either ineffective in partial seizures (5,6) or contraindicated in severe complex partial seizures (7) argues that sodium valproate 'can be described as the sole drug in previously untreated partial epilepsies' on the basis of his own findings and experience.

Dean and Penry (8), following a retrospective study of 30 patients with partial seizures who received sodium valproate following a lack of response or allergic reaction to carbamazepine or phenytoin, noted an 'improvement' or 'control' in 22 patients, but nevertheless recommended a double-blind controlled trial with sodium valproate in patients with partial seizures.

The Lancet (9) in a leading article acknowledges that 'the use of sodium valproate monotherapy in partial epilepsy is less well established' and 'there is insufficient hard evidence in support of valproate as a first line drug in partial epilepsy'.

Comparative trials between sodium valproate and carbamazepine have been few, but in spite of this, a common practice that has emerged has been that sodium valproate is recommended for generalized seizures while carbamazepine is recommended for partial seizures.

It is against this uncertain background that we organized this multicentre trial on the long term efficacy and side-effect profiles of sodium valproate and carbamazepine in the commoner forms of epilepsy seen in paediatric outpatients. A similar study in adult outpatients started just prior to our own study, and the experiences thus far from this other trial are to be reported later on this morning.

Support amongst paediatric neurologists and paediatricians has been overwhelming. By the close of recruitment in December 1987, over 80 clinicians at 64 centres in the UK and Ireland (Fig. 1) had entered patients. A full list of all these participants is included in the Appendix to this paper.

Fourth international symposium on sodium valproate and epilepsy, edited by David Chadwick, 1989; Royal Society of Medicine Services International Congress and Symposium Series No. 152, published by Royal Society of Medicine Services Limited.

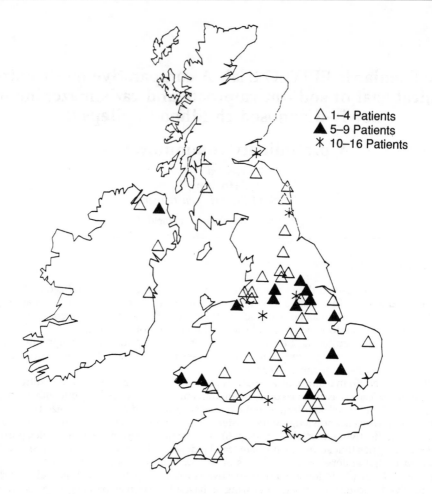

Figure 1 *Paediatric EPITEG trial recruitment centres.*

We would like to present today our initial experiences with the study: a review of the patient population involved, some comments on the seizure classification, an overview of patient progress, and a brief analysis of events other than efficacy which have influenced this progress. A report on the final outcome, with a full analysis of seizure control cannot be made before 1991 when all patients will have completed the three-year trial period.

METHODS

The study is an open randomized multicentre comparative trial of sodium valproate and carbamazepine in the treatment of newly diagnosed generalized or partial seizures in children with epilepsy. We planned to recruit at least 125 patients on each drug with, whenever possible, each centre recruiting 5–10 patients. Each patient if possible will be followed up for three years. Patients who fail because of poor seizure control and/or side-effects on the first drug are changed on to the alternative drug. Further treatment for patients who fail on both drugs is at the investigating clinician's discretion, but the clinician is asked to continue documenting follow-up for the remainder of the three-year trial period to ensure a full analysis of all patients entered.

Allocation to treatment regime was randomized in accordance with a computer-generated minimization programme stratified for sex, age, centre and seizure type.

Table 1 *Inclusion criteria*

1. Ages between 5 and 16 years
2. Attending normal school
3. Newly diagnosed epilepsy
4. At least two generalized tonic-clonic seizures, or partial seizures with or without generalization, in the previous six months
5. Children who would routinely have been treated with either sodium valproate or carbamazepine

Table 2 *Exclusion criteria*

1. Accompanying disorder other than epilepsy
2. Abnormal liver function tests, platelet counts below $150 \times 10^9/l$ or other blood dyscrasia on entry
3. Absences (simple or complex) or myoclonic jerks alone
4. Pregnancy, risk of pregnancy, or on contraceptive medication

Table 3 *Permitted seizure types*

1. Primary generalized (generalized from onset)
2. Complex partial seizures without generalization
3. Complex partial seizures with generalization
4. Simple partial seizures without generalization
5. Simple partial seizures with generalization

The progress of each patient over the three-year trial period has been monitored by assessment at intervals that we believe to be in accordance with the follow-up procedures of the majority of paediatric physicians.

Our entry criteria are summarized in Table 1 and our exclusions in Table 2.

The classification of seizure types has, in the first instance, been undertaken by the investigating physicians on the basis of clinical histories, seizure descriptions and reported electroencephalograph (EEG) findings. Classification (Table 3) has been in accordance with the proposed Revised Classification of the International League against Epilepsy (10). Patients have been entered into the trial on the basis of the investigating clinician's own classification of seizure type and the primary analysis of the data will be made on this basis.

An independent assessment of these seizure classifications has been done by an independent clinician (GH) on the basis of the seizure description given in the Case Record Forms, and the results of this analysis will be summarized later on in this presentation. In addition, a further independent classification by a clinical neurophysiologist based on the history and the original EEG record is also in progress, but this is not yet completed.

Laboratory investigations have been kept to a minimum. Haematology and biochemical screening were done before entry into the trial, and repeated (with the parent's consent) at three and 12 months after start of treatment if part of the clinician's normal routine. Similarly, plasma drug levels were done during follow-up to monitor compliance if part of the Investigator's normal practise. EEG examinations were done before entry (or as soon as possible thereafter) by the investigating physician's usual centre. A summary of the clinical and laboratory monitoring of patients in the study is given in Table 4.

Table 4 *Assessment schedule*

	Pre-entry visit	Entry visit	Follow-up visits (months after entry)							
			1	3	6	9	12	18	24	36
Patient history	X	X								
Seizure chart		X	X	X	X	X	X	X	X	X
Side-effects			X	X	X	X	X	X	X	X
Serum drug levels				X			X			
Haematology	X			X			X			
Biochemistry	X			X			X			
EEG recording	X									

Table 5 *Pretreatment variables*

	Sodium valproate	Carbamazepine	Total
Number of patients	130	130	260
Male	60	62	122
Female	70	68	138
Age 5–10 years	77	78	155
Age 11–16 years	53	52	105

All investigating physicians obtained the approval of their respective Ethical Committees before taking part in the trial. Informed consent was obtained from the parent or guardian (in writing) and from the child (where appropriate) before acceptance into the trial.

RESULTS

Patient population

Recruitment commenced in January 1986 and was completed in December 1987: 260 children from 64 centres in the United Kingdom and Ireland had been entered by the close of recruitment. The results of the randomization of the children entered are summarized in Table 5 and Fig. 2.

a . *Seizure classification*: over half of the patients entered were reported as having primary generalized seizures on entry. Complex partial with generalization was the next commonest seizure category (17%), with lesser proportions of complex partial without generalization (13%), simple partial with generalization (9%) and simple partial alone (5%). Two patients entered as having generalized seizures were subsequently shown to have absence seizures only.

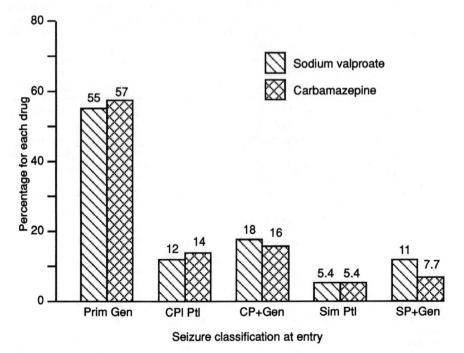

Figure 2 *Seizure classification at entry: (A) original investigator's classification.*

b . *Age at entry*: Patients from all ages from 5 to 15 are well represented in the trial, with approximately equal numbers in each age group being randomized to each trial drug.

c . *Sex*: Slightly more girls (138) than boys (122) were recruited into the trial, but overall and within each stratum, treatment allocation was well-balanced.

Independent assessment of seizure type

We have been able, at this stage of the trial, to compare the investigating physician's clinical classification of seizure types with that of an experienced paediatric neurologist. In most cases, investigating physicians had EEG reports available on children entered into the study, and with this the opportunity to make their classifications on the basis of both clinical descriptions and EEG comments.

A comparison between the original clinical classification and the independent assessment based on seizure description and EEG summary is given in Tables 6 and 7.

The high incidence of 'unclassified' entries in the independent assessments needs some comment. Clinicians were not given this category, which was available only to the independent clinician, and was used by him to classify patients with clearly epileptiform seizures, but inadequate clinical data to be certain about the seizure type. If this particular group is excluded, there is overall a reasonable match between the investigating clinician's assessment and that of the independent physician. Perhaps the most significant difference between the two assessments is in the relative proportions of primary generalized tonic-clonic seizures and secondarily generalized seizures. The importance of any features indicating partial origin to the seizures (auras, 'funny feelings', etc.) and hence classification as 'secondarily generalized' may not be as well appreciated as it should be.

Patients with 'unclassified' seizures were usually children with seizures that could not in the opinion of the independent clinician be classified into one specific group. This was largely because of a lack of adequate clinical details relating to attacks. This in itself is not

Table 6 *Comparison of seizure classifications*. Results based on seizure descriptions received for 221 patients in the trial

Paediatric neurologist's assessment	Original investigator's assessment					
	Primary generalized	Complex partial alone	Complex partial with generalization	Simple partial alone	Simple partial with generalization	Total
Primary generalized	40	0	3	0	4	47
Complex partial	1	19	3	5	1	29
Complex partial with generalization	16	0	22	0	4	42
Simple partial	0	0	0	4	0	4
Simple partial with generalization	2	2	6	2	10	22
Absences only	2	0	1	0	0	3
Unclassified	51	5	1	0	2	59
Query epilepsy	8	2	3	2	0	15
Total	120	28	39	13	21	221

Table 7 *Independent assessment of seizure type: summary*

	No. of patients	%
Agreement with investigator	95	43
Disagreement—different seizure type	49	22
absences only	3	1
probably not epilepsy	15	7
Unclassified[a]	59	27
Total assessed	221	100%

[a]*Diagnosis of a seizure disorder not disputed, but insufficient information for definitive classification.*

to say that investigating clinicians were dilatory or lax with the details recorded, but rather that greater detail on attacks was not available to clinicians, to increase the certainty of the diagnosis.

Adverse event review

The investigating clinician was asked to record all adverse events reported by the patients while on drug treatment. A preliminary analysis of these events has now been completed.

This analysis has been done on follow-up data corresponding to over 1500 months' treatment with sodium valproate, and over 1800 months' treatment with carbamazepine as first drug (Table 8). Over this period, we have recorded 190 events on the first drug employed and 209 when first and second drugs are combined. To simplify the presentation,

Table 8   *Total treatment periods on each drug (first drug only)*

	Sodium valproate	Carbamazepine
No. of patients	108	122
Mean period per patient	14.8 months	14.9 months
Total (all patients)	1594 months	1823 months

only those events occurring while the patient was on the first drug have been included here. The patterns, whether it is reported in relation to the first drug or the second drug that is employed, are very similar. Where patients reported more than one event each visit, all are included. If however the patient reported the same adverse event at several visits, this event is only included once in the analysis.

Overall incidence of adverse events

Table 9 summarizes the most commonly reported adverse events (defined as being reported by five or more patients) for the two drugs, sodium valproate and carbamazepine, when employed as the first drug.

For sodium valproate, appetite increase (nine reports) and weight increase (nine) appear to be the most specific effects. Non-specific abdominal pain and anorexia were reported by several patients (five reports each), but these effects were noted also by patients on carbamazepine (two reports each). Similarly, 'somnolence' was a frequent adverse event on both valproate (nine reports) and more especially on carbamazepine (20 reports), as were headache (five and six respectively) and nausea (five and three respectively). Rather unexpectedly, there were only three reports of alopecia on valproate (and two on carbamazepine). This finding, together with the relatively high incidence reported from previous studies suggests that this phenomenon is dose-related, and is unlikely to be of any great clinical importance with the relatively low doses needed by most paediatric patients attending outpatient clinics.

In this trial, specific side-effects of carbamazepine treatment appeared to be somnolence (20), fatigue (10), rash (8), dizziness (7), and insomnia (5).

Table 9   *Adverse events reported on first drug.* Events reported by 5 or more patients during treatment

Sodium valproate		Carbamazepine	
Appetite increase	(9)	Somnolence	(20)
Weight increase	(9)	Fatigue	(10)
Somnolence	(9)	Rash	(8)
Abdominal pain	(5)	Dizziness	(7)
Anorexia	(5)	Headache	(6)
Nausea	(5)	Insomnia	(5)
Fatigue	(5)	Weight increase	(5)
Headache	(5)		

(.) Number of patients reporting event.

Table 10 *Adverse events within the first three months (first drug).* The four most common adverse events on each drug in the first three months of treatment were:

Sodium valproate		Carbamazepine	
Appetite increase	(5)	Somnolence	(14)
Anorexia	(3)	Rash	(8)
Fatigue	(3)	Fatigue	(7)
Headache	(3)	Dizziness	(5)
All events	(34)	All events	(71)

(.) Number of patients reporting event.

Table 11 *Adverse events after the first three months (first drug).* The four most common adverse events on each drug after the first three months of treatment were:

Sodium valproate		Carbamazepine	
Somnolence	(7)	Somnolence	(6)
Weight increase	(7)	Weight increase	(4)
Nausea/ABD pain	(6)	Fatigue	(3)
Appetite increase	(4)	Insomnia	(3)
All events	(50)	All events	(35)

(.) Number of patients reporting event

Time of adverse event

We were interested in identifying whether the adverse events reported in this trial occurred 'early'—i.e. within the first three months'—or 'later', after three months treatment. Table 10 summarizes the 'early' adverse events while Table 11 reports the 'late' adverse events.

There were in total 71 'early' adverse events reported in patients taking carbamazepine and 34 on those taking sodium valproate; after three months there were 35 adverse events on carbamazepine and 50 on sodium valproate.

For valproate, there were no obvious 'early' adverse effects—the reports of appetite increase, weight gain and other adverse effects being roughly evenly distributed during and after the first three months. In contrast, all the reports on rashes with carbamazepine, and most of the reports of somnolence, fatigue and dizziness occurred in the first three months.

Summary of patient progress

Clinical progress is summarized in Table 12. Most patients are still in the trial and still on their first drug. Forty patients have failed on first drug, and seven of these on both drugs. Six patients have had their treatment withdrawn by the clinicians concerned in accordance with their normal clinical practice after two years' freedom from seizures on the first drug allocated.

One major problem with long-term multicentre trials is the high incidence of patient dropout, most often due to patients failing to re-attend follow-up clinics. In the present

Table 12 *Summary of clinical progress Jan. 1989*

Status	No. of patients
Still on first drug	175
Failed on first drug: now on second drug	33
Failed on both drugs	7
Treatment stopped after two years[a]	6
Awaiting data	22
Lost to follow-up	17
Total	260

[a]*Treatment stopped by Investigators in accordance with their normal practice after two years' freedom from seizures on first drug.*

Table 13 *Patients lost to follow-up:*

Status	No. of patients
No attendance since entry	2
No attendance after 6 months	4
Moved/emigrated	1
Encephalopathy diagnosed after entry	1
Violation of entry criteria[a]	5
No data available	4
Total	17

[a]*Two patients with absences alone, one patient with abnormal liver function tests on entry, one patient with weight below the stated minimum on entry.*

Table 14 *Treatment failure on first drug*

Poor seizure control	17
Adverse events	11
Both poor control and adverse events	6
Possible adverse events[a]	2
Parental pressure[b]	1
Total	37

[a]*Doubt expresses by Investigators on causality of the adverse event.* [b]*Treatment changed at parental request following mild mood changes.*

trial, I am very pleased to report that to date, very few patients have been lost to follow-up, as shown in Table 13.

The reasons given for changing treatment for 37 of the patients who failed on the first drug are summarized in Table 14. As shown, 17 of these patients failed because of poor seizure control, and 11 because of severe adverse events on the first drug. For six patients, both poor control and adverse events appeared responsible.

Rash (either alone or in combination with other adverse event) was the commonest adverse event warranting treatment change, and weight increase was at least partially responsible for treatment change in three children, and non-specific abdominal pain and nausea in two others. Most withdrawals for adverse events occurred in the first three months of treatment.

DISCUSSION

The majority of clinicians taking part in the study are responsible for busy general paediatric clinics, and do not have the facilities for detailed clinical investigations on their patients. Many of these physicians have asked the question as to which drug is most suitable for their patients, particularly in regard to partial seizures, and their involvement in this trial reflects their own uncertainty about the best drug for particular patients and/or seizure type.

We are encouraged that such a large number of clinicians have wished to support the study, which because of their active involvement ranks as one of the largest studies yet established to compare the efficacy and tolerability of two well-known antiepileptic drugs used in childhood. The study is large by any standards, and in January this year, data corresponding to over 350 patient-years of drug treatment had already been collected (Table 8).

It is confidently expected that this study will answer a wide range of outstanding questions. We anticipate that knowledge of the efficacy of the two drugs in the trial will be considerably increased, and at the same time we will be able to build up a detailed picture of the long-term tolerability of the two drugs.

Success, however, is dependent upon the continued support of investigating clinicians and their willingness to continue to at least the same extent as has been achieved thus far.

REFERENCES

(1) Jeavons PM, Clark JE, Maheshwari MC. Treatment of generalised epilepsies of childhood and adolescence with sodium valproate (Epilim). *Dev Med Child Neurol* 1977; **19**: 9–25.
(2) Shakir RA. Sodium valproate, phenytoin and carbamazepine as sole anticonvulsants. In: Parsonage MJ, Caldwell ADS, eds. *The place of sodium valproate in the treatment of epilepsy.* London: Royal Society of Medicine International Congress and Symposium Series, No. 30, 1980; 7–16.
(3) Callaghan N, Kenny RA, O'Neill B, Crowley M, Groggin T. A prospective study between carbamazepine, phenytoin and sodium valproate as monotherapy in previously untreated and recently diagnosed patients with epilepsy. *J Neurol Neurosurg Psych* 1985; **48**: 639–44.
(4) Loiseau P. Rational use of valproate: Indications and drug regimen in epilepsy. *Epilepsia* 1984; **25** (Suppl 1): 565–72.
(5) Haigh D, Forsythe WI. The treatment of childhood epilepsy with sodium valproate. *Dev Med Child Neurol* 1975; **17**: 743–8.
(6) Heathfield K, Dunlop D, Karanjia P, Retsa SS. The long-term results of treating 36 patients with intractable epilepsy with sodium valproate (Epilim). In: Legg NJ, ed. *Clinical and pharmacological aspects of sodium valproate (Epilim) in the treatment of epilepsy.* Kent: MCS Consultants, 1976; 165–70.
(7) Marescaux C, Warter JM, Micheletti G, Rumbach L, Coquillat G, Kurtz D. Stuperous episodes during treatment with sodium valproate: Report of seven cases. *Epilepsia* 1982; **23**: 297–305.
(8) Dean JC, Penry JK. Valproate monotherapy in 30 patients with seizures. *Epilepsia* 1988; **29**: 140–4.
(9) Editorial. Sodium valproate. *Lancet* 1988; **ii**: 1229–31.
(10) Parsonage M. The classification of epilepsies. In: Laidlaw J, Richens A, eds. *Textbook of epilepsy*, 2nd edn. Edinburgh and London: Churchill-Livingstone, 1982; XIII–XVII.

Appendix

Clinicians participating in the trial

National Co-ordinator:
Dr G. Hosking — Ryegate Children's Centre — Sheffield

Clinical consultant
Dr G. Stores — Park Hospital — Oxford

Statistical adviser
Dr A. L. Johnson — MRC Biostatistics Unit — Cambridge

Regional co-ordinators

Dr E. Hicks	Royal Belfast Hospital for Sick Children	Belfast
Dr I McKinley	Royal Manchester Children's Hospital	Manchester
Dr J. B. McMenamin	Our Lady's Hospital for Sick Children	Dublin
Dr D. Mellor	City Hospital	Nottingham
Dr R. W. Newton	Pendlebury/Booth Hall	Manchester
Dr M. J. Noronha	Pendlebury/Booth Hall	Manchester
Dr L. Rosenbloom	Alder Hey Children's Hospital	Liverpool
Dr S. Wallace	University Hospital of Wales	Cardiff

Other clinicians participating in the trial

Dr R. S. Ackroyd	Children's Hospital	Cheltenham
Dr N. K. Agarwal	Morriston Hospital	Swansea
Dr J. M. T. Alexander	General Infirmary	Pontefract
Dr W. A. Arrowsmith	Royal Infirmary	Doncaster
Dr P. Barbor	Queen's Medical Centre	Nottingham
Dr W. Barry	Royal Hospital for Sick Children	Brighton
Dr D. Bates	Royal Victoria Infirmary	Newcastle
Dr R. Beach	Norfolk and Norwich Hospital	Norwich
Dr M. Bommen	Queen Mary's Hospital	Roehampton
Dr A. M. Butterfill	County Hospital	Hereford
Dr T. L. Chambers	Southmead Hospital	Bristol
Dr T. K. R. Chandran	Leighton Hospital	Crewe
Dr S. A. Clarke	Royal Preston Hospital	Preston
Dr M. Clarke	Duchess of York Hospital	Manchester
Dr A. F. Conchie	Royal Infirmary	Doncaster
Dr C. Corkey	Daisy Hill Hospital	Newry
Dr A. J. Cottrell	General Hospital	Bishop Auckland
Dr C. E. Cramp	St Helens Hospital and Whiston Hospital	St Helens/Liverpool

Dr M. J. Crawford	Pilgrim Hospital	Boston, Lincs
Dr M. A. Cresswell	Chesterfield & N. Derbyshire Royal Hospital	Chesterfield
Dr A. J. Cronin	Freedom Fields Hospital	Plymouth
Dr D. A. Curnock	City Hospital	Nottingham
Dr M. B. Duggan	Northern General Hospital	Sheffield
Dr W. D. Elliott	North Tyneside General Hospital	North Shields
Dr H. M. Fleet	General Hospital	Amersham
Dr N. Fraser	County Hospital	Hereford
Dr S. J. Ghulam	Royal Hospital	Chesterfield
Dr A. Goodwin	West Wales General Hospital	Carmarthen
Dr A. Habel	West Middlesex Hospital	Isleworth
Dr F. M. Howard	Frimley Park Hospital	Frimley
Dr J. Inglis	Royal Infirmary	Doncaster
Dr D. Jefferson	Royal Infirmary	Derby
Dr J. G. Jenkins	Waveney Hospital	Ballymena
Dr R. W. A. Jones	Freedom Fields Hospital	Plymouth
Dr V. Joss	General Hospital	Milton Keynes
Dr P. K. Lakharni	General Hospital	Milton Keynes
Dr M. M. Liberman	Northwick Park Hospital	Harrow
Dr J. Lim	Waveney Hospital	Ballymena
Dr M. F. Lowry	District General Hospital	Sunderland
Dr M. J. Maguire	Prince Charles Hospital	Merthyr Tydfil
Dr P. A. Manfield	Good Hope General Hospital	Sutton Coldfield
Dr I. G. Mannall	General Hospital	Halifax
Dr J. P. McClure	Seafield Hospital	Ayr
Dr P. I. McFarlane	District General Hospital	Rotherham
Dr H. McKinnon	Whittington Hospital	London N19
Dr P. K. A. McWilliam	General Infirmary	Pontefract
Dr D. Mellor	City Hospital	Nottingham
Dr R. Miles	Hinchingbrooke Hospital	Huntingdon
Dr J. P. Osborne	Royal United Hospital	Bath
Dr A. Palit	Withybush General Hospital	Haverfordwest
Dr B. L. Priestley	Children's Hospital	Sheffield
Dr R. E. Pugh	Leighton Hospital	Crewe
Dr M. Quinn	Altnagelvin Hospital	Londonderry
Dr C. Rajagopal	Duchess of Kent Military Hospital	Catterick
Dr B. Reynolds	District General Hospital	Grimsby
Dr I. F. Roberts	Chesterfield & N. Derbyshire Royal Hospital	Chesterfield
Dr. C. Rolles	General Hospital	Southampton
Dr S. H. Roussounis	General Infirmary	Leeds
Dr P. T. Rudd	Royal United Hospital	Bath
Dr C. Sainsbury	Torbay Hospital	Torquay
Dr S. A. W. Salfield	District General Hospital	Rotherham
Dr J. E. Shorland	District General Hospital	Rotherham
Dr B. A. M. Smith	Northern General Hospital	Sheffield
Dr M. L. Smith	Bradford Children's Hospital	Bradford
Dr G. D. Stark	Royal Hospital for Sick Children	Edinburgh
Dr C. Steer	Victoria Hospital	Kirkcaldy
Dr. D. A. Sutherland	Glan Clwyd Hospital	Bodelwyddan
Dr L. S. Taitz	Children's Hospital	Sheffield
Dr M. J. Tarlow	East Birmingham Hospital	Birmingham
Dr G. Taylor	Royal Cornwall Hospital	Truro
Dr P. J. Todd	Arrowe Park Hospital	Upton
Dr P. Tomlin	Royal Preston Hospital	Preston
Dr R. M. Tyler	Chesterfield & N. Derbyshire Royal Hospital	Chesterfield
Dr M. J. Vaizey	Pilgrim Hospital	Boston, Lincs.
Dr C. M. Verity	Addenbrookes Hospital	Cambridge
Dr C. M. Weaver	University Hospital of Wales	Cardiff
Dr A. J. Williams	Glan Clywd Hospital	Bodelwyddan
Dr L. H. P. Williams	Bassetlaw District General Hospital	Worksop
Dr T. D. Yuille	Glan Clwyd Hospital	Bodelwyddan

A prospective randomized comparative monotherapy clinical trial in childhood epilepsy

M. de Silva[1], B. McArdle[1], M. McGowan[1], B. G. R. Neville[2], A. L. Johnson[3] and E. H. Reynolds[1]

[1]Department of Neurology, King's College Hospital, London, [2]Department of Paediatric Neurology, Guy's Hospital, London, [3]MRC Biostatistics Unit, Cambridge, UK

INTRODUCTION

There has been increasing evidence of the value and potential of monotherapy, especially in newly diagnosed patients with epilepsy (1–3). This has emphasized the need for prospective comparative trials of the major antiepileptic drugs, used as monotherapy. Such trials have so far only been undertaken in adult epileptic patients (4–7). We here report preliminary findings in a prospective randomized comparative trial of four major antiepileptic drugs (phenobarbitone, phenytoin, carbamazepine and sodium valproate) in newly diagnosed epileptic children referred to the departments of neurology at King's College Hospital and paediatric neurology at Guy's Hospital.

PATIENTS AND METHODS

One hundred and sixty-seven previously untreated newly diagnosed epileptic children entered the study between December 1980 and September 1987.

Criteria for entry to trial

We recruited children aged between 3–16 years, with generalized tonic-clonic seizures or with partial seizures with or without secondary generalization, who had had two or more attacks or an episode of status epilepticus in the year preceding entry to the trial, and who had not received anticonvulsant drugs. Febrile seizures, other seizure types and progressive cerebral disease, i.e. tumours or degenerative disorders, were excluded.

Trial design

After stratification for seizure classification, and presence or absence of neurological and/or mental handicap, the children were randomized to one of the four trial drugs, i.e. phenobarbitone, phenytoin, carbamazepine or sodium valproate. Seizure classification was based on clinical information available at the time of entry. Treatment began with a small dose of the starting drug (Table 1), administered twice daily with regular monitoring of blood levels. If seizures continued despite good compliance the dose was increased by small increments until blood levels were within the upper half of the optimum range (Table 2). No changes were made to dosage unless seizures recurred. Patients who had two or more seizures despite blood levels in the upper half of the optimum range were considered to have failed to respond to the initial drug. In the event of unacceptable

Fourth international symposium on sodium valproate and epilepsy, edited by David Chadwick, 1989; Royal Society of Medicine Services International Congress and Symposium Series No. 152, published by Royal Society of Medicine Services Limited.

Table 1 *Starting dose of anticonvulsant drugs*

Drug	Dose (mg/kg/day)
Phenobarbitone	3
Phenytoin	5
Carbamazepine	8
Sodium valproate	15

Table 2 *Optimum blood anticonvulsant drug ranges*

Drug	Range (μg/ml)
Phenobarbitone	20–40
Phenytoin	10–20
Carbamazepine	4–10
Sodium valproate	50–100

side effects the offending drug was withdrawn and treatment restarted with an alternative drug. Both the monotherapy failure group and the group withdrawn because of side effects continued to be followed up. Analysis is based on the policy of intention to treat and therefore the first drug used.

Measurements

All children had a detailed clinical examination, haematological and biochemical screening, skull X-ray, EEG and CT scan of head prior to the start of treatment. Psychometric assessments were carried out in children over five years of age.

RESULTS

Characteristics of children in the trial

Of the total of 167 entered, 78 were recruited from King's College Hospital and 89 from Guy's Hospital. The age range at the time of randomization was 3–15.9 years (mean age 10.3). There was an almost equal sex distribution, with 86 boys and 81 girls. Seventy-eight patients had generalized tonic-clonic seizures and 89 had partial seizures ± generalized seizures; 32 patients had additional handicaps (eight with generalized tonic-clonic seizures and 21 with partial ± generalized seizures).

Distribution of drugs

Ten patients were randomized to phenobarbitone, 54 to phenytoin, 54 to carbamazepine and 49 to sodium valproate. Phenobarbitone was withdrawn from the trial in October 1982 because of a high incidence of side effects (Table 3) and because some participating

Table 3 *Side effects leading to drug withdrawal (n) (%)*

Drug	Side effects
Phenobarbitone (6) (60%)	Behavioural problems (5)
	Drowsiness (1)
Phenytoin (5) (9%)	Rash (1)
	Neutropenia/thrombocytopenia (1)
	Hirsutism (1)
	Drowsiness (2)
Carbamazepine (2) (4%)	Neutropenia (1)
	Drowsiness and memory impairment (1)
Sodium valproate (2) (4%)	Tremor (1)
	Behavioural problems (1)

Table 4 *Patients remaining seizure free by duration of follow up*

Drug	Patients (n) (%)[a]		
	6 Months	12 Months	24 Months
Phenobarbitone	4 (40)	4 (40)	2 (20)
Phenytoin	25 (46)	21 (38)	13 (25)
Carbamazepine	16 (30)	15 (28)	11 (21)
Sodium valproate	19 (39)	15 (32)	12 (25)

[a]*Actuarial percentages in brackets*

Table 5 *Patients achieving one year remission by duration of follow up*

Drug	Patients (n) (%)[a]		
	12 Months	24 Months	36 Months
Phenobarbitone	4 (40)	6 (60)	7 (70)
Phenytoin	19 (36)	39 (73)	43 (80)
Carbamazepine	14 (26)	28 (52)	37 (68)
Sodium valproate	13 (27)	33 (67)	38 (78)

[a]*Actuarial percentages in brackets*

paediatricians were unwilling to randomize further children to this drug. This accounts for the small number in the group. Data were collected until the end of March 1988. The period of follow-up ranged from six months to 88 months (median 44 months).

Withdrawals from the trial

Fifteen patients (9%) were withdrawn because of adverse effects (including six of the 10 patients treated with phenobarbitone) (Table 3). Two patients emigrated and one died following a drug overdose. A further 23 patients violated the protocol and discontinued treatment, but six of them later restarted treatment.

Patients remaining seizure free by duration of follow-up

At six months the overall recurrence rate (i.e. first seizure after treatment) was 62% and by 12 months it was 67%, at 24 months 76% and at 48 months 82%. The highest recurrence rate was in the first six months of treatment, with approximately two-thirds of all patients relapsing during that time. No significant difference was noted between the four drug groups (Table 4).

Patients in six months and one year remission

Overall 35% of children achieved a six month remission at six months of follow-up, 65% by 12 months, 79% by 24 months and 84% by 36 months. Thirty-one percent of patients achieved a year's remission at 12 months of treatment, 63% by 24 months and 74% by 36 months. There were no significant differences in remission rates between the four drug subgroups as is illustrated for one year remission rates in Table 5.

DISCUSSION

For the series of 167 children as a whole the prognosis was good. One-third remained seizure free from the start of treatment to one year of follow-up. At three years of follow-up 84% had achieved six months remission and 74% had experienced a one year remission. These observations are similar to those reported for newly diagnosed adult patients with epilepsy treated with monotherapy (4–7). As in the adult studies the highest recurrence rate was in the first six months to one year after the start of treatment which has been suggested to be the most critical period in the drug treatment of epilepsy (3,8). Despite the high initial recurrence rate most children subsequently achieved long periods of remission.

We have found no significant difference in outcome between the four drug subgroups for any measure of seizure control. This is similar to the study by Mattson *et al.* (5) as well as our own study in adults (7) in whom no differences in efficacy between four drugs, utilized as monotherapy, were found. The four drugs evaluated in these studies were similar with the exception that Mattson *et al.* (5) included primidone, but not sodium valproate. Turnbull *et al.* (6) found no difference in efficacy between phenytoin and valproate in a two year prospective study in newly diagnosed adult patients. Callaghan *et al.* (4) compared carbamazepine, phenytoin and sodium valproate in 181 patients followed for a median of 14 months and also found a good prognosis with all three drugs in newly diagnosed adult epilepsy.

The choice of drug for newly diagnosed generalized tonic-clonic or partial seizures with or without secondary generalization will therefore to a large extent be influenced by considerations of toxicity. Overall 9% of the children were withdrawn from the randomized treatment because of unacceptable side effects, but this included six (60%) out of the 10 patients treated with phenobarbitone. For the three other drugs the incidence of withdrawals because of toxicity was between 4% and 9%.

SUMMARY

In a prospective randomized study of 167 newly diagnosed previously untreated children with at least two tonic-clonic or partial seizures with or without secondary generalization and followed for a median of 44 months (range 6 to 88 months), no differences in efficacy were found between phenobarbitone, phenytoin, carbamazepine or sodium valproate. Nine percent of the children developed unacceptable side effects including six of 10 patients who were randomized to phenobarbitone, which was therefore withdrawn from the study. The overall prognosis in these children was good and similar to that reported in previously untreated newly diagnosed adult patients with epilepsy.

ACKNOWLEDGMENTS

We are grateful to the consultant paediatricians, King's College Hospital, St George's Hospital and St Thomas' Hospital, London, The Kent and Canterbury Hospital, Canterbury, Farnborough Hospital, Kent and Pembury Hospital, Tunbridge Wells for referring patients for inclusion in the study; to Miss Judy Kelly for her assistance in co-ordinating the study; to the Medical Research Council and The Health Promotion Trust and to Sanofi UK Limited, Ciba-Geigy and Parke-Davis for financial support.

REFERENCES

(1) Reynolds EH, Chadwick D, Galbraith AW. One drug (phenytoin) in the treatment of epilepsy. *Lancet* 1976; i: 923–6.
(2) Reynolds EH, Shorvon SD. Monotherapy or polytherapy for epilepsy? *Epilepsia* 1981; **22**: 1–10.
(3) Reynolds EH. Early treatment and prognosis of epilepsy. *Epilepsia* 1987; **28** (2): 97–106.
(4) Callaghan N, Kenny RA, O'Neill B, Crowley M, Goggin T. A prospective study between carbamazepine, phenytoin and sodium valproate as monotherapy in previously untreated and recently diagnosed patients with epilepsy. *J Neurol Neurosurg Psych* 1985; **48**: 639–44.
(5) Mattson RH, Cramer JA, Collins JF, *et al.* Comparison of carbamazepine, phenobarbital, phenytoin and primidone in partial and secondarily generalized tonic-clonic seizures. *N Engl J Med* 1985; **313**: 145–51.
(6) Turnbull DM, Howell D, Rawlins MD, Chadwick DW. Which drug for the adult epileptic patient: phenytoin or valproate? *Br Med J* 1985; **290**: 815–19.
(7) Heller AJ, Chesterman P, Elwes RDC, *et al.* Monotherapy for newly diagnosed adult epilepsy: a comparative trial and prognostic evaluation. Presented to the XVIIIth International Epilepsy Congress, New Delhi, India, 1989.
(8) Reynolds EH, Elwes RDC, Shorvon SD. Why does epilepsy become intractable? Prevention of chronic epilepsy. *Lancet* 1983; ii: 952–4.

Discussion after Drs Hosking and de Silva

on paediatric clinical trials

Interactive question from Dr Hosking

In your opinion	Response
1 The EEG is essential in diagnosis	30%
2 The EEG is not essential in diagnosis but is for accurate classification	55%
3 The EEG is of little value either for diagnosis or classification	15%

Dr Hosking *(Sheffield, UK):* I totally agree with that interactive response.

Dr Abraham *(London, UK):* This is a question for Dr Hosking. I was surprised by the number of people that the independent assessor said did not have epilepsy, compared with the answer from the clinical investigators.

Dr Hosking: Taking the unclassified section, in a significant number there was not enough information relating to the attacks to put them fairly confidently into one clinical category or another. A large number of children within that context had attacks predominantly at night, and in those cases there were very poor eye witness accounts of the attack and the characteristics. As to the other part of your question, those children that did not have seizures, we are talking about one person's opinion against others. There was not a 'don't know' category but if the clinicians did not think the child had epilepsy, they should not have entered the child into the study.

Dr Verity *(Cambridge, UK):* Dr de Silva, one of the striking things about your graphs is that the curves follow similar trajectories. You clearly did not have a no-treatment group. I wonder whether, if you did have a no-treatment group, they would have shown a similar trend.

Dr de Silva *(London, UK):* It is a difficult question to answer. For ethical reasons it is not easy to design a trial with a no treatment group. Therefore, it is hard to say what they would have done without treatment. But looking through the various remission and relapse rates that have been reported in the literature, perhaps a small percentage would remain seizure free without treatment, but I think the great majority would have gone on to have further seizures.

Dr Verity: I think that is good support for Dr Chadwick's proposed trial of early treatment. Clearly it is difficult to have a no-treatment group, but designing a trial where you can compare early with later treatment might enable you partly to answer that question.

Professor Dam *(Copenhagen, Denmark):* A question to Dr Hosking. Could you give me a good argument for not making such a trial blind? I understand it was an open trial, so I would hesitate in trusting the results, despite the large number of patients in the trial. Dr de Silva, could you elaborate a little more on the one patient who died in your trial. It was due to an overdosage of which drug?

Dr de Silva: She committed suicide by taking an overdose of her antiepileptic drug, sodium valproate.

Dr Hosking: I am not sure what the advantages would be of a blind trial in this context. We are comparing two already established antiepileptic drugs and it is an independent randomization. I am not sure what advantages can accrue from it being blind.

Dr Schutt *(Bristol, UK):* A question to Dr de Silva about compliance. Children and parents are capable of making up their own minds on how long to continue the treatment. To what extent did compliance influence your data, and were you able to look at that?

Dr de Silva: About half of the 23 patients who violated the protocol had treatment for more than six months, then discontinued at some later stage. But one of them had completed treatment with two year's remission.

Dr Jivani *(Blackburn, UK):* Dr Hosking, were the investigators in the study always paediatric neurologists?

Dr Hosking: The majority of the investigating clinicians were paediatricians.

A study of valproate in infants with West syndrome

F. Kotlarek[1], U. Rübenstrunk[1], V. Raemakers[1], G. Groß-Selbeck[2],
K. Kellermann[3], K. Rheingans[3], W. Mortier[4], R. Pothmann[4], H. von Bernuth[5],
and U. Schauseil-Zipf[6]

[1]Department of Paediatrics, Klinikum RWTH, Aachen, [2]Department of Neuropaediatrics, Städtische Krankenanstalten, Düsseldorf-Gerresheim, [3]Department of Paediatrics, Städtisches Kinderkrankenhaus, Köln, [4]Department of Paediatrics, Städtische Krankenanstalten, Wuppertal, [5]Department of Paediatrics, Städtische Krankenanstalten, Bielefeld, [6]Department of Paediatrics, University of Köln, FRG

SUMMARY

In a prospective multicentre study of 79 infants presenting with infantile spasms and hypsarrhythmic EEG patterns, the efficacy of monotherapy with high dose valproate (VPA) has been evaluated. An initial dose of 50 mg/kg/day was administered to all infants over a 10 day period. Those infants not responding to the initial dose received VPA up to a dose of 100 mg/kg/day in a subsequent phase of 10 days. After a trial of 4 weeks, the group of infants in whom VPA did not control the seizures, have been treated with ACTH while VPA was phased out gradually.

Complete cessation of seizures and hypsarrhythmia has become established amongst 21 out of a total of 79 infants treated with VPA. Relapses occurred in only two cases during the course of VPA treatment. Based on the underlying aetiology infants have been classified into three groups. The best response rate to VPA has been noticed in five out of seven infants belonging to the idiopathic group, who showed a prompt response within two weeks after introduction of VPA. Compared to the idiopathic group a lower response rate to VPA has been documented amongst 14 out of 68 cases with symptomatic aetiology defined as neurological deficits due to various pre-, peri- and postnatal insults. Two out of four children with tuberous sclerosis responded only at the highest dose of VPA following a time interval of five weeks. Valproate had to be discontinued in six out of 79 cases because of serious side-effects. Although the immediate cause of death could not be attributed directly due to VPA toxicity, two infants died during the course of treatment with VPA. In conclusion, monotherapy with high dose VPA appears to possess potent anticonvulsive action in a number of infants with West syndrome, particularly in the so-called idiopathic cases, but also in a limited number of cases with organic brain injuries. However, the relative efficacy of valproate and ACTH in the management of West syndrome still remains to be established.

INTRODUCTION

Adrenocorticotropin (ACTH) and dexamethasone have become established as therapy of first choice in infantile spasms since they have been proved to be the most potent anticonvulsant drugs in controlling seizures and the hypsarrhythmic EEG pattern (3,5). However, the serious side-effects of hormone therapy demand a search for equally effective but safer drugs. Since 1981 several authors have reported valproate (VPA) as an effective

Fourth international symposium on sodium valproate and epilepsy, edited by David Chadwick, 1989; Royal Society of Medicine Services International Congress and Symposium Series No. 152, published by Royal Society of Medicine Services Limited.

alternative drug in the control of infantile spasms (1,2,4,6). In the present study we report the results of a prospective multicentre study with high dose VPA as monotherapy in West syndrome.

PATIENTS AND METHODS

A total of 79 infants with West syndrome entered the study. All previously ineffective drugs (such as benzodiazepines and barbiturates) had been discontinued before VPA monotherapy was started. Children pretreated with ACTH or dexamethasone were excluded from the present study.

The infants were subdivided into three main groups according to aetiology. The first group, defined as the idiopathic group ($n=7$), included children with a normal history and development before the onset of seizures and in whom no neurological abnormalities have been found. The computed tomography (CT) brain scan was normal. The second symptomatic group ($n=68$) consisted of infants with neurodevelopmental delay before the onset of seizures who suffered from various pre-, peri- or postnatal insults. In these children a high proportion of abnormal CT-scans has been found. The third group comprised cases with tuberous sclerosis ($n=4$).

DESIGN OF THE STUDY

VPA was increased within three days up to a dose of 50 mg/kg/day, in two divided doses. If VPA failed to control seizures after a trial of ten days, it was increased to a maximum dose of 100 mg/kg/day. If seizures stopped, treatment with VPA monotherapy was continued (with either 50 or 100 mg/kg/day). If VPA failed to control seizures, small doses of ACTH (3 IU/kg/day) were introduced. Following initiation of ACTH treatment, the dose of VPA was reduced gradually within four weeks and then stopped. If no response was documented within 10 days following small doses of ACTH, the dose was further increased to 6 IU/kg/day.

The following laboratory investigations have been performed prior to and at 1, 2, 3, 4, 5, 6, 9 and 12 months after starting VPA: haemoglobin, white cell count, platelet count, liver transaminases, alkaline phosphatase, amylase and coagulation studies (prothrombin time, partial thromboplastin time and fibrinogen levels).

RESULTS

At present the follow-up period for all infants is a minimum of six months. The overall results of the present study show that 21 out of 79 infants (i.e. 26.6%) responded to VPA monotherapy and became completely seizure-free within five weeks. In all responders the hypsarrhythmic EEG pattern disappeared.

Considerable differences in response rate to VPA have been observed between the three subgroups (Table 1). In the idiopathic group, five out of seven infants responded promptly

Table 1 *Results of valproate therapy (VPA) in treatment of children with idiopathic and symptomatic aetiology and in four cases with tuberous sclerosis (TS)*

	Idiopathic ($n=7$)	Symptomatic ($n=68$)	TS ($n=4$)
Seizure free on VPA			
—50 mg/kg/day	4	10	
—100 mg/kg/day	1[a]	4	2
Responders/total	5/7	14/68	2/4
Number of relapses	1[a]	1	

[a]*Idiopathic case relapsing after initial improvement on 50 mg/kg/day, but remaining seizure free at the highest dose of 100 mg/kg/day.*

to VPA within a short time interval of two weeks. Among the symptomatic group, only 14 out of 68 patients responded to VPA. Compared to the symptomatic group a significantly higher proportion of patients belonging to the idiopathic group responded to VPA (chi-square test; $p<0.01$). Two of the four children with tuberous sclerosis responded only after treatment with the highest doses of VPA (i.e. 100 mg/kg/day).

Table 1 shows the distribution of patients in each group who responded to either 50 or 100 mg/kg/day. Fig. 1 shows that all responders did so within five weeks after VPA was started. Seizure control in the idiopathic group tended to manifest earlier (within two weeks) compared to either the symptomatic group or children with tuberous sclerosis.

Relapse of spasms occurred in one patient of the idiopathic group, who subsequently became seizure-free after elevation of VPA up to 100 mg/kg/day. In the symptomatic group relapse of spasms occurred in only one out of 14 children after initial successful control with VPA. Relapse of spasms also occurred in the two children with tuberous sclerosis responding first to VPA.

Some of the non-responders to VPA have been successfully treated with ACTH. The two non-responders in the idiopathic group became seizure-free on the lowest dose of ACTH. Further control of seizures was possible in 24 out of 48 non-responders belonging to the symptomatic group. Six symptomatic cases were not treated with ACTH because of the extent of major handicaps.

Severe side-effects leading to discontinuance of VPA occurred in two children with severe thrombocytopenia (platelets below 30 000/mm³), two children with pancytopenia and two children with lethargy and vomiting after introduction of VPA.

Two out of 79 children treated with VPA died. The immediate cause of death in one child was attributed to severe dehydration. Postmortem liver biopsy did not show characteristic histopathological features consistent with VPA toxicity. Sudden infant death syndrome was diagnosed in another child who died suddenly at the age of 11 months after VPA had been administered for more than five months.

DISCUSSION

Our results show that high-dose VPA monotherapy can achieve seizure control in most of the patients within the idiopathic group of cases of the West syndrome, while a substantial but smaller number of patients within the symptomatic group respond to VPA within a time interval of four weeks. Two patients with tuberous sclerosis became seizure-free after five weeks of treatment.

Compared to ACTH (3,5) administration of VPA seems to provoke far less serious side-effects. Published data on limited numbers of patients show that lower doses of VPA achieved similar rates of seizure control from 22:2 to 33.3% (1,2,4). However, the numbers of treated patients in these studies are small and differences with respect to patient populations exist between the various studies.

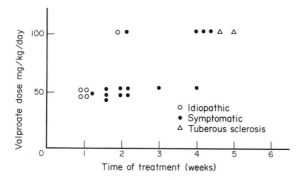

Figure 1 *Response to VPA (i.e. seizure-free) indicating dose and time interval to control spasms in each of the subgroups.*

Siemes *et al.* (6) treated 22 children with infantile spasms with high doses of VPA up to 100 mg/kg/day (6). Despite the small number of patients, Siemes *et al.* achieved far better seizure control among 72.7% of their patients. After four weeks of treatment with VPA, 11 out of 22 (or 50%) became seizure-free. This is in marked contrast to our study where only 24.1% responded after four weeks of drug therapy.

Possible differences in number and definition of subgroups might impose important statistical hazards when studies are compared.

In accordance with Siemes's study we also found a better response in the idiopathic group of cases of West syndrome than in symptomatic cases. We think a trial with VPA is worth while, especially amongst idiopathic cases. More studies are needed to investigate the place of VPA in treatment of West syndrome, to determine other outcomes such as neurodevelopmental progress, cognitive function and epilepsy in later life.

REFERENCES

(1) Bachmann DS. Use of valproic acid in treatment of infantile spasms. *Arch Neurol* 1982; **39**: 49–52.
(2) Dulac O, Arthuis M. Open trials with valproate in epilepsy. *Epilepsia*, 1984; **25** (Suppl 1): S23–S31.
(3) Fois A, Malandrini F, Balestri P, Giorgi D. Infantile spasms—long term results of ACTH treatment. *Eur J Pediatr* 1984; **142**: 51–5.
(4) Pavone L, Incorpora G, La Rosa M, Li Volti S, Mollica F. Treatment of infantile spasms with sodium dipropylacetic acid.*Dev Med Child Neurol* 1981; **23**: 454–461.
(5) Riikonen R. A long-term follow-up study of 214 children with the syndrome of infantile spasms. *Neuropediatrics* 1982; **13**: 14–23.
(6) Siemes H, Spohr HL, Michael Th, Nau H. Therapy of infantile spasms with valproate: Results of a prospective study. *Epilepsia* 1988; **29**: 553–60.

Valproate in juvenile myoclonic epilepsy

W. Christe

Klinikum Rudolf Virchow, Department of Neurology, Free University of Berlin, FDR

INTRODUCTION

Juvenile myoclonic epilepsy (JME) is the most specific of the epileptic syndromes with age-dependent generalized seizures listed in the classification proposed by the ILAE-Commission (1). Herpin (2) in 1867 provided the first extensive report of a patient with JME, while Janz and Christian (3) published the first systematic description of this syndrome in 1957 in a study comprising 47 patients. Janz suggested the term 'impulsive petit mal' for this syndrome which has received relatively little attention in the English language literature until the early 1980s.

Juvenile myoclonic epilepsy represents approximately 4–5% of all cases of epilepsy and 20 to 30% of idiopathic generalized epilepsies (Table 1). The age of onset of seizures is most often between the ages of 12 and 18 years, and the sex ratio is equal. Seizures in this syndrome are characteristically sudden bilateral myoclonic jerks affecting mainly the shoulders and the arms. They occur singly or repetitively in irregular intervals, usually in the morning on awakening. Consciousness is always preserved (4): 90% of the patients also have generalized tonic-clonic seizures (GTCS), and about 10% of patients have additional absences of the juvenile type with infrequent recurrences (5). Precipitating factors are sleep deprivation and premature awakening. The typical EEG pattern of epileptic discharges comprises bilateral symmetric polyspike-wave complexes faster than 3 Hz with fronto-central accentuation (6,7). More than 30% of patients are photosensitive (8). The aetiology is unknown, though there is evidence for a considerable hereditary predisposition (9,10). The response to appropriate antiepileptic drug treatment is good (Table 2).

Complete seizure control was reported by a number of different authors with valproate, primidone, and phenobarbital, either in monotherapy or in combination, in 55–94%

Table 1 *Juvenile myoclonic epilepsy*

Prevalence	4–5% of all types of epilepsy 20–30% of idiopathic generalized epilepsies
Age of onset	12–18 years
Sex ratio	Equal
Seizure types	Sudden shock-like jerks affecting mainly shoulders and arms, bilateral, isolated or repeated. Consciousness preserved. Additional GTCS frequent (90%), additional absences less frequent (10%)
Chronobiology	Mainly in the morning on awakening
Precipitating factors	Sleep deprivation, premature awakening
EEG	Bilateral symmetric polyspike-wave-complexes (>3/sec), fronto-central accentuation, photosensitivity frequent (30.5%)
Aetiology	Unknown, genetic disposition
Therapy	Valproate, primidone
Prognosis	Good

Fourth international symposium on sodium valproate and epilepsy, edited by David Chadwick, 1989; Royal Society of Medicine Services International Congress and Symposium Series No. 152, published by Royal Society of Medicine Services Limited.

Table 2 *Treatment of epilepsies with juvenile myoclonic jerks. Results of clinical studies*

Authors	n	Medication	Seizure-free	
			n	%
Janz (4) (1969)	156	PRM, PB, AED	120	77
Jeavons (16) (1982)	17	VPA	13	76
Covanis (12) (1982)	45	VPA	31	69
Feuerstein (14) (1983)	17	VPA	14	77
Asconapé (11) (1984)	11	VPA	6	55
Delgado (13) (1984)	40	VPA, AED	32	80
Franzen (15) (1988)	97	VPA, PRM, AED	91	94
Obeid (17) (1988)	50	VPA, CNZ, AED	42	84

Table 3 *VPA monotherapy in juvenile myoclonic epilepsy*

Authors	Patients	n	Seizure-free		Study design
			n	%	
Covanis et al. (12) 1982	22/45 photosensitive some pretreated	45	31	69	open trial
Feuerstein et al. (14) 1983	15/17 IPM + GM some pretreated	17	14	77	open trial
Asconapé & Penry (11) 1984	9/11 IPM + GM some pretreated	11	6	55	case report
Franzen (15) 1988	27/29 IPM + GM 18/29 pretreated	29	28	97	open trial

of patients (4,11–17). Valproate (VPA) has gained favour as the drug of first choice in JME over the past 10 years.

There are no controlled studies of VPA monotherapy in the current literature (Table 3). In an open trial of VPA monotherapy Covanis et al. (12) reported complete control in 31 of 45 patients (69%), of whom 22 were photosensitive. It is not possible to determine how many of these patients suffered also grand mal seizures. Treatment results were similarly good in the report published by Feuerstein et al. (14), Franzen (15) found that 28 of 29 patients (97%) were free of seizures under treatment with VPA. The majority of patients in these studies had already been treated with other anticonvulsants.

PATIENTS

The present study summarizes the clinical courses of 22 newly diagnosed, previously untreated patients (10 male, 12 female) with JME, treated with VPA monotherapy in our department during the period from 1980 to 1988 (Table 4). Mean age at onset of epilepsy was 15.7 years (12.1–36.8) and therapy was instituted at a mean age of 19.3 years (15.3–71.5). Mean duration of disease until treatment was 3.6 years (0.4–34.7). All patients had

Table 4 *VPA monotherapy in juvenile myoclonic epilepsy. Clinical data*

Patients:	$n = 22$ (12f, 10m), previously untreated
Age:	19.3 years (range, 15.3–71.5)
Age of onset:	15.7 years (range, 12.1–36.8)
Seizure types:	19/22 IPM + GTCS 3/22 IPM + GTCS + Abs 6/22 photosensitive
GTCS-frequency:	1.6 (range, 1–6)
Dosage:	1650 mg (range, 900–3500) 24.8 mg/kg (range, 15.5–56.5)
Plasma-levels:	86.4 μg/ml (range, 58.2–109.6)
Follow-up:	4.6 years (range, 2.2–8.8)

Table 5 *VPA monotherapy in juvenile myoclonic epilepsy. Results*

		Seizure-free	
Patients	n	n	%
Previously untreated IPM + GTCS	22	21	95

Table 6 *Discontinuation of antiepileptic drug treatment in idiopathic generalized epilepsies. Prognosis (Janz et al., 1983) (19)*

		Seizure-free	Relapses
Type of seizure	n	%	%
GTCS	86	84	58
Absences + GTCS	113	60	65
IPM + GTCS	49	75	91

myoclonic jerks and GTCS on awakening, while three had additional infrequent simple absences, and six were photosensitive. An average of 1.9 (1–6) GTCS was reported before initiation of treatment. The average daily dose of VPA was 1650 mg (900–3600), which represents 24.8 mg/kg (15.5–56.5). Mean duration of follow-up was 4.6 years (2.2–8.8).

RESULTS

All patients were advised to regulate their sleeping habits. Those who were photosensitive were instructed to avoid potential stimuli. Three patients, who had initially tried to control seizures without medication ultimately requested medical treatment after finding that continual avoidance of precipitating factors was more restrictive than was regular ingestion of antiepileptic drugs.

Twenty-one of 22 patients (95%) became free of seizures during the follow-up period (Table 5), which lasted for a minimum of 26 months. Separate evaluation of major and minor seizures revealed that there was complete control of myoclonic jerks (22/22) and absences (3/3). Twenty-one patients were also free of GTCS, while the remaining patient experienced a reduction in frequency of seizure but not complete control.

Although all 21 of these patients have been free of seizures for at least two years and some for more than five years, no patient has discontinued treatment with VPA. We have not encouraged patients to discontinue their medication, since relapse may occur in up to 90% (Table 6), more than in any other form of epilepsy (18,19).

CONCLUSION

In summary, our study confirms the available data derived from open trials demonstrating that monotherapy with VPA is very effective in JME. The drug is also effective in other forms of idiopathic epilepsy with primarily generalized seizures (20–23). Treatment should be initiated with VPA alone, since combination treatment with other drugs always entails the possibility of drug interactions (24). Monotherapy results also in more rapid achievement of therapeutic serum levels and desired clinical effects. However, effective treatment of JME is not equivalent to definitive recovery. The risk of relapse is very high when medication is reduced or withdrawn. For this reason JME may be described as a 'benign' condition in regard to therapeutic success but not in regard to the risk of relapse.

Table 7 *Trials of antiepileptic drug treatment in different epileptic syndromes*

—Seizure frequency
—Specific effects on different seizure types
—Long-term effects
—Tolerance
—Effects on the EEG
—Relapse rate following drug withdrawal

Currently available information on VPA is concerned primarily with its effect on seizures in various forms of epilepsy. Future trials should concentrate more on clinical syndromes (Table 7). One such study might attempt to define whether the drug has specific effects on different types of seizures in a given epileptic syndrome. Improved estimates of treatment prognosis will require information on long-term clinical effects, tolerance, effects on the EEG, and rates of relapse following reduction and termination of treatment in various clinical syndromes.

REFERENCES

(1) Commission on Classification and Terminology of the International League Against Epilepsy. Proposal for classification of epilepsies and epileptic syndromes. *Epilepsia* 1985; **26** (3): 268–78.
(2) Herpin TH. *Des accès incomplets d'épilepsie.* Paris: Baillière, 1867.
(3) Janz D, Christian W. Impulsiv-Petit mal. *Dtsch Z Nervenheilk* 1957; **176**: 346–86.
(4) Janz D. *Die Epilepsien.* Stuttgart: Thieme, 1969.
(5) Wolf P. Juvenile myoclonic epilepsy. In: Roger J, Dravet C, Bureau M, Dreifuss FE, Wolf P, eds. *Epileptic syndromes in infancy, childhood and adolescence.* London: Libbey, 1985: 247–58.
(6) Janz D. Epilepsy with impulsive petit mal (juvenile myoclonic epilepsy). *Acta Neurol Scand* 1985; **72**: 449–59.
(7) Tsuboi T. Primary generalized epilepsy with sporadic myoclonias of myoclonic petit mal type. Stuttgart: Thieme, 1977.
(8) Goosses R. Die Beziehung der Fotosensibilität zu den verschiedenen epileptischen Syndromen. Thesis, Free University of Berlin, 1984.
(9) Beck-Mannagetta G, Anderson VE, Doose H, Janz D. *Genetics of the epilepsies.* Berlin, Heidelberg: Springer, 1989.
(10) Tsuboi T, Christian W. On the genetics of the primary generalized epilepsy with sporadic myoclonias of the impulsive petit mal type. *Humangenetik* 1973: **19**: 155–82.
(11) Asconapé J, Penry K. Some clinical and EEG aspects of benign juvenile myoclonic epilepsy. *Epilepsia* 1984; **25** (1): 108–14.
(12) Covanis A, Gupta AK, Jeavons PM. Sodium valproate: monotherapy and polytherapy. *Epilepsia* 1982; **23**: 693–720.
(13) Delgado-Escueta AV, Enrile-Bascal F. Juvenile myoclonic epilepsy of Janz. *Neurology* 1984; **34**: 285–94.
(14) Feuerstein J, Revol M, Roger J, *et al.* La monothérapie par le valproate de sodium dans les épilepsies de l'enfant. *Sem Hôp Paris* 1983; **59**: 1263–74.
(15) Franzen S. Die medikamentöse Behandlung der Epilepsien mit Impulsiv-Petit mal. Thesis, Free University of Berlin, 1988.
(16) Jeavons PM. Myoclonic epilepsies: therapy and prognosis. In: Akimoto H, Kazamatsuri H, Seino M, Ward A, eds. *Advances in epileptology: XIIIth Epilepsy International Symposium.* New York: Raven Press, 1982.
(17) Obeid T, Panayiotopoulos CP. Juvenile myoclonic epilepsy: a study in Saudi Arabia. *Epilepsia* 1988; **29** (3): 280–2.
(18) Baruzzi A, Procaccianti G, Tinuper P, Lugaresi E. Antiepileptic drug withdrawal in childhood epilepsy: preliminary results of a prospective study. In: Faenza C, Prati GL, eds. *Diagnostic and therapeutic problems in pediatric epileptology.* Amsterdam: Elsevier Science Publishers, 1988: 117–23.
(19) Janz D, Kern A, Mössinger HJ, Puhlmann U. Rückfall-Prognose nach Reduktion der Medikamente bei Epilepsie-behandlung. *Nervenarzt* 1983; **54**: 525–9.
(20) Bourgeois B, Beaumanoir A, Blajev B, *et al.* Primäre generalisierte Epilepsien. *Therapiewoche* 1987; **26**: 2573–7.
(21) Christe W, Janz D. Sodium valproate in idiopathic generalized epilepsies. *Boll Lega It Epil* 1988; **61**: 11–15.
(22) Dulac O, Steru D, Rey E, Perret A, Arthuis M. Sodium valproate in childhood epilepsy. *Brain Develop* 1986; **8**: 47–52.
(23) Groß-Selbeck G. Valproat—ein risikoreiches Medikament? *Epilepsie-Blätter* 1988; **1** (1): 7–13.
(24) Henriksen O, Johannessen SI. Valproate monotherapy. *Epilepsia* 1988; **25** (Suppl 1); S73–S77.

Paediatrician to neurologist—how to hand on the patient successfully?

H. J. Heggarty

York District Hospital, York, UK

The predicament in which the patient and the paediatrician find themselves at the time of 'handing over' to the neurologist is well known, and the question of how to do this successfully is a difficult subject. Each city or district has its own arrangements, each patient has his unique problem. The predicaments are therefore unique, and there is no single answer. Sometimes the problem or predicament is amusing, but the question nevertheless remains, who will be the advocate on behalf of the adolescent with epilepsy?

Many, if not most, adolescents have major areas of concern about their appearance, peer group conformity, ability to participate in sports and driving motor cars. The epileptic adolescent has these 'normal' anxieties to contend with as well as difficulties perhaps caused by insufficient sleep or alcohol excess, fatigue, discos, and possibly drug abuse. Self esteem is a major problem. I would strongly disagree with anyone who feels that there is now no stigma attached to epilepsy. Anybody who has taken physically or mentally retarded children who have seizures to a smart restaurant for tea, or to the local swimming baths, will know that the stigma does still exist.

There are constraints on the career choices of these children and many of them need special help and extra tuition to help them with examinations. The educational difficulties of some children with epilepsy constitute an enormous subject, and much helpful literature has been produced by experts such as Thompson, Corbett and Reynolds (1–3).

Many of these epileptic young people are misunderstood by teachers and therefore the links between the paediatrician, the School Medical Officer and the teachers are crucial. I do my best to strengthen these on every occasion and often visit ordinary schools to discuss such children with the staff.

The choice of future marriage partners may be restricted by society or by the patient himself, and potential problems of genetics or teratogenic risk should also be discussed with the patient and his family.

Sadly in my experience, what wrecks families and pulls them apart is not necessarily the primary handicap, but the behaviour problems which ensue. To attempt to prevent or ameliorate behaviour problems in epileptic children while they are young, and before they reach the adult neurologist or general physician is a great challenge to paediatricians and one which, so far, we are failing to meet.

In those children with cerebral palsy or mental handicap with epilepsy as a complicating factor, the behaviour and educational problems are often much more difficult to deal with than the seizures. I suspect that they are a particularly abandoned class: there seems no-one to be their buffer and their advocate when they outgrow the paediatric age range.

Some of the problems with these children arise either through misdiagnosis or a lack of communication, both between doctors and between doctor and patient. For instance, one young boy of about 11 years of age developed giggling incontinence but was not suspected of having epilepsy until the diagnosis was made by a clinical psychologist who witnessed one of these episodes. Another boy had the problem of acquired epileptic aphasia and it was not until I heard a description of this problem during a lecture given by

Fourth international symposium on sodium valproate and epilepsy, edited by David Chadwick, 1989; Royal Society of Medicine Services International Congress and Symposium Series No. 152, published by Royal Society of Medicine Services Limited.

David Mellor in York that I was able to help the child and his teachers understand, if not overcome, the difficulty. The sad case of a mother with tuberous sclerosis, whose three children also suffer from this condition, highlights the tragic consequences of failure to make the primary diagnosis, failure to give genetic advice, and failure to offer counselling about future pregnancies.

Adult physicians often accuse paediatricians of mollycoddling their patients. That may be so, but nevertheless a number of our adolescent epileptic patients come back to us after attending the adult out-patient clinic. Adolescents often oscillate emotionally for a year or two between adulthood and childhood, and it is no surprise therefore if they do the same with their doctors. Perhaps this is an argument for shared clinics. At the District Hospital in York we have simplified the handover of asthmatics, cystic fibrosis children, diabetic and spina bifida children by the use of combined clinics, shared between orthopaedic surgeon, paediatrician, psychologist, adult physician with a special interest, a neurosurgeon and a urologist. We have not yet included epilepsy in this system but I believe that we should do so.

Adolescents whose epilepsy is well controlled and in whom there are no major problems are generally cared for by their family doctors. Some are transferred at the age of 15–18 years, depending on the patient's wishes, to a general physician with a CNS interest. At this stage it is important to pass on the fullest possible details of the patient.

For young adults with mental retardation and/or cerebral palsy with epilepsy as a complicating factor, I arrange the hand-over to the Community Mental Handicap Team via a clinic held in special schools where both the consultant in mental handicap and I visit. The presence of genuine psychiatric problems in this group is important, and his skills are very relevant. Moreover, we overlap in the care of these patients when they are 16–18 years old. He has an out-patient clinic in the children's centre and his team and I are able to meet informally (over coffee) and discuss the patients' problems. The involvement of a psychologist is particularly valuable when we need to discuss vocation, jobs, marriage etc. A consultant in adolescent psychiatry is also available but I feel that if mental retardation is the underlying problem then the orthodox child and adolescent psychiatry services are less interested. One of the most helpful people that we have in York is our occupational therapist, Dorothy Penso, who has written books on learning difficulties, and career problems (4) and is an advocate for these 'problem children' from the point of view of examination difficulties and future employment. Uniquely perhaps in York we have members of the Neuropsychiatric Unit, neurophysiologist Tony Da Costa and neurologist Ernie Spokes, who are willing to take on long-term follow-up of young adults with particularly difficult problems of epilepsy.

Nevertheless, there remains a hard core of young people with epilepsy whom I feel we fail to help. Particular problem groups such as epileptics in prison, or gypsies, are difficult to help, and patients with temporal lobe epilepsies and behavioural problems can prove intractable. Young adults who attend adult training centres often seem to have no-one to turn to when they leave the paediatric clinic. There is no specific major helping agency, and although a social worker or a senior clinical medical officer could fill the gap, the time and persistence needed to obtain the help is sometimes more than the patient can cope with.

Our out-patient clinics sometimes seem to be clinics for crisis management only. What the adolescents with epilepsy need is time—time for regular contact with someone they can trust and relate to; time for repeated and careful explanations; time to give information, for constant encouragement, for arranging optimal educational opportunity; time to aim for a stable personality in a growing child and to enlighten the attitudes of parents, peers, teachers and prospective employers.

It is important to involve the Education Department Special Careers Officer long before the child approaches school leaving age. The School Medical Officer should be deeply involved when the child is at secondary school. Many adolescents, of course, are apathetic, even when the service is perfect and it is sometimes helpful to arrange meetings of such children after school or at clubs. Our Asthma Swimming Club model could perhaps be extended to those with seizures, and the diabetics have also formed a similar adolescent group.

Continuing medical presence and medical contact is necessary because changes occur as children grow into adults. The dangers of alcohol abuse and barbiturate suicide attempts are more likely in this age group and the possibility of deteriorating epilepsy in an adolescent being evidence of a rare slow growing tumour has to be borne in mind.

The need for involvement of a number of professions to help the adolescent epileptic suggest that it would be reasonable to propose an adult neurological rehabilitation service in each Health District. There are of course problems in finance, resources and leadership, and the way in which the Health Service now works militates against the primary need of the adolescent epileptic—the doctor's time.

The recurring question in my paper is, who will be the advocate for these young people when they leave the care of the paediatrician? A child and a young adult has the right to dream of a job, sport, marriage, leisure and a sense of mattering to someone. Any such advocate needs a sense of humour to cope with the variability and unpredictability of both epilepsy and adolescence. The young people require a balance between excessive parental control and privacy, yet I feel that we can and should mix both optimism and realism, and generally strive for the fulfilment of the precepts of the good physician—

> To cure, sometimes
> To ease, often
> To console, always

REFERENCES

(1) Thompson PJ, Trimble MR. Anticonvulsant drugs and cognitive function. *Epilepsia* 1982; **33**: 531–4.
(2) Corbett JA, Trimble MR, Nichol TC. Behavioural and cognitive impairment in children with epilepsy. The long-term effects of anticonvulsant therapy. *J Am Acad Child Psych* 1985; **24**: 17–23.
(3) Reynolds EH. Chronic antiepileptic toxicity. A review. *Epilepsia* 1975; **16**: 319–52.
(4) Penso DE. *Occupational therapy for children with disabilities*. London: Croom Helm, 1987.

Discussion after Drs Raemakers, Christe and Heggarty

Professor Dreifuss (*Chairman*): Thank you very much Dr Heggarty, I think your patients are very lucky that you have nobody to hand them over to.

Interactive question from Dr Christe

What is the risk in recurring seizures after withdrawal of therapy in patients with JME free of seizures for 2 years?	Response
1 10%	8%
2 40%	27%
3 60%	35%
4 90%	30%

Dr Christe (*Berlin, FDR*): The relapse risk in fact is very high, it is 90%.

Dr Robinson (*Manchester, UK*): Dr Raemakers, was the child who died with the infection neutropenic?

Dr Raemakers (*Aachen, FDR*): No.

Professor Dreifuss: The mortality of the severe myoclonic epilepsies in childhood which incorporate the symptomatic West syndrome is extraordinarily high.

Dr Raemakers: Can I make another comment: this was a child who had very severe fetal embyropathy, with intracranial calcifications, failure to thrive and who was microcephalic. We had to choose between hormone treatment and valproate. We started him on valproate, but we had to increase the dose as the mother was reluctant to give her child hormones. The child tolerated the medication well for about 12 months but then he died at home suddenly within 24 h. The parents did not permit a full autopsy, but allowed us to take a liver biopsy, and the typical changes due to valproate toxicity were not found in this child. The changes we found have been attributed to early prenatal infections. We had no serological evidence as to the cause, but the mother remembers that she had a 'flu' infection in early pregnancy.

Dr Verity (*Cambridge, UK*): It is difficult to accept a recommendation to change to the use of valproate without any longer term follow-up information, as to how these children do subsequently. Secondly, the group that you recommend as being most likely to respond to valproate is relatively small. Could you compare the outcome of valproate as opposed to ACTH or no treatment at all in that group.

Dr Raemakers: One may talk about no treatment, but I do not think anybody in the audience would refuse to treat idiopathic cases. But after valproate treatment, long term effects on cognitive function, mental handicap and epilepsy have still to be defined. The study has been going on since 1984 and we will follow-up these patients, but the short term effects are that these children have normal development following response to valproate; their EEG is improved and in idiopathic cases only one had some non-specific abnormalities left.

Dr Gram *(Dianalund, Denmark):* A question for Walter Christe. You showed that valproate controls seizures in 90–95% of patients with juvenile myoclonic epilepsy. What would you recommend with regard to treatment in the last 5–10% of patients?

Dr Christe: When valproate does not work, I would change to primidone therapy, which has been shown to be highly effective in juvenile myotonic epilepsy. There is a problem with the combination of primidone and valproate, since it may avoid the achievement of therapeutic serum levels and clinical effects.

Dr Gram: Is there any definite proof that primidone is superior to phenobarbitone in this situation?

Dr Christe: No, there is no convincing proof that phenobarbitone is more effective than primidone. One reason for prescribing primidone might be that it is impossible to commit suicide with that drug.

Dr Eeg-Olofsson *(Sweden):* I have two questions to Dr Raemaker about his cases of West syndrome. What plasma levels of valproate did you obtain in your children? I ask that because according to the results from other authors, you obtained the same results as those who gave their children a low dose of 20–30 mg/kg/day. The second question is, which type of ACTH preparation did you use?

Dr Raemakers: The plasma levels were monitored but were sometimes very high; we found peaks above the therapeutic range without toxic symptoms. We monitored plasma levels carefully and also the clinical reaction and biochemical parameters. In most patients the problems were transient thrombocytopenia, often associated with febrile infections. We would then admit the patient and reduce the dose; the platelets would go up and we increased the dose after the infection had subsided. The ACTH we used was the pork derived ACTH. In Germany this was withdrawn from the market and we now use the synthetic synecthen which has enormous side effects. If we use the same amount of international units as the natural product we can reduce the dose of synecthen by a half, but we feel that the synthetically derived ACTH is more potent and produces more hypertension and cardiomyopathy.

Dr Abraham *(London, UK):* This is a question to the paediatricians. When I take over children from our paediatric epileptologist into my epilepsy clinic, I am impressed with the number of patients that you do not treat but just watch. We heard earlier about the unethical nature of not treating. What percentage in your experience do you not treat?

Dr Heggarty *(York, UK):* Of the overall referrals to a general paediatric clinic, with one seizure or perhaps two seizures? I would leave almost all of them untreated.

Dr Abraham: Do you always treat your complex partial seizures?

Dr Heggarty: Yes.

Delegate: I have a question to Dr Raemakers. The design of your study was such that ACTH treatment was put in first after non-response to valproate. Have you considered whether delay of treatment with ACTH effects outcome in that group? Could that be improved if you had a design where a group started with ACTH treatment? The dosage we commonly use in Sweden is much higher than yours, and we do not encounter the mortality rates that you do.

Dr Raemakers: We always start with a small dose of ACTH, three units per kilo, per day. If children do not respond on that dose then we increase it to six and then to nine as the highest dose. We also feel that the synthetically derived ACTH has more side effects, but we do not know why that is. As to the delay in treatment with hormones, if we do not see a response after four weeks we would start ACTH. I know of people who wait for a longer time, and there is a debate about whether the delay in effective treatment impairs outcome and control.

I would not recommend all patients to be treated with valproate. We had such a good response in the idiopathic group that I think a trial of two or three weeks is worthwhile, but we still have to identify which patients in the symptomatic group are likely to respond to valproate and which patients are not. Valproate has other advantages, in that there is more serious toxicity with ACTH and you can treat patients for longer periods of time with valproate. But we have to select patients more carefully, and we need more results of long term outcome to be able to select those patients who would do better on valproate and those who would do better with ACTH.

SESSION III

ADULT EPILEPSY

Chairman: J. Oxley

INTRODUCTION

I am going to exercise the Chairman's prerogative and ask a few questions. I edit a magazine for general practitioners and one of my functions is to pass on relevant expertise to those physicians who are treating patients with epilepsy. In this session we are going to hear about partial seizures so I am going to ask you one or two questions.

1. My treatment of choice for partial seizures in males is: **Response**

   1 Phenytoin   12%
   2 Carbamazepine   78%
   3 Sodium valproate   10%

2. My treatment of choice for partial seizures in females of childbearing potential is: **Response**

   1 Phenytoin   5%
   2 Carbamazepine   85%
   3 Sodium valproate   10%

3. If you could choose only one drug with which to treat partial seizures in all age groups what would you choose?   **Response**

   1 Phenytoin   5%
   2 Carbamazepine   65%
   3 Sodium valproate   30%

4. Sodium valproate is an effective drug against partial seizures?   **Response**

   1 Agree   63%
   2 Disagree   27%
   3 No view   10%

Therapy of partial epilepsy.
A multicentre study* on
monotherapy with sodium valproate

G. Scollo-Lavizzari

Department of Neurology, Basle University Hospital, Basle, Switzerland
*Collaborative Study Group: A. Beaumanoir, B. Blajev, C. Bucher, P. A. Despland, B. Geudelin, S. Hotz, E. Ketz, S. De Meuron, H. Matthis, G. Scollo-Lavizzari, F. Vassella, S. Zagury

INTRODUCTION

Many clinical investigations have established that treatment of primary generalized epilepsy with sodium valproate (VPA) leads to good results. Complete freedom from seizures is found in 72–95% of patients with this type of seizure under VPA monotherapy (1–5).

By contrast, the efficacy of VPA for focal seizures is controversial. Also VPA has been described as inactive in temporal lobe epilepsy (6–7), but it can be shown that, as additional medication it brings about improvement in therapy-resistant focal seizures in 55% of children (8) and in 25–45% of adult patients (9–11).

VPA monotherapy has proven to be as effective as carbamazepine (12) and phenytoin (13–16) in patients with various types of seizures, including partial seizures, who were not previously treated.

Dean and Penry (17) investigated VPA monotherapy in 30 patients with focal seizures, who showed resistance to therapy or side effects under other anticonvulsants. VPA monotherapy was very effective, especially in patients who showed focal attacks with secondary generalization. Twenty-two of 30 patients (73%) became free of seizures. Ten patients had a decrease of the seizure frequency of over 50%; only in eight patients was there minimal or no reduction of the seizure frequency.

In our study the efficacy of VPA was investigated in different forms of partial epilepsy.

METHODS

A multicentric open study was carried out. Altogether 64 patients with different forms of partial epilepsy were investigated. There were 27 men and 37 women. The youngest patient was less than one year old, the oldest was 68 years old. Age was between five and 20 years in 20% of the patients, between 21 and 30 in 44%, and over 30 years in 33%. The average age was 28 years.

The distribution according to the simplified International Classification of Epileptic Seizures (1981) was as follows:
(a) partial seizures with elementary symptoms (without loss of consciousness)
(b) partial seizures with complex symptoms (with initial loss of consciousness)
(c) development in the direction of a secondary generalized seizure (with or without grand mal symptomatology) (loss of consciousness, altered respiration and blood circulation, sometimes with tonic or tonic clonic movements, seizure of more than 3 s duration).

Only patients who had experienced two seizures at least 24 h apart within a period of two months, were taken into the study. The patients were previously untreated or had continued seizures or adverse effects under the previous medication.

Fourth international symposium on sodium valproate and epilepsy, edited by David Chadwick, 1989: Royal Society of Medicine Services International Congress and Symposium No. 152, published by Royal Society of Medicine Services Limited.

Table 1   *Case material (patients with partial seizures)*

Simple partial seizures without generalization	10 = (16%)
Complex partial seizures without generalization	12 = (19%)
Simple and complex seizures without generalization	5 = (7%)
	42%
Simple and complex seizures with generalization	10 = (16%)
Complex partial seizures with generalization	25 = (39%)
Simple and complex seizures with generalization	2 = (3%)
	58%
Total patients	64 = 100%

The administration of medication was carried out gradually until a constant blood level of 50–100 mg/litre (350–700 μmol/l) was attained. Samples were taken approximately 2 h after dosing, the drug being given at supper-time. During the further course the VPA blood levels were no longer systematically measured. VPA was administered in two doses daily. A two-month period of evaluation followed. Seizure frequency, changes of the seizure type, effect on the electroencephalogram (EEG), influence on physiological parameters and clinical tolerability were registered. A similar assessment was carried out after a further four months. With satisfactory results for this observation time of six months, the patient entered an 18-month therapy phase. If the results were not satisfactory (i.e. further fits sometimes occurred but at irregular intervals) further therapeutic measures were undertaken; the patient was withdrawn from the study and was counted as a therapeutic failure. Unacceptable side effects also led to exclusion from further investigation.

Patients with no EEG changes during or between seizures were excluded from the study. Patients with therapy-resistant epilepsy of more than five years' duration were considered unsuitable. Further exclusion criteria were the presence of a cerebral illness with a progressive course (for example, brain tumour), poor compliance, severe psychic disturbances, pregnancy or the desire to have children. The presence of previous significant gastrointestinal tract, heart, liver, blood or kidney disease also were exclusion criteria.

Table 1 shows the distribution of the seizure types of partial epilepsy in our case material: 42% of the patients had partial seizures without generalization, 58% of the patients showed focal seizures with generalization.

RESULTS

The patients (or their relatives) had to note their seizures meticulously in a special diary, comprising time of occurrence, duration of the seizure, type of seizure, marked by special symbols, and in respect of female patients, time relationship to their menstrual cycle. A comparison of these records before and after treatment with VPA showed that VPA monotherapy in 64 patients with focal seizures resulted in freedom from seizures in 39% of the patients. A further 39% showed improvement of the seizure disorder with a decrease of the frequency of more than 50%; 22% of the patients had to be classified as 'not improved'. The success rate with the various seizure forms are given in detail in Table 2.

Table 2   *Results of treatment*

	Controlled	Improved	Unimproved
Simple partial seizures	5 = 50%	4 = 40%	1 = 10%
Complex partial seizures	5 = 42%	3 = 25%	4 = 33%
Simple and complex	2 = 40%	2 = 40%	1 = 20%
Simple with generalization	2 = 20%	4 = 40%	4 = 40%
Complex with generalization	10 = 40%	11 = 44%	4 = 16%
Simple and complex seizures with generalization	1 = 10%	1 = 10%	0 = 0%
Total patients with seizures	25 = 39%	25 = 39%	14 = 22%

Table 3 *Overall results*

	Controlled	Improved	Unimproved
Only partial seizures	12 = 44%	9 = 33%	6 = 22%
controlled + improved	77%		
Partial with generalization	13 = 35%	16 = 43%	8 = 22%
controlled + improved	78%		
All patients	25 = 39%	25 = 39%	14 = 22%

In our case material of 64 patients, 27 exhibited focal seizures without generalization. Thirty-seven patients (58%) had focal seizures with generalization. Focal attacks without generalization showed a better success rate (44% free of seizures, 33% improved) than focal attacks with generalization (35% free of seizures, 43% improved). The EEGs in our patients demonstrated no correlation between EEG abnormalities and the duration of improvement or the degree of seizure control. Dean and Penry (17) noted the same results.

Side-effects of VPA occurred in 14 (22%) of 65 patients. They led only in one case to interruption of therapy (due to massive weight gain). Seven patients showed mild weight gain, of whom one patient had epigastric pain in addition. Three patients reported tiredness, which was accompanied by epigastric pain in one patient. Three patients had tiredness and mild weight gain.

DISCUSSION

VPA monotherapy was previously employed mainly in generalized epilepsies, especially in absence epilepsy. However, VPA shows, in our experience, good activity in focal epilepsies. Other authors also came to this conclusion (3,15–19).

Dean and Penry (17) found in 22 of 30 (73%) patients with focal seizures freedom from seizures or improvement with VPA monotherapy. Interestingly, 15 of 17 patients with secondarily generalized epilepsy were found in this group. They expressed the idea that focal seizures with secondary generalization responded better to VPA monotherapy than focal seizures without secondary generalization.

In this respect we obtained different results. Fifty of 64 (78%) patients, (with and without secondary generalization) were free from seizures or showed a decrease of seizure frequency of over 50%. In this case material this occurred in 77% of patients with exclusively focal seizures and in 78% of patients with focal seizures with secondary generalization (Table 3). Thus no difference was seen between the focal epilepsies without generalization and the focal epilepsies with secondary generalization.

Callaghan *et al*. (16) found that anticonvulsants (carbamazepine, VPA, phenobarbitone) are less successful with focal attacks (44% of 79 patients seizure-free) than with primary generalized seizures (59% of 102 patients seizure-free). The response of various seizure forms was comparable under monotherapy with carbamazepine, VPA and phenobarbitone.

The known advantages of VPA speak for its choice in the treatment of focal seizures.

VPA demonstrates good tolerability. To be emphasized is—in contrast to the other anticonvulsants—its lack of or only minor impairment of cognitive function. VPA exhibits a wide therapeutic margin which considerably simplifies the adjustment of the medication. The retard tablets permit a simple dosage scheme. Further it should be mentioned that VPA does not lead to induction of liver enzymes; the effect of ovulation inhibitors and many other medications is therefore not impaired.

REFERENCES

(1) Penry JK, Dean JC. Valproate monotherapy in partial seizures. *Am J Med* 1988; **84** (Suppl 1A): 14–16.
(2) Bourgeois B, Beaumanoir A, Blajev B, *et al*. Monotherapy with valproate in primary generalized epilepsies. *Epilepsia* 1987; **28** (Suppl 2): 8–11.
(3) Covanis A, Gupta AK, Jeavons PM. Sodium valproate: monotherapy and polytherapy. *Epilepsia* 1982; **23**: 693–720.

(4) Dulac O, Steru D, Rey E, Arthuis M. Monotherapie par le valproate de sodium dans les epilepsies de l'enfant. *Arch Fr Pediatr* 1982; **39**: 347–52.

(5) Feuerstein J. A long-term study of monotherapy with sodium valproate in primary generalized epilepsy: *Br J Clin Pract* 1983; **27** (Suppl): 17–23.

(6) Haigh D, Forsythe WJ. The treatment of childhood epilepsy with sodium valproate. In: Legg NS, ed. *Clinical and pharmacological aspects of sodium valproate (Epilim) in the treatment of epilepsy.* Tunbridge Wells: MCS Consultants, 1976: 52–5.

(7) Heathfield K, Dunlop D, Karanjia P, Retras S. The long-term results of treating thirty-six patients with intractable epilepsy with sodium valproate (Epilim). In: Legg NS, ed. *Clinical and pharmacological aspects of sodium valproate (Epilim) in the treatment of epilepsy.* Tunbridge Wells: MCS Consultants, 1976: 165–70.

(8) Sherard ES Jr, Steiman GS, Couri D. Treatment of childhood epilepsy with valproic acid: results of the first 100 patients in a 6-month trial. *Neurology* 1980; **30**: 31–55.

(9) Simon D, Penry JK. Sodium di-N-propylacetate (DPA) in the treatment of epilepsy. A review. *Epilepsia* 1975; **16**: 549–73.

(10) Pinder RM, Brogden RN, Speight TM, Avery GS. Sodium valproate: a review of its pharmacological properties and therapeutic efficacy in epilepsy. *Drugs* 1977; **13**: 81–123.

(11) Mattson RH, Cramer JA, Williamson PD, Novelly RA. Valproic acid in epilepsy: clinical and pharmacological effects. *Ann Neurol* 1978; **3**: 20–5.

(12) Shakir RA. Sodium valproate, phenytoin and carbamazepine as sole anticonvulsants. In: Parsonage MJ, Caldwell ADS, eds. *The place of sodium valproate in the treatment of epilepsy.* RSM International Congress and Symposium Series No. 30. London: Royal Society of Medicine, 1980: 7–15.

(13) Shakir RA, Johnson RH, Lambie DG, Melville ID, Nanda RN. Comparison of sodium valproate and phenytoin as single drug treatment in epilepsy. *Epilepsia* 1981; **22**: 27–33.

(14) Turnbull DM, Rawlins MD, Weightman D, Chadwick DW. A comparison of phenytoin and valproate in previously untreated adult epileptic patients. *J Neurol Neurosurg Psych* 1982; **45**: 55–9.

(15) Loiseau P. Rational use of valproate: indications and drug regimen in epilepsy. *Epilepsia* 1984; **25** (Suppl 1): 65–72.

(16) Callaghan N, Kenny RA, O'Neill B, Crowley M, Goggin T. A prospective study between carbamazepine, phenytoin and sodium valproate as monotherapy in previously untreated and recently diagnosed patients with epilepsy. *J Neurol Neurosurg Psych* 1985; **48**: 639–44.

(17) Dean JC, Penry JK. Valproate monotherapy in 30 patients with partial seizures. *Epilepsia* 1988; **29**: 140–4.

(18) Henriksen O, Johannessen SI. Clinical and pharmacokinetic observations on sodium valproate—a 5-year follow-up study in 100 children with epilepsy. *Acta Neurol Scand* 1982; **65**: 504–23.

(19) Porter RJ. Clinical efficacy and use of antiepileptic drugs. In: Woodbury DM, Penry JK, Pippenger CE, eds. *Antiepileptic drugs.* New York: Raven Press, 1982: 167–75.

The Adult EPITEG trial: A comparative multicentre clinical trial of sodium valproate and carbamazepine in adult onset epilepsy

Part 1: Description of trial and demographic data

Presented on behalf of the Participants by
N. E. F. Cartlidge

Department of Neurology, Royal Victoria Infirmary, Newcastle upon Tyne, UK

INTRODUCTION

Over the last 10 years the approach towards anticonvulsant therapy has changed dramatically (1). In particular, it has now become apparent that a single drug is capable of controlling as many as three-quarters of adult outpatients with epilepsy (2). Nevertheless, there have been few studies on single anticonvulsants involving previously untreated patients. Furthermore, there have been few comparative trials of anticonvulsants to determine if one particular drug produces better control of a seizure or has better short-term tolerance (3–6).

In the light of this it was decided in 1982 to undertake a prospective study to compare the anticonvulsants sodium valproate and carbamazepine in adult onset epilepsy. Twenty-two out patient clinics in the United Kingdom participated in the study (footnote) and by 1987 300 patients had been included.

This paper presents the objectives and design of the study and such demographic data as is available. A subsequent paper deals with adverse effects noted in the trial patients.

OBJECTIVES

The aims of the study were to compare the efficacy and tolerance of sodium valproate and carbamazepine in the treatment of generalized and partial adult epilepsy. It was also proposed to examine the suggested therapeutic range for sodium valproate when administered as monotherapy and to determine if a relationship exists between dose, serum level and seizure control in this group of patients.

Participants:
Dr D. Bates, Royal Victoria Infirmary, Newcastle; Dr G. Boddie, North Staffordshire General Infirmary, Stoke; Dr N. Cartlidge, Royal Victoria Infirmary, Newcastle; Dr C. Clarke, St. Bartholomew's Hospital, London; Dr P. Cleland, District General Hospital, Sunderland; Dr R. Corston, New Cross Hospital, Wolverhampton; Dr R. Cull, Royal Infirmary, Edinburgh; Dr W. Cumming, Withington Hospital, Manchester; Dr D. Davidson, Ninewells Hospital, Dundee; Dr G. Ellis, General Hospital, Poole; Dr A. Gupta, Dudley Road Hospital, Birmingham; Dr M. Harrison, Middlesex Hospital, London; Dr G. Harwood, Greenwich District Hospital; Dr D Jefferson, Derbyshire Royal Infirmary, Derby; Dr C. Kennard, London Hospital, London; Dr L. Loizou, Pinderfields General Hospital, Wakefield; Dr P. Millac, Royal Infirmary, Leicester; Dr P. Newman, District General Hospital, Middlesbrough; Dr V. Patterson, Royal Victoria Hospital, Belfast; Prof. A. Richens (Principal Investigator), University Hospital of Wales, Cardiff; Dr D. Shepherd, North Manchester General Hospital, Manchester; Dr J. Wilson, Royal Free Hospital, London.

Fourth international symposium on sodium valproate and epilepsy, edited by David Chadwick, 1989: Royal Society of Medicine Services International Congress and Symposium No. 152, published by Royal Society of Medicine Services Limited.

DESIGN

The study was planned to be a randomized open controlled comparative trial of sodium valproate and carbamazepine in the treatment of adults presenting with epilepsy. Inclusion criteria were as follows:
(a) Male and female patients over the age of 16.
(b) Patients with newly diagnosed epilepsy requiring anticonvulsant medication or patients with recurrence of seizures after withdrawal of anti-convulsant medication: such patients must not have received anticonvulsant medication in the previous six months.
(c) At least two generalized tonic-clonic or partial seizures with or without generalization in the previous six months; diagnosis in accordance with international classification on the basis of reliable historic evidence from the patient or a witness.
Exclusion criteria including the following:
(a) Patients with an accompanying disorder other than epilepsy.
(b) Patients with abnormal liver function tests or blood dyscrasias.
(c) Patients who have previously reacted adversely to sodium valproate or carbamazepine.
(d) Patients who were pregnant or lactating or who were positively planning to become pregnant during the course of the study.
(e) Patients with absences or myoclonic jerks alone.
Informed consent was obtained from all patients.

TREATMENT ALLOCATION

Patients were randomized on entry to either sodium valproate or carbamazepine by a computerized minimization programme stratified in accordance with age, sex, seizure type and centre. Randomization was organized through the medical department at Sanofi UK Limited by Dr Derrick Easter.
   Age stratification was as follows:
(a) 16–25 years
(b) 26–65 years
(c) above 65 years
   Stratification by seizure type was as follows:
(a) generalized seizures
(b) complex partial seizures without generalization
(c) complex partial seizures with generalization
(d) simple partial seizures without generalization
(e) simple partial seizures with generalization

DOSAGE

Medication for both drugs was taken twice daily, in the morning and the evening.

CARBAMAZEPINE

Patients began therapy at 100 mg twice a day, increasing by the second week to 200 mg twice a day. Further increases were made at a rate of 200 mg per day at fortnightly intervals until control of seizures had been achieved with serum levels in the therapeutic range or until signs of toxicity ensued.

SODIUM VALPROATE

Patients began therapy at 200 mg twice a day and the dose was increased at a rate of 200 mg twice a day at weekly intervals until control of seizures with blood levels within the therapeutic range had been achieved or toxic symptoms ensued.

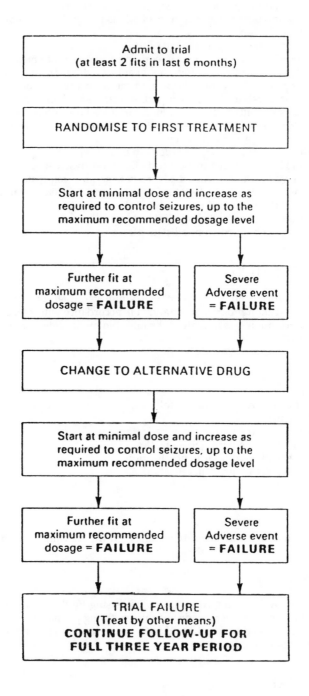

Figure 1 *Summary of trial procedures.*

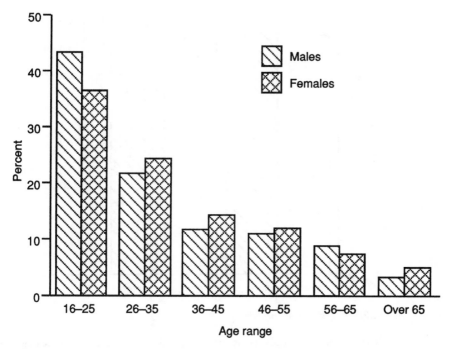

Figure 2 *Age ranges for patients in the trial.*

INVESTIGATIONS

Routine haematology and liver function tests were carried out on entry to the trial and at three months and then at the discretion of the clinician. Plasma drug levels were determined at each visit. Electroencephalograms (EEGs) were carried out on entry to the trial and then at the discretion of the clinician. Patients were followed at three monthly intervals for the first two years following entry to the trial and thereafter at six monthly intervals or at the discretion of the clinician.

Seizure control was assessed by the patient being asked to keep a seizure diary for the duration of the study.

END POINTS

The end points for the trial were as follows:
(a) *Poor control* Patients who continued to have seizures with a serum drug level in the upper part of the therapeutic range were regarded as treatment failures.
(b) *Severe adverse events* Patients were classed as treatment failures if they had side effects of sufficient severity to warrant discontinuation of their current treatment.

TREATMENT FAILURES

Patients who were regarded as treatment failures on one drug were then switched to the alternative anticonvulsant and followed up for the remainder of the three-year trial period.

PATIENT POPULATION

Three hundred patients have been included in the study from twenty-three neurological centres in the United Kingdom. With this number of patients (150 per group, 300 total) the trial is capable of detecting an overall difference in seizure recurrence rate of 15–20% between

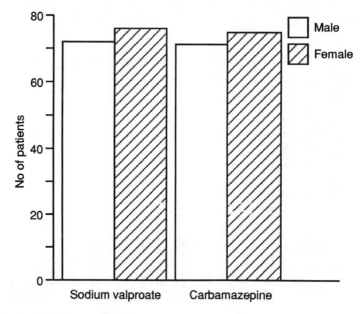

Figure 3 *Adult EPITEG trial: sex distribution*

treatments with a type I error rate (false positives) of 5% and a type II error rate (false negatives) of 0.2 (80% power). The age and sex distribution of the patients in the study are summarized in Figs. 2 and 3. There were no differences in these parameters. Age and sex distribution between patients receiving sodium valproate and carbamazepine were similar (Fig. 3).

A qualitative assessment was made in all patients of intellectual status and this appeared to be similar in the two treatment groups (Fig. 4). Similarly, other baseline variables did not significantly differ between the two groups (Table 2).

The investigators' classification of seizure type on entry to the study is presented in Fig. 5. Half of the patients were thought to have primary generalized seizures and the seizure type distribution did not differ between the two treatment groups. Figure 6 presents the results of the EEGs performed at entry to the study and reported to the clinician by the EEG department concerned. The EEGs showed similar findings in both treatment groups (Fig. 6).

Table 3 presents a comparison of the investigators' assessment of seizure type at entry with the EEG. As might be expected, a significant number of patients who were thought clinically to have primary generalized epilepsy were found on EEG to have focal abnormalities.

As many as possible of the EEGs were sent to an independent assessor and thus far records from 119 patients have been examined. Table 4 compared the investigators' and the independent assessors' classification of the seizure type.

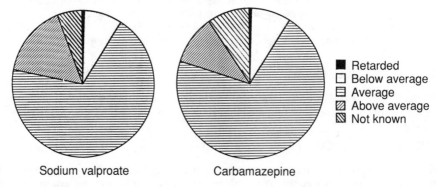

Figure 4 *Adult EPITEG trial: IQ distribution.*

Table 2 *EPITEG trial: other baseline variables history*

	Sodium valproate	Carbamazepine	Total
Birth injury	3	4	7
Birth anoxia	1	2	3
Febrile convulsions	6	2	8
Head injury	18	10	28
Family history	1	5	6
Previous history	4	3	7
Childhood epilepsy	3	4	7
Other illness	7	5	12
No known history	98	102	200
No data	8	14	22
Total	149	151	300

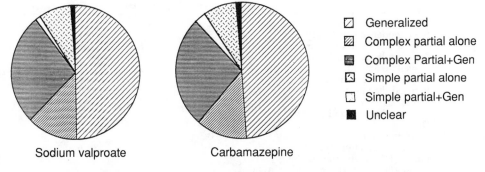

Generalized
Complex partial alone
Complex Partial+Gen
Simple partial alone
Simple partial+Gen
Unclear

Sodium valproate   Carbamazepine

Figure 5 *Adult EPITEG trial: Seizure classification at entry (A) investigators' classification.*

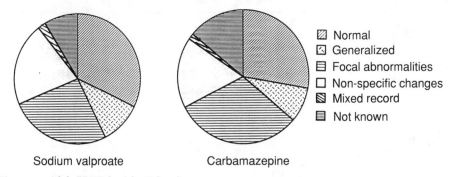

Normal
Generalized
Focal abnormalities
Non-specific changes
Mixed record
Not known

Sodium valproate   Carbamazepine

Figure 6 *Adult EPITEG trial: EEG coding on entry.*

Table 3 *EPITEG trial: Seizure classification and EEG at entry*

EEG abnormalities

Seizure type at entry	Normal	Gen	Focal S/W	Non-spec	Mixed	Not known	Total
Primary generalized	50	20	24	20	2	22	148
Complex partial	7	1	18	10	1	1	38
Comp PTL+2[ary] gen	25	7	24	14	2	8	80
Simple partial	1	0	4	1	0	0	6
Simple PTL+2[ary] gen	5	1	14	2	0	2	24
Unclear	2	0	1	0	0	1	4
Total	90	29	85	57	5	34	300

Table 4   *Adult EPITEG trial: Independent EEG assessments*

		Epileptiform records					
Investigators' assessment	Normal record	Prim gen	Sec gen	PTL	Unclass only	N/S	Total
Primary gen	29	4	3	9	4	4	52
Complex PTL	6	0	0	8	0	2	17
Complex PTL+gen	9	0	0	12	4	4	29
Simple PTL	2	0	0	1	0	1	4
SP+gen	7	0	0	2	6	0	15
Unclear	1	0	0	0	1	0	2
Total	54	4	3	32	15	11	119

Excludes one patient with ambulatory monitoring only and 7 patients whose EEG records are still to be assessed

Table 5   *Adult EPITEG trial: Withdrawal analysis*

	No. of patients		
	Sodium valproate	Carbamazepine	All
No data since entry	2	1	3
No attendance since entry	3	4	7
No attendance in first 6 months	2	6	8
No attendance after 6 months	2	1	3
Moved/emigrated	1	2	3
Uncooperative patients	4	2	6
Refused diagnosis	1	0	1
Wrong diagnosis	0	1	1
Tumour diagnosed after entry	2	1	3
Died	2	0	2
Entry violation	0	1	1
No follow up after 2 years	3	3	6
Lost to follow up after reaching endpoint (poor control and/or ADR) on first drug	4	4	8
Total	26	26	52

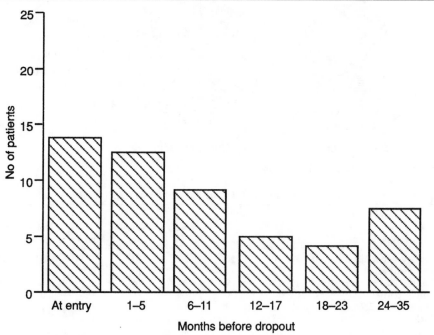

Figure 7   *Time of drop out.*

Overall 52 patients have been lost or withdrawn from the study (Table 5) and drop-out has occurred at variable times following randomization (Fig. 7).

SUMMARY

The results from this study when available should provide important information regarding the efficacy and short-term side-effects of the anticonvulsant drugs sodium valproate and carbamazepine in adult onset epilepsy. Analysis of efficacy will become available within the next year.

ACKNOWLEDGMENTS

Three other contributors to this study deserve mention—Dr Colin Binnie who provided the independent EEG analysis, Dr Tony Johnson who advised on the analysis of the data and Dr Derrick Easter from Sanofi UK Ltd who coordinated the whole project.

REFERENCES

(1) Shorvon SD, Birdwood GFB. *Rational approaches to anti-convulsant drug therapy*. Bern, Stuttgart, Vienna: Hans Huber, 1984.
(2) Shorvon SD. Problems in anti-convulsant trial design. In: Clifford-Rose F, ed. *Research progress in epilepsy*. London: Pitman International, 1983: 384–401.
(3) Shakir R, Johnson R, Lambie D, Melville I, Nanda R. Comparison of sodium valproate and phenytoin as single drug treatment in epilepsy. *Epilepsia* 1981; **22**: 27–33.
(4) Hakkarainen H. Carbamazepine and phenytoin as monotherapy or in combination in the treatment of adult epilepsy. *13th epilepsy international symposium, Kyoto, Japan*. New York: Raven Press, 1981: 140 [Abstract].
(5) Turnbull D, Rawlins M, Weightman D, Chadwick D. A comparison of phenytoin and valproate in previously untreated adult epileptic patients. *J Neurol Neurosurg Psych* 1982; **45**: 55–9.
(6) Shorvon SD, Reynolds EH. Early prognosis of epilepsy. *Br Med J* 1982; **285**: 1699–701.

The Adult EPITEG trial: A comparative multicentre clinical trial of sodium valproate and carbamazepine in adult onset epilepsy

Part 2: Adverse effects

Presented on behalf of the Participants by

D. L. W. Davidson

Section of Neurology, Department of Medicine, Ninewells Hospital and Medical School, Dundee, UK

INTRODUCTION

The selection of an anticonvulsant drug depends on the efficacy in control of seizures, and on the frequency and severity of adverse reactions. This study reports the adverse events during treatment with sodium valproate (VPA) or with carbamazepine (CBZ) in a multicentre trial carried out by clinicians* in 22 outpatient clinics in the UK and Northern Ireland. Three hundred adult patients with newly-diagnosed primary generalized or partial epilepsy (with or without generalization) were randomized to either VPA or CBZ by a computerized stratified minimization programme based on age, sex and seizure (see Part 1 for details). Patients who fail on the first treatment (poor seizure control and/or severe adverse events) are crossed over to the alternative treatment. All patients are being followed up for three years after entry.

Adverse event reports were received from all the clinicians participating in this multicentre trial, and this interim review is based on all reports received by the end of January 1989 for treatment on the first drug only, corresponding to 3350 patient months on sodium valproate treatment and 2952 patient months on carbamazepine treatment.

METHODS

Patients were randomized to treatment with VPA (Epilim® enteric-coated tablets) or to CBZ, as described in Part 1. The recommended starting regimens were as follows: VPA 200 mg b.d., increasing by 200 mg/day at weekly intervals until control of the seizures or adverse effects; CBZ 100 mg b.d. for the first week, 200 mg b.d. for the second week, then increasing by 200 mg/day at two-weekly intervals until seizures were controlled or adverse effects occurred.

---

*Participants

Dr D. Bates, Royal Victoria Infirmary, Newcastle; Dr G. Boddie, North Staffordshire General Hospital, Stoke; Dr N. Cartlidge, Royal Victoria Infirmary, Newcastle; Dr C. Clarke, St Bartholomew's Hospital, London; Dr P. Cleland, District General Hospital, Sunderland; Dr R. Corston, New Cross Hospital, Wolverhampton; Dr R. Cull, Royal Infirmary, Edinburgh; Dr W. Cumming, Withington Hospital, Manchester; Dr D. Davidson, Ninewells Hospital, Dundee; Dr G. Ellis, General Hospital, Poole; Dr A. Gupta, Dudley Road Hospital, Birmingham; Dr M. Harrison, Middlesex Hospital, London; Dr G. Harwood, Greenwich District Hospital, London; Dr D. Jefferson, Derbyshire Royal Infirmary, Derby; Dr C. Kennard, London Hospital, London; Dr L. Loizou, Pinderfields General Hospital, Wakefield; Dr P. Millac, Royal Infirmary, Leicester; Dr P. Newman, District General Hospital, Middlesbrough; Dr V. Patterson, Royal Victoria Hospital, Belfast; Professor A. Richens (Principal Investigator), University Hospital of Wales, Cardiff; Dr D. Shepherd, North Manchester General Hospital, Manchester; Dr J. Wilson, Royal Free Hospital, London.

Fourth international symposium on sodium valproate and epilepsy, edited by David Chadwick, 1989: Royal Society of Medicine Services International Congress and Symposium No. 152, published by Royal Society of Medicine Services Limited.

Table 1 *Total numbers of patients with adverse drug reactions*

	Valproate	Carbamazepine
Number of patients	149	151
Number reporting adverse events	69	76
Percentage with adverse event	46%	50%
Percentage of adverse events occurring in first three months	42%	62%

Table 2 *Numbers of adverse events reports*

Number of adverse events reported	Valproate		Carbamazepine	
Neurological				
Fatigue	9	(6%)	12	(8%)
Somnolence	9	(6%)	17	(11%)
Dizziness	3	(2%)	10	(7%)
Migraine/headache	3	(2%)	9	(6%)
Ataxia/incoordination	1	(1%)	3	(2%)
Tremor	7	(5%)	2	(1%)
Amnesia	6		2	
Depression	2		4	
Malaise	1		3	
Thinking abnormal	2		0	
Impaired concentration	2		0	
Euphoria	0		1	
Anxiety	0		1	
Dysphasia/speech disorder	2		2	
Emotional lability	0		1	
Nystagmus	1		0	
Insomnia	0		1	
Extrapyramidal disorder	1		0	
Behavioural change	1		1	
Impotence	0		1	
Dermatological				
Rash	2	(1%)	19	(13%)
Alopecia	4		1	
Pruritis	1		1	
Gastroinestinal				
Abdominal pain	1		2	
Abnormal hepatic function	1		2	
Nausea, vomiting, dyspepsia	8	(5%)	12	(8%)
Constipation	0		1	
Diarrhoea	1		0	
Endocrine/metabolic				
Weight gain	20	(13%)	2	(1%)
Appetite gain	4		0	
Decreased appetite	0		1	
Thirst/polyuria	1		3	
Menstrual disorder	0		1	
Decreased libido	0		1	
Haematological				
Anaemia	1		0	
Leucopenia	0		1	
Thrombocytopenia	1		1	
Cardiorespiratory				
Cardiac failure/dyspnoea	2		0	
Syncope/hypotension	0		3	
Flushing	0		1	
Miscellaneous				
Pregnancy	0		5	
Arthralgia/arthritis	0		2	
Fever/viral infection	1		2	
Respiratory tract infection	2		1	
Furunculosis	1		0	
Total	101		132	

Each patient was followed up in the outpatient clinic, with visits 1, 3, 6, 9, 12, 18, 24 and 36 months after entry wherever possible. Patients who failed on both trial drugs were also followed up for the full three-year trial period, on any alternative treatment decided by the individual Investigator.

Blood samples were taken for full blood count and liver function tests before entry, at three months, and subsequently if required clinically.

Any adverse events reported by the patient were recorded at each visit as were the current drug dose and plasma drug level (if available). The adverse events were defined according to the terminology of the WHO classification for International Monitoring of Adverse Reaction to Drugs. For completeness, all reported adverse events have been included in this review, whether or not the event was attributable to the trial drug or other possible cause.

RESULTS

Adverse events reported

The numbers of patients with adverse events on the first drug are shown in Table 1, and the total numbers of adverse events are shown in Table 2. The adverse events that were severe enough to require anticonvulsant withdrawal are shown in Table 3. Many patients reported more than one adverse event. The same adverse events reported by the patient at repeat visits were only included once in this analysis.

The overall prevalence was similar in the two groups with 46% reporting adverse events on VPA and 50% on CBZ. 62% of adverse events occurred in the first three months of treatment with CBZ and 42% of adverse events occurred in the initial three months of treatment with VPA.

Table 3 *Numbers withdrawn because of ADRs*

	Valproate		Carbamazepine	
Number of patients				
Number of patients withdrawn	14	(9%)	23	(15%)
Number reporting more than one adverse event at withdrawal	4		9	
Mean time of withdrawal (months)	11.1		3.2	
Adverse events reported in patients withdrawing from treatment				
Rash	1		14	(9%)
Tiredness/malaise/fatigue	4		4	
Nausea/vomiting	2		3	
Tremor	4		0	
Dizzy/ataxia/blurred vision	1		3	
Weight gain	3		0	
Abnormal hepatic function	1		1	
Depression	0		2	
Headache	0		2	
Somnolence	0		2	
Cardiac failure	1		0	
Personality change	1		0	
Nervousness	1		0	
Diarrhoea	1		0	
Alopecia	1		0	
Abdominal pain	1		0	
Flatulence	1		0	
Insomnia	0		1	
Fever/flu-like symptoms	0		1	
Arthralgia	0		1	
Amnesia	0		1	
Appetite increase	0		1	
Total	24		35	

There were more neurological adverse events on CBZ (70) than on VPA (48). The differentiation between fatigue, malaise, somnolence, impaired concentration or thinking, abnormal behaviour and depression was difficult, and detailed studies of cognitive function were not performed. Many of the central effects of CBZ were mild and transient. Dizziness was relatively common on CBZ treatment (7%) while tremor was more frequent with VPA treatment (5%) than with CBZ.

The commonest non-neurological adverse event was weight gain in 20 patients (13%) on treatment with VPA but only two treated with CBZ. Rashes were reported in 19 patients (13%) on CBZ but only two on VPA. Both treatment groups had a similar prevalence of nausea, vomiting or dyspepsia (7% on VPA, 8% on CBZ). One interesting observation was that five patients on CBZ became pregnant (not always intentionally) during the trial period. Four patients developed alopecia on VPA, and one reported curly hair on regrowth. Other adverse events were less frequently reported.

Adverse events causing anticonvulsant withdrawal

More patients withdrew from CBZ than from VPA within the first three months of treatment, as shown in the frequency histogram (Fig. 1). The larger number of withdrawals on CBZ (23) compared to VPA (14) was predominantly due to rashes (14 on CBZ, one on VPA). Dizziness, ataxia and blurred vision were additional vauses of early withdrawal of CBZ.

Weight gain, tremor, nervousness or personality change warranting drug withdrawal were reported as later adverse effects on VPA. One patient on VPA was withdrawn because of abnormal liver function after 16 months' treatment, but at the time this patient also had cardiac failure, Parkinsonism and exacerbation of a pre-existing tremor. One patient withdrew with a platelet count of $103 \times 10^9/l$ but had been taking a large dose of VPA at 3 g/day.

Haematology and biochemistry

Haematology results are summarized in Table 4. There was a small decrease in the white cell count on treatment with CBZ which was statistically but not clinically significant. The numbers of patients with abnormally high or low results either at entry or during follow-up are also shown in Table 4. The frequency distributions of white cell counts and serum glutamic-pyruvate transaminase (SGPT) at entry and at three months are shown in Figs 2 and 3. Biochemistry results are summarized in Table 5. There were no significant changes in the concentrations of total serum proteins, albumen, and bilirubin during treatment.

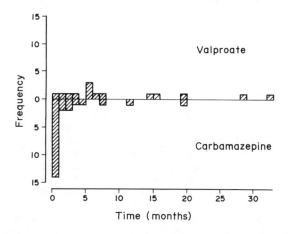

Figure 1 *The time of onset of adverse events on treatment with valproate and carbamazepine.*

Table 4 *Haematology results*

	Valproate	Carbamazepine
Haemoglobin		
Normal range 12.5–17.5 g/dl		
Hb at entry±SD	14.4±1.4	14.3±1.4
HB at review±SD	14.1±1.0	14.1±0.7
n	108	95
Numbers with abnormal results		
At entry: high	1	0
low	3	3
Treatment: low at review	5	4
White blood cell count		
Normal range 3.5–10.5×10⁹/l		
WBC at entry±SD	7.2±2.1	7.5±2.2
WBC at review±SD	6.8±1.8	6.7±1.9
n	108	95
Numbers with abnormal results		
High: at entry	6	11
at review	3	4
Low: at entry	2	1
at review	2	0
Platelet count		
Normal range 150–400×10⁹/l		
Plat at entry±SD	266±65	270±50
Plat at review±SD	263±61	274±50
n	99	88
Numbers with abnormal results		
High: at entry	4	6
at review	6	5
Low: at entry	1	1
at review	5	2

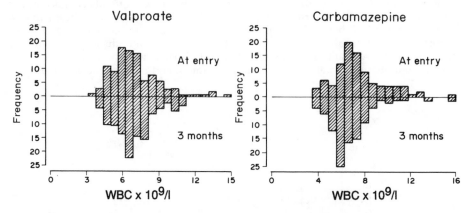

Figure 2 *The white cell counts at entry and at 3 months on valproate and carbamazepine.*

Interpretation of serum liver enzyme results is more difficult, since the normal ranges for alkaline phosphatase, SGPT, and serum glutamic-oxaloacetic transaminase (SGOT) varied in several laboratories. As the main concern has been to establish whether clinically significant changes occur the mean activities of alkaline phosphatase, SGOT and SGPT are shown before and on treatment. There were no significant changes. The number of patients with SGOT levels above their reference range declined by three on CBZ and was unchanged on VPA. The total number of patients with raised alkaline phosphatase and SGOT fell at review and there was a small increase from nine to 11 in the number of patients with high SGPT levels. The largest increases in serum enzyme activities were in two patients

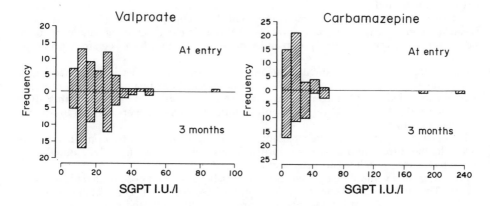

Figure 3 *SGPT at entry and at 3 months on valproate and carbamazepine.*

Table 5 *Liver function tests*

	Valproate	Carbamazepine
Alkaline phosphatase		
Normal levels vary, 100–130 IU/l		
AP at entry ± SD	97.2 ± 63.6	104.4 ± 73.1
AP at review ± SD	93.8 ± 25.9	112.3 ± 32.4
n	107	93
Numbers with abnormal results		
High: at entry	15	17
at review	11	15
normal→high	7	6
SGOT		
Upper limits vary, < 30–45 IU/l		
SGOT at entry ± SD	21.0 ± 8.7	29.0 ± 55.2
SGOT at review ± SD	19.5 ± 8.4	20.3 ± 55.3
n	69	60
Numbers with abnormal results		
High: at entry	3	7
at review	3	3
normal→high	2	1
SGPT		
Upper limits vary, 25–45 IU/l		
SGPT at entry ± SD	22 ± 13	19 ± 11
SGPT at review ± SD	20 ± 10	29 ± 40
n	57	44
Numbers with abnormal results		
High: at entry	6	9
at review	3	11
normal→high	1	7

treated with CBZ in whom the SGPT increased from 36 and 19 at entry to 191 and 231 IU/l at three months. One of these patients was reported to have nausea, vomiting and pharyngitis and was changed to VPA. The other patient had no adverse events reported.

DISCUSSION

In this trial, response to a general question (e.g. 'Has the treatment affected you in any way?') was used to gather information on adverse events. Specific questions or a structured questionnaire (1) would have given a higher response rate, but without a control group of placebo-treated patients, an unacceptably high rate of non-drug related effects could have been expected.

The overall prevalence of adverse events with VPA (46%) and CBZ (50%) in this trial is similar to previous reports and reviews (2–7). Although about half of the patients reported side-effects there was no control group and some symptoms may have been from unrelated events.

Patients treated with VPA exhibited predominantly toxic effects reflecting pharmacological actions other than the drug's desired therapeutic effect. Weight gain, the extent of which was not recorded, was the commonest adverse event with VPA. Although this effect occurred in 20 patients (13%) on VPA, only in four cases was it severe enough to warrant treatment change.

Tremor was reported by seven patients on VPA (5%) but only two on CBZ. Where available, the corresponding serum valproate levels were also high (506–1279 μmol/l), and this effect is clearly related to drug levels.

Patients treated with CBZ exhibited both toxic reactions and non-dose-related idiosyncratic effects. The latter occurred early in treatment. Rashes occurred in 19 (13%) of patients on CBZ which is somewhat higher than the range of 5–10% reported elsewhere.

The prevalence of gastrointestinal adverse events was similar on the two drugs and to previous reports (6,7). There were no reports of pancreatitis on either drug.

The sedative side-effects, dizziness, ataxia and/or inco-ordination occurred earlier in the CBZ treated group than with VPA treatment.

The pregnancies in five patients treated with CBZ may have been a consequence of enhanced metabolism and hence reduced effectiveness of oral contraceptives by CBZ. This emphasizes the need for oral contraceptive doses to be increased when given in combination with CBZ.

The most important adverse events were those causing anticonvulsant withdrawal. Fourteen patients withdrew from CBZ treatment because of rashes and three because of dizziness, ataxia or blurred vision. Other causes with withdrawal of CBZ therapy were less frequent.

The reasons for withdrawal of VPA were diverse, most commonly non-neurological adverse effects such as rash, hepatic dysfunction, nausea, vomiting, weight gain, cardiac failure and alopecia. Several adverse events occurred in combination in the same patients. These adverse events resolved on withdrawal of drug treatment. Cardiac failure is not a previously reported adverse event with VPA and because it occurred as part of a more complex medical problem the relationship of cardiac failure to VPA is very doubtful.

There were very few changes in haematology or biochemistry during treatment and these findings do not suggest that routine monitoring of full blood counts and liver function tests is useful. The slight reduction in white cell count on CBZ was not clinically significant. Similarly, there were no overall changes in platelet counts on either drug. One patient developed thrombocytopenia (103×10^9/l platelets) on a large dose of VPA at 3 g/day, in keeping with a dose-related effect. The only evidence for a clinical bleeding problem was in one patient who became anaemic with a bleeding ulcer at one month, in which the rôle of VPA in this event, if any, is unclear. Abnormalities of platelet aggregation (8) and of fibrinogen concentrations (9) have been reported elsewhere, but these parameters were not measured in this study.

The adverse event profiles for VPA and CBZ reported here are similar to those reported elsewhere. The study is sufficiently large to provide useful information on the prevalence of adverse effects when treating adult patients with monotherapy with VPA or CBZ in a neurological outpatient clinic.

REFERENCES

(1) Harranz JL, Arteaga R, Armijo JA. Side effects of sodium valproate in monotherapy controlled by plasma levels: A study in 88 patients. *Epilepsia* 1982; **23**: 203–14.

(2) Davidson DLW. A review of the side-effects of sodium valproate. In *Third International Symposium on Sodium Valproate. Br J Clin Pract* 1983; **27** (Suppl): 79–85.

(3) Dreifuss FE, Langer DH. Side effects of valproate. *Am J Med* 1988; **84** (Suppl 1A): 34–41.
(4) Harranz JL, Armijo JA, Arteaga R. Clinical side effects of phenobarbital, primidone, phenytoin, carbamazepine and valproate during monotherapy in children. *Epilepsia* 1988; **29**: 794–804.
(5) Collaborative Group for Epidemiology of Epilepsy. *Epilepsia* 1988; **29**: 787–93.
(6) Covanis A, Gupta AK, Jeavons PM. Sodium valproate: Monotherapy and polytherapy. *Epilepsia* 1982; **23**: 693–720.
(7) Collaborative Study Group. Monotherapy with valproate in primary generalised epilepsies. *Epilepsia* 1987; **28** (Suppl 2): S8–11.
(8) Richardson SGN, Fletcher DJ, Jeavons PM. Sodium valproate and platelet function. *Br Med J* 1976; **1**: 221–2.
(9) Dale BM, Purdie GH, Rischbith RH. Fibrinogen depletion with sodium valproate. *Lancet* 1978; **i**: 316–7.

Discussion after Professor Scollo-Lavizzari, and Drs Cartlidge and Davidson

Dr Oxley *(Chairman):* I would now like to ask about monitoring liver function tests.

Interactive questions from Dr Oxley

1. In your own country, in official publications, is it recommended that you should do regular liver function tests after starting patients on valproate? **Response**
   1 Yes — 50%
   2 No — 30%
   3 Don't know — 20%

2. Do you routinely do liver function tests after starting somebody on valproate? **Response**
   1 Yes — 55%
   1 No — 45%

Professor Dam *(Hvidovre, Denmark):* It was stated that the side effects of carbamazepine were mainly seen in the first or initial phase of the trial. I would therefore like to know the dosage regimen and the starting doses of carbamazepine and valproate. Normally we increase the dose of carbamazepine by 100 mg every second day over 10 days to the full dose, whereas we start with a full dose with valproate. Could you comment on that?

Dr Cartlidge *(Newcastle, UK):* The recommendations that we had were that carbamazepine should be started at 100 mg twice a day for the first week, increasing to 200 mg twice a day for the second week, thereafter further increased being made at fortnightly intervals, increases being of the order of 100 mg twice a day. So it would be 300 mg twice a day at four weeks etc.

Dr Davidson *(Dundee, UK):* I should add that a lot of the early withdrawals were because of rash, which is an idiosyncratic rather than a dose-related effect. One might argue that some of the sedative effects, the dizziness and drowsiness, might have been avoided by slow drug introduction, but certainly not the larger group of idiosyncratic reactions.

Dr Gram *(Dianalund, Denmark):* First, have you calculated the Type 2 error in this trial? Second, could you elaborate on the cases developing a rash during valproate treatment. This is extremely infrequent.

Dr Davidson: With regard to the rash it is infrequent on valproate, I do not have a full description because the accounts come from multiple centres which simply described the occurrence of a rash. It is difficult to know whether the rash on valproate was from an intercurrent illness.

Dr Johnson *(Cambridge, UK):* The definition of Type 2 error is the power to detect a difference in a study, given that such a difference exists. The power, of course, will vary according to the difference you think is clinically important, that the trial should detect. The adult

EPITEG trial does have an 80% power to detect something like 20% differences in efficacy, measuring differences in terms of recurrence rates, but again the calculation of power does depend upon the end point that you are using in the analysis. So far we have not presented data on efficacy for this trial or for any of the other trials that were reported early this morning. You are quite right that the power of some of those studies is reduced, but as the studies have been reported in two forms, one for children and one for adults, the studies can of course be combined when it comes to assessing relative efficacy. Numbers in excess of 500 give very high power indeed to detect clinically important differences between treatments, in order of between 10% and 15%.

Mr Price *(Leeds, UK):* I would like to ask you why you limited your maximum daily dose to 800 mg of carbamazepine and 2 g of valproate. Some of us are using up to twice that amount, and it may be that you would be more likely to find a difference between the drugs if you were prepared in some patients to give higher doses.

Dr Cartlidge: The maximum dose of carbamazepine was between 1.6 and 2 g/day, and the maximum dose of valproate was of the order of 2 to 2.5 g/day. We certainly do not intend to go higher than 2.5 g/day of valproate.

Dr Brodie *(Glasgow, UK):* Could you clarify how you used the serum anticonvulsant concentrations; did the patient tell you that the concentration was toxic, or did the biochemist?

Dr Davidson: The biochemist does not tell us.

Dr Brodie: I had the impression that if the concentration was above a certain limit, you reduced the dose. Is that correct?

Dr Davidson: No, this is left to the discretion of the individual neurologist.

Dr Reynolds *(London, UK):* Our comparative monotherapy trial with four drugs in children has been reported earlier, and we have been doing an exactly similar study with the same drugs in adults. We have follow-up data on some 241 adults for up to four years of follow-up. So far there are no differences in efficacy between these four drugs. Dr Johnson has said, it will be possible to combine the data from our childhood and adult trials to increase the power.

With both trials of newly diagnosed patients we have been able to look at many different factors influencing long-term prognosis, and out of both the adult and the paediatric trial the most important prognostic factor was the number of seizures prior to entry to the trial. Whether these were tonic-clonic seizures or partial seizures, the more seizures—the worse the long-term prognosis. This is probably a real finding since it has emerged as the most significant finding in both studies and it adds yet more evidence to the concept that the most important thing is not which drug you choose to treat the patient, but how soon you treat the patient, how quickly you arrest the seizures.

Dr Pearce *(Hull, UK):* In view of the vastly different pharmacokinetics of valproate and carbamazepine and in particular the half lives of the two drugs, what steps have you taken to ensure that you are getting maximum efficacy within the total stated dosage?

Dr Cartlidge: We have followed the protocol as I have outlined and we carefully monitored the increases with the drug levels to get them into the upper end of the therapeutic range as fast as possible.

Dr Alving *(Dianalund, Denmark):* I think that it should be stated clearly in the protocol whether you stop when you have reached the upper end of the so-called therapeutic range, or if the treatment is a failure only after you reached the level where clinically intolerable side effects emerge. It is also interesting that you have a low incidence of side effects with carbamazepine, 50% compared with the Scandinavian study which in a double blind trial showed that 75% of patients on carbamazepine monotherapy had side effects. Maybe the lower side effects you found in your patient sample compared with the Scandinavian study is partly explained by the fact that some patients have not fully benefited from the trial. Some patients can tolerate, and need, levels which are higher than the so-called therapeutic level.

Dr Cartlidge: We increased the levels of the anticonvulsants until we reached the upper end of the therapeutic range, rather than until toxic symptoms appeared. Obviously in some instances symptoms of what we interpreted as toxicity came in before we reached the upper end of the therapeutic range.

Dr Rai (*Zurich, Switzerland*): In the case of valproate patients with neurological side effects such as tremors, have you found a correlation with increased plasma levels?

Dr Davidson: It is too small a number to draw firm conclusions. The levels were fairly high but not dramatically so, but I do not think we can say more than there was a tendency for higher levels to be present in those with tremor.

Dr Hosking (*Sheffield, UK*): Were your data on rising valproate levels taken from a whole cohort of patients on valproate or from individual patient monitoring?

Dr Davidson: Those were cumulative data for all the patient population.

Dr Brodie: There is no therapeutic range for valproate and the therapeutic range for carbamazepine is very tenuous indeed. For both drugs there are variations of about 100% in concentration within a dosage interval in twice daily dosage and I do not think you can compare these two drugs for this trial.

Dr Oxley (*Chalfont St Peter, UK*): Drawing this discussion to a close, I will now take a vote on it.

Interactive question from Dr Oxley

The EPITEG study will yield clinically useful and scientifically reliable information.	**Response**
1 Agree	55%
2 Disagree	18%
3 Don't know	27%

Epilepsy in the elderly

R. Tallis

Department of Geriatric Medicine, Hope Hospital, Salford, UK

INTRODUCTION

My title itself speaks volumes: could one imagine a quarter hour presentation at an international meeting entitled 'Epilepsy in the young?' Such a talk would be superficial to say the least. It is an unfortunate truth, however, that our knowledge of epilepsy presenting in the aged patient is scanty. I will begin by mapping our ignorance. Table 1 lists some of the questions to which we have no, or incomplete, answers at the present time.

I propose to deal briefly with some of these questions. Dr Pedersen will deal with the vitally important topic of drug treatment. Before I begin my reconnaissance, it may be worthwhile reflecting on why we are comparatively ignorant about epilepsy presenting for the first time in old age. I suspect it arises from several misconceptions. The first is that epilepsy matters less in the elderly. So much is going wrong anyway that the odd fit or two hardly counts. Nothing, of course, could be further from the truth. The precise diagnosis and careful management of epilepsy in this age group is as important as, if not more important than, its precise diagnosis and careful management in younger patients. Uncontrolled fits in the elderly present a greater danger due to the increased risk of fractures. Prolonged postictal states and inappropriate use of anticonvulsants are also more dangerous. Another reason for the comparative lack of information is the belief that epilepsy in the biologically aged patient is essentially the same as that in the younger patient so that we can extrapolate from the knowledge we have gained about the latter to the former. This, too, may be incorrect. Although the principles of management are the same, their application is slightly different—for example, when to treat, and how far to investigate likely causes.

Finally, the tradition that epilepsy presenting for the first time in old age is relatively uncommon is one that dies hard. It is based on an even more venerable tradition—that of observing elderly patients with a lesser degree of care than would be acceptable for younger patients. As a result, epilepsy is often lost in the rather noisy background of changes due to ageing and diseases that occur more commonly with advancing age. The relative indifference towards epilepsy in the elderly is well illustrated by the observations in the National General Practice Study of Epilepsy (NGPSE) (1). Whereas only 4%

Table 1 *Epilepsy in old age: some unanswered questions*

How common are seizures in old age?
What is the relative importance of different causes?
How do elderly patients view seizures?
What is the psychological impact of seizures in old age?
What is the prognosis of elderly onset seizures?
When should treatment begin?
Choice of drug, ideal dosage, blood level?

Fourth international symposium on sodium valproate and epilepsy, edited by David Chadwick, 1989: Royal Society of Medicine Services International Congress and Symposium No. 152, published by Royal Society of Medicine Services Limited.

of cases of epilepsy in younger patients were not referred to hospital, this figure was 20% in elderly patients. Correspondingly, there was a higher proportion of 'uncertain' as opposed to 'definite' cases.

INCIDENCE AND PREVALENCE

What then do we know about prevalence and incidence of epilepsy in the elderly? Hauser and Kurland (2) observed a steep rise in both the incidence and prevalence of epilepsy above the age of 50. In their study, the annual incidence of epileptic seizures rose from 12 per 100 000 in the 40–59 age range to 82 per 100 000 in those over 60. This latter figure is remarkably close to the incidence observed in Luhdorf's (3) which included all patients over 60 in a well-defined population and arrived at an incidence of 77 per 100 000. The National General Practice Study of Epilepsy (1), a prospective community-based study, identified 1200 patients with newly diagnosed or suspected epilepsy in its three-year study period (1984–87): 24% of new cases of definite epilepsy were over the age of 60, indicating an excessive representation of elderly people.

Hauser and Kurland (2) also showed a rise in prevalence for older subjects: 7.3 per thousand in the 40–59 age range to 10.2 per thousand for those over 60.

WHAT TYPE OF FITS DO ELDERLY PATIENTS HAVE?

To answer this question, there is little point in looking at the series that have emanated from neuro-medical or other referral centres in which elderly patients tend to be under-represented. The most reliable answers we have at present come from Luhdorf's study and from the NGPSE. Luhdorf found that 51% of elderly onset patients apparently had primary tonic-clonic seizures, 42% partial or secondary generalized seizures and 6% unclassifiable seizures. Of those with apparent primary tonic-clonic seizures, however, 38% had focal abnormalities on the EEG. In total, over 70% of their subjects had seizures which were either clinically or electrically partial or partial in origin. In the NGPSE the proportions of different seizures for the overall population were: partial or secondary generalized 52%; generalized from the outset 43%; and unclassified 7%. In the elderly cases, however, the proportions were: partial or secondary generalized 73%; primary generalized 17%; and unclassified 10%. This confirms the tendency for fits in elderly patients to be of focal origin, reflecting their relationship to focal cerebral pathology. Except in those cases where fits are due to some systemic cause, such as a metabolic disturbance or a drug lowering the convulsive threshold, it is probable that elderly onset seizures are, with very few exceptions, focal in origin. Certainly, the harder one looks, the more one is likely to find a potential focal cause.

PRESENTATION OF EPILEPSY IN OLD AGE

Epilepsy may present in a bewildering variety of guises at any age and old age is no exception. Diagnostic problems may be even greater, however, in an elderly patient who may offer an incomplete history and may have concurrent cardiac and primary cerebral causes for episodic loss or disturbance of consciousness. Since cerebral anoxia associated with syncope may itself cause convulsions and complex partial seizures may present with autonomic features, and since furthermore non-specific abnormalities are often seen in the EEG of elderly patients and transient cardiac arrythmias unconnected with the patient's clinical problems may be recorded on 24-h tapes, one is often left with an irresolvable uncertainty as to whether the 'turns' or 'spells' originate from the heart or the head. In many cases even after a careful history, examination and appropriate investigations, one may simply have to wait and see. A therapeutic trial of anticonvulsants as a diagnostic test is not usually recommended as it will rarely produce a clear answer and will add the burden of possibly unnecessary drug therapy to the patient's troubles.

It has to be remembered that, due to age-related changes in the brain and the fact that fits usually takes place against the background of cerebral damage, post-ictal states may be prolonged in elderly people. This may be another source of confusion. At least 14% of patients in one series (4) suffered a confusional state lasting over 24 h; in some cases it may persist as long as a week. This may well cause diagnostic problems where the history is incomplete. A focal postictal paresis (Todd's Palsy) is also more frequent in elderly patients. This may lead to misdiagnosis of stroke, and such patients have been referred to stroke units (5). This is especially likely to happen where fits occur against a background of known cerebrovascular disease, when a recurrent stroke may be incorrectly diagnosed (6).

CAUSES OF EPILEPSY IN THE ELDERLY (Table 2) (1,3,7–9)

The number of possible causes of epilepsy in elderly patients is, of course, legion. There is time only to emphasize one or two points.

As the Table shows, it is becoming increasingly recognized that cerebrovascular disease is the main cause of epilepsy in the elderly. It accounts for an even higher proportion of those cases in which a definite cause is established. The more carefully cerebrovascular disease is sought in epileptic patients, the more frequently is it found. Shorvon and colleagues (10) compared the CT scan appearances of patients with late onset epilepsy and no evidence of cerebral tumour with those of age- and sex-matched controls. There was an excess of ischaemic lesions in epileptic patients. In half of those epileptic patients who were found to have CT evidence of vascular disease, clinical examination was normal.

Epilepsy commonly follows stroke and may also precede it. In Marquardsen's series (11), epilepsy occurred in 8% of hemiplegic stroke patients. Cocito (12) examined the incidence of post-stroke epilepsy in patients with angiographically proven carotid or middle cerebral artery occlusive disease and found that fits occurred in 17% of the former and 11% of the latter in a three year follow-up. Conversely, studies have shown an excess of previous epilepsy in patients admitted to hospital with acute stroke compared with controls suggesting that in some elderly patients epilepsy may be the earliest manifestation of cerebrovascular disease (13).

Clinicians are often concerned that very late onset epilepsy may indicate a cerebral tumour. Most series suggest that this applies only to the minority of cases, ranging from 2–14% in different series (1,3,7–9). This enormous variation is due to different populations being studied (reflecting different referral patterns), the different extent to which patients are investigated, and related to this, the different proportion of cases in which no definite cause is found. In most cases, tumours are either metastatic, or (inoperable) gliomas, though a few meningiomas are found. Until there is information in adequately documented, adequately investigated and sufficiently large population-based series, one cannot be certain what proportion of cases of very late onset epilepsy are due to treatable and non-treatable tumours. At any rate, treatable tumour does not appear to have the aetiological importance attached to it in traditional teaching.

Some seizures are attributed to non-vascular cerebral degeneration. Again the data are inadequate and will remain so until large series with uniform access to CT scanning facilities

Table 2 *Causes of epilepsy in the elderly as reported in the literature*

	Series				
	Hildick-Smith %	Schold %	Godfrey %	Luhdorf %	NGPSE %
Cerebrovascular disease	42(48)	30(60)	44(52)	32	50(76)
Cerebral tumour	10	2	12	14	13
Senile dementia/ cerebral atrophy	14	NR	7	2	NR
Toxic/metabolic	12	10	6	12	NR

Figures in brackets are percentages of those cases in which a cause was found.
NR=figures Not Reported for this cause.

are reported. Subdural haematoma is a rare but remediable cause. Direct brain damage due to head injury is a relatively uncommon cause of elderly-onset epilepsy. Epilepsy may rarely follow severe central nervous system infections.

Recent series have reminded us of the importance of toxic and metabolic causes of seizures in the elderly and they appear to account for between 10 and 15% of cases. As alcohol abuse is becoming increasingly prevalent amongst the elderly, this will continue to be a major aetiological factor. Dam (14) found that 25% of patients with late onset epilepsy had alcohol or alcohol withdrawal as the main cause.

A wide range of drugs has been suspected of causing convulsions. Drug-induced seizures are particularly likely to occur when the drug is given in high dosage or parenterally or to patients with impaired drug handling. This especially applies to biologically aged patients who will have alterations in the distribution, metabolism and excretion of some drugs.

Finally, one very occasionally encounters a patient whose seizures may be idiopathic, presenting for medical help for the first time in old age. Such patients sometimes have a lifetime of untreated epilepsy. Without such a long history it is difficult to sustain the diagnosis of idiopathic epilepsy.

INVESTIGATIONS

There is insufficient time to touch on this topic more than cursorily. I should like to make a comment or two about the electroencephalogram (EEG) and about the use of computerized tomography.

The value and limitations of the EEG are well known. The range of normal increases with age so that discriminating normal from abnormal becomes more difficult in an elderly patient. Moreover, non-specific abnormalities, or abnormalities that are not related to seizures, are also more common in the elderly. It follows from this that the general rule that a diagnosis of epilepsy should not be made on EEG findings alone applies even more to elderly patients. Very occasionally, the patient with non-convulsive seizures may present with neuropsychiatric symptoms. In such cases, the EEG may be especially useful, in particular if it shows ictal discharges.

Financial constraints imply that computerized tomography cannot be offered to all patients who have seizures, even in those in whom there is a suspicion that the fits may be related to a cerebral lesion. CT scanning is of course an extremely powerful method of identifying structural lesions of the brain. Moreover, there is a good deal of evidence from the literature that the older the patient the greater the change of a positive scan (15). As many as 60% of very late onset patients with epilepsy may show a structural lesion on a CT scan. These facts would support routine scanning of elderly onset epileptic patients, however, only if the identification of such lesions were of benefit to the patient. The discovery of a space occupying lesion amenable to neurosurgical removal would be an obvious case in point. However, in only a minority of patients with elderly onset epilepsy is a neoplasm or subdural haematoma the cause and in only a small proportion of tumour cases would neurosurgical intervention be appropriate (16,17). Tumours are more likely to be gliomas or metastases than meningiomas and even where a meningioma is diagnosed, neurosurgical treatment may not always be indicated. There is an impression that some meningiomas in old age may be relatively inert and there is no doubt that craniotomy is often tolerated poorly by elderly patients. Even so, it is sometimes useful to have a definitive diagnosis though treatment for the underlying condition may be not available or considered in appropriate. Arguable indications for CT scanning are given in Table 3.

Table 3 *Indications for computerized tomography in elderly patients with seizures*

Strong indications
Unexplained focal neurological signs
Progressive or new neurological symptoms or signs
Poor control of fits not attributable to poor compliance

Less strong indications
Clear-cut focal fits
Focal slow wave abnormality on the EEG

CONCLUSION

The topic of epilepsy in the elderly should be a large one. Unfortunately, as yet it boasts only a small autonomous literature. This, however, is growing and the kind of information obtained from the studies of Luhdorf and colleagues and the National General Practice Study of Epilepsy are advancing our knowledge. Certainly, elderly onset epilepsy is an area ripe for much further investigation. In particular, it is to be hoped that elderly patients will not be overlooked in the future as they have been in the past, especially in trials of newer anticonvulsants.

Note

I am very grateful to Dr Simon Shorvon and colleagues for permission to refer to the data obtained in the National General Practice of Study of Epilepsy.

REFERENCES

(1) Hart Y, Shorvon S. Personal communication of unpublished data from the National General Practice Study of Epilepsy.
(2) Hauser WA, Kurland LT. The epidemiology of epilepsy in Rochester, Minnesota 1935 through 1967. *Epilepsia* 1975; **16**: 1–16.
(3) Luhdorf K, Jensen LK, Plesner A. Etiology of seizures in the elderly. *Epilepsia* 1986; **27**(4): 458–63.
(4) Godfrey JW, Roberts MA, Caird FI. Epileptic seizures in the elderly: 2. Diagnostic problems. *Age Ageing* 1982; **11**: 29–34.
(5) Norris JW, Hachinski VC. Mis-diagnosis of stroke. *Lancet* 1982; **i**: 328–31.
(6) Fine W. Post hemiplegic epilepsy in the elderly. *Br Med J* 1967; **1**: 199–201.
(7) Hildick-Smith M. Epilepsy in the elderly. *Age Ageing* 1974; **3**: 203–8.
(8) Schold C, Warnell PR, Earnest NP. Origin of seizures in elderly patients. *JAMA* 1977; **238**: 1177–8.
(9) Roberts MA, Godfrey JW, Caird FI. Epileptic seizures in the elderly: 1. Aetiology and type of seizure. *Age Ageing* 1982; **11**: 24–8.
(10) Shorvon SD, Gilliatt RW, Cox TC, Yu YL. Evidence of vascular disease from CT scanning in late onset epilepsy. *J Neurol Neurosurg Psych* 1984; **47** (3): 225–3.
(11) Marquardsen J. The natural history of acute cerebrovascular disease. A retrospective study of 769 patients. *Acta Neurol Scand* 1969; **45** (Suppl 38): 150–2.
(12) Cocito L, Favale E, Reni L. Epileptic seizures in cerebral arterial occlusive disease. *Stroke* 1982; **13** (2): 189–95.
(13) Shinton RA, Gill JS, Zezulk AV, Beevers DJ. The frequency of epilepsy preceding stroke. *Lancet* 1987; **1**: 11–13.
(14) Dam AM. Late onset epilepsy, etiologies, types of seizure and value of clinical investigation, EEG and CT Scan. *Epilepsia* 1985; **26**: 227–31.
(15) Ramirez-Lassepas M, Cipolle RJ, Morillo LR, Gumnit RJ. Value of computed tomography scan in the evaluation of adult patients after their first seizure. *Ann Neurol* 1984; **15** (6): 436–43.
(16) Young AC, Costanzi JB, Mohr PD, Forbes WS. Is routine computerised axial tomography in epilepsy worthwhile? *Lancet* 1982; **ii**: 1446–7.
(17) Chadwick D. How far to investigate the elderly patient with epilepsy. In: Tallis RC. ed. *Epilepsy and the elderly*. London: Royal Society of Medicine, 1988.

Treatment of epilepsy in old age

B. Pedersen and G. Anderson

Department of Neurology, Aalborg Sygehus, Aalborg, Denmark

INTRODUCTION

The age composition of the population in western societies is shifting towards a larger share of old people. Many old age pensioners live a very active and independent life. Therefore, treatment of epilepsy in patients over 60 years of age ought to command the attention of neurologists, geriatricians and general practitioners.

Can epilepsy in elderly patients be treated in accordance with the guidelines in use when treating young people or are there some special problems to deal with in the care of elderly patients?

MATERIAL AND METHODS

A retrospective study comprising patients over 60 years of age seen either as inpatients or outpatients in our department between 1 January 1986 and 31 December 1988 with one or more fits has been undertaken. Ninety-eight patients were identified, 11 of whom were excluded as they did not have a minimum observation time of three months or were not followed up in our clinic. Nine patients had malignant cerebral tumours and were excluded.

Thirteen of the patients had only a single generalized seizure and were not on antiepileptic medication. The sex distribution of the remaining 65 patients is shown in Table 1. Median

Table 1 *Sex distribution of patients*

	%	n
Male	63	41
Female	37	24
	100	65

Table 2 *Aetiology of fits*

	%	n
Stroke	38	25
Dementia	19	12
Status epilepticus	6	4
Other	9	6
Unknown	28	18

Fourth international symposium on sodium valproate and epilepsy, edited by David Chadwick, 1989: Royal Society of Medicine Services International Congress and Symposium No. 152, published by Royal Society of Medicine Services Limited.

Table 3 *First choice of drug*

	%	n
Carbamazepine	77	50
Valproate	8	5
Phenytoin	5	3
Phenobarbitone	2	1
Combination of 2 drugs	8	6
		65

age was 69 years (range 61–88 years). The aetiology of the fits is seen in Table 2. In four patients the fits started with convulsive or non-convulsive status epilepticus and the aetiology could not be found by EEG and CT-scan. Only 43% of the patients had no known concomitant disease and 35% had heart disorders. In all patients a CT-scan was performed. Only 28% of the scans were normal and in 68% infarction, atrophy or both were found. The epilepsy was of partial type in all patients and 88% suffered from complex partial seizures with secondary generalization. Table 3 lists the drugs which patients were already taking at admission or were given as first choice drug after admission. In patients with unacceptable seizure control or side-effects, medication was changed to a second drug.

RESULTS

The first choice of antiepileptic drug is shown in Table 3. None of the patients were treated with more than two drugs. Table 4 shows that although 74% of the patients became seizure-free only 42% were without side-effects. In 43% the side-effects were unacceptable and the medication had to be changed to the second drug. The choice can be seen in Table 5. When on the second drug a further 17% of patients became seizure-free and the side-effects decreased as 23% got rid of their complaints (Table 6). Overall 91% became totally seizure-free and 85% were on monotherapy. Carbamazepine was the first drug of choice in 75% of the patients; when a change was necessary the second choice was most often oxcarbazepine or valproate. None of the 14 patients on valproate either as first or second drug changed medication and all of them were on mono-dose and monotherapy. The types of side-effects which occurred with all drugs are listed in Table 7.

Table 4 *Seizure frequency and side-effects on first choice drug*

	%	n
Seizure frequency		
Seizure-free	74	48
Acceptable	18	12
Unacceptable	8	5
Side-effects		
None	42	27
Acceptable	15	10
Unacceptable	43	28

Table 5 *Second choice of drug*

	%	n
Carbamazepine	6	4
Oxcarbamazepine	12	8
Valproate	17	11
Phenytoin	2	1
Clonazepam	2	1
Combination of 2 drugs	6	4
		27

Table 6 *Seizure frequency and side-effects on second day*

	%	n
Seizure frequency		
Seizure-free	17	11
Acceptable	25	16
Unacceptable	0	0
Side-effects		
None	23	15
Acceptable	19	12
Unacceptable	0	0

Table 7 *Side-effects with all drugs*

	%	n
Tiredness	14	9
Dizziness	22	14
Both	8	5
Skin rash	14	9
Gastrointestinal problems	2	1

DISCUSSION

In this retrospective study consisting of 65 patients over 60 years of age with epilepsy and on antiepileptic drug therapy we found that the sex distribution, aetiology, seizure type and result of CT-scan were in accordance with other studies concerning epilepsy in old age (1). We found that seizure control was easily established in 74% with the first drug and an additional 17% became seizure-free on the second drug. The main factor limiting treatment was side-effects. Forty-three per cent had to be changed from the first drug due to side-effects. On both first and second drugs 85% of the patients were on monotherapy and no patients received more than two drugs.

Compliance was poor when patients took their medication divided into two or more doses per day, perhaps because many were also receiving other types of medication. Side-effects such as tiredness and dizziness also enhanced non-compliance.

Fourteen patients received valproate either as first or second choice in mono-dose and monotherapy. In none of these patients was medication changed either due to unacceptable seizure frequency or side-effects. Compliance was high in this group. The number of patients on valproate does not allow statistical analysis but it may be that valproate should be used more often as the first drug in treating epilepsy in patients over 60 years of age because of good control of seizure frequency, the low rate of side-effects and good compliance when given as monotherapy in a single dose.

REFERENCES

(1) Luhdorf K, Jensen LK, Plesner AM. Etiology of seizures in the elderly. *Epilepsia* 1986; **27** (4): 458–63.

Discussion after Professor Tallis and Dr Pedersen

Interactive question from Dr Oxley

Sodium valproate is a good drug for elderly patients with epilepsy because of its relative lack of side-effects.	**Response**
1 Agree	48%
2 Disagree	24%
3 No view	28%

Dr Poole *(Oxford, UK):* There is one problem with someone who has had a fit in association with acute stroke or cardiac dysrhythmia and a different problem if the stroke patient has attacks a few months later. Does that represent an incremental infarct, temporary impoverishment, or a continued seizure tendency? Your therapeutic decision might be different in those settings. As far as EEG is concerned the people that I see in a post-stroke situation have fewer episodic EEG abnormalities than those without this type of history.

Professor Tallis *(Salford, UK):* One has to distinguish between a seizure occurring, say, in association with an acute event and a tendency to recurrent seizures i.e. epilepsy. Many patients who have epilepsy on the background of cerebrovascular disease may not have had an overt stroke. In those where there is a relation to stroke, the fits may develop following the stroke or some time after it. I would not regard someone who has a single fit in association with a stroke as suffering from epilepsy.

Dr Pedersen *(Aalborg, Denmark):* In our studies 13 patients had only one fit and were not put on medication; the patients on medication had more than one fit over a period of time. EEGs were performed in all our patients, but the results were not interesting. In this age group we do not use the EEG on a routine basis.

Dr Nasar *(Bridlington, UK):* If you had a patient of 70 years of age on phenytoin and phenobarbitone whose fits were still not controlled, what would you do in that situation?

Professor Tallis: First I would establish whether or not the patient is taking the medication. I would not be happy with a patient on two anticonvulsants; it may be that he is suffering the effects of intoxication, and anyway everyone is persuaded that a single anticonvulsant is preferable in the vast majority of cases. If one found that the person was taking the medication as prescribed and the blood levels indicated that they were in the so-called therepeutic range then there would be a case for changing to another drug, and that is what I would do, assuming that there was not some other remediable underlying predisposing factor causing fits—alcohol for example.

Dr Nasar: What would you do about somebody on phenobarbitone for 10 years in whom there was no real diagnosis and what dose do you go up to before you changed to a second drug?

Professor Tallis: Withdrawing anticonvulsants in the elderly is a tricky business because often the original indication for anticonvulsants has been lost in the mists of time. I personally have had the experience of withdrawing phenytoin 100 mg daily from an elderly patient who did not appear to have a good reason to be taking it and who arrived in the casualty department in status epilepticus four weeks later, so I am a little nervous about anticonvulsant withdrawal. However, if there is no good reason for anticonvulsant therapy, one has to bite the bullet and withdraw medication with extreme care, very slowly; there is no rush to withdraw.

Dr Pedersen: In answer to that last question—how far the serum level rose before we changed the drug—we used the drug to the maximum serum combination before entering the toxic range.

Dr Besag *(Surrey, UK):* I have to treat many cases of status epilepticus in a younger age group and, of course, we can treat with quite large doses and quite rapidly; but my brief experience with elderly patients is that they are acutely sensitive to intravenous diazepam and we might do great harm by giving what in other age groups would be considered to be a very modest dose. I would be interested in the comments of the speakers on the treatment of status epilepticus in the elderly.

Dr Pedersen: If the seizures cannot be stopped by small doses of diazepam the routine procedure in our department is loading by phenytoin which is well tolerated in this age group. The advantage of using phenytoin is that you do not get depression in respiration which is troublesome in these patients and often causes several days on a respirator and artificial ventilation.

Dr Hildick-Smith *(Canterbury, UK):* Dr Pedersen and Professor Tallis are talking about two different populations. It is commonplace of geriatric medicine that patients aged 60 to 75 are a volunteer group, not a patient group, and Dr Pedersen's study is largely of younger patients from whom we cannot generalize when we are talking about the increasing problem that we have to face for the future which is the over 75 age group. Could I ask Dr Pedersen to give a breakdown of her 100 over 60 age group, in ages?

Dr Pedersen: The median age was 69, but of the 65 patients I cannot give you the exact figures in the different age groups.

Dr Brodie: As general physicians we see a lot of strokes, but not many patients having fits. Those we do see can come in in status epilepticus or they have serial seizures; then they recover and they have no neurological deficit. I wonder whether there is any family history in these people; have they a low seizure threshold that is suddenly triggered after 60 or 70 years of life?

Professor Tallis: It is an interesting question, but we have no relevant information on that.

Dr Voskuil *(The Netherlands):* I want to comment on two things; first the value of EEG. A few years ago a study was published of 9 elderly patients who had never had any epilepsy and then started with non-convulsive status epilepticus when they were over 60. When older people start to behave in a strange way you should do an EEG. Stroke patients followed up for a few years were found to have a good prognosis, so one can consider because of the age whether or not you should treat these patients for a long time or try to stop the medication after one or two years.

Professor Tallis: You are quite right. There was a series of papers in the 1970s which looked at neuropsychiatric presentations of epilepsy in the elderly. If somebody is behaving oddly in a paroxysmal way, against a background of cerebrovascular disease, even if you do not see anything particularly helpful on the EEG, there is a dangerous temptation to carry out a therapeutic trial on the assumption that the acute behavioural psychiatric disturbance is epileptic in origin.

You referred to post-stroke epilepsy and I wondered if you were referring to a recent series that distinguished between fits occurring immediately after a stroke and those that occurred at an interval after a stroke. It appeared that the seizures had a different prognosis in the two cases. It was an interesting observation, and, although there was only a small number of patients in each group, I think it is important to be aware of the difference between late onset and early onset post-stroke epilepsy. Clearly, if earlier onset fits have a good prognosis, it may be inappropriate to start chronic medication.

Dr Poole: I can certainly confirm petit mal status-type disorder in the elderly. A therapeutic trial of anticonvulsants in a systematic way in the elderly has the important advantage that, although the diagnosis may be more uncertain because of the various possible contributing factors, the use of anticonvulsants need not create the same problems over work and driving as will occur with a therapeutic trial in a younger group.

SESSION IV

UNWANTED EFFECTS

Chairman: A. Richens

INTRODUCTION

This session will deal mainly with the unwanted effects of anti-epileptic drugs.

There is a picture which looks rather like a spike wave complex in an excellent and entertaining book on clinical pharmacology by Professor Desmond Laurence. It was in fact intended to signify what happened to a new drug after its introduction. The top of the spike represents the enthusiasm that we all show for using new drugs, then subsequently a spate of bad reports come out and the use of the drug plummets to the trough; thereafter, common sense takes over and we begin to weigh up the advantages and disadvantages and we reach a point where we can say that we have achieved a balance of risks and benefits. I think we have now reached that point with sodium valproate; in the UK it has been on the market since 1973 and we have now reached more or less that steady state point where we know what it does therapeutically and what it does not do. We know for instance, that valproate, phenytoin and carbamazepine are not very different when treating partial or secondary generalized seizures. Therefore, our choice of drug often depends not on therapeutic efficacy but on the balance of adverse reactions in the particular patient that we wish to treat. These, then, are the subjects of this part of the meeting.

The first topic in this session is enzyme induction. You are all well aware that the traditional anti-epileptic drugs have the major disadvantage of inducing not only their own metabolism but that of other drugs. This is something that we have looked towards new drugs not to have.

Disinduction of valproate metabolism: Timing and magnitude of change

R. H. Mattson,[1,2] **J. A. Cramer,**[1,2] **R. D. Scheyer,**[1,2] and **J. M. Hochholzer**[1,2]

[1]Department of Neurology, Yale University School of Medicine, New Haven, CT, USA and [2]Epilepsy Center, Veterans Administration Medical Center, West Haven, CT, USA

INTRODUCTION

Drug interactions can result in pharmacodynamic actions not expected when drugs are used alone. Usually, these are a consequence of pharmacokinetic changes (1). Properties of drugs that make interactions probable include relative insolubility of compounds that make formulation difficult, high protein binding, and biotransformation mediated by the microsomal cytochrome P450 oxidizing enzyme systems. Most antiepileptic drugs share one or more of these characteristics. Interactions with valproate (VPA) are exceedingly common (1,2). VPA is highly protein bound and can displace other protein bound drugs such as carbamazepine (CBZ) and phenytoin (PHT) with potentially clinically important consequences (3,4,5,6). Enzyme inhibition by VPA can cause increased levels of antiepileptic drugs, including phenobarbital (PB) (1,3,7,8,9), PHT (6,10), primidone (PRM) (11), and ethosuximide (12,13) leading to toxicity and/or greater efficacy.

An interaction of particular importance when using VPA is enzyme induction caused by CBZ (14), PB (8), PHT (3), or PRM (11). VPA clearance is increased during polytherapy compared to its use as monotherapy (15,16). Consequently, it is necessary to administer greater VPA dosage to achieve desired blood levels. Doses need to be given more often or large changes can be expected between peak and trough. Thus, the expense of treatment increases and compliance may worsen (17). In addition, the induction may enhance omega oxidation of VPA to produce the potentially hepatotoxic 4-en-VPA metabolite in susceptible individuals (18,19).

Although these types of interactions have become increasingly well appreciated over the past decade, their magnitude and timing have not been fully investigated. For this reason, we have recently reviewed the VPA blood levels in patients also receiving either CBZ or PHT during conversion to VPA monotherapy. These observations allowed some determinations of the time course and magnitude of disinductive effect of CBZ and PHT withdrawal.

METHODS

Seventeen patients taking VPA plus CBZ ($n = 6$) or PHT ($n = 11$) have been studied during a single dose interval when at steady state. Hourly samples were obtained for 8–12 h. The samples were obtained before conversion to VPA monotherapy at one or two weekly intervals during the crossover, and until monotherapy steady state was reached with VPA. Prior to and after conversion, extended studies of minimal and maximal total and free VPA, CBZ or PHT levels were performed at times of trough and peak.

RESULTS

Magnitude of disinductive effect

Mean trough VPA levels rose an average of 44% after discontinuation of CBZ or PHT. The magnitude of change was greater after stopping PHT, averaging 74%. The lowest dose

Fourth international symposium on sodium valproate and epilepsy, edited by David Chadwick, 1989; Royal Society of Medicine Services International Congress and Symposium Series No. 152, published by Royal Society of Medicine Services Limited.

Table 1 *Valproate serum concentrations. Mean (SD) µg/ml*

On PHT	Off PHT	Increase
58 (7)[a]	101 (17)	74%
On CBZ	Off CBZ	Increase
85 (21)[a]	103 (18)	21%
All Poly	All Mono	Increase
71[a]	102	44%

PHT, $n=11$; CBZ, $n=6$. [a]$p<.001$.

Table 2 *Illustrative case of valproate disinduction during phenytoin decrease*

DAY	PHT (mg/d)	PHT (µg/ml)	VPA (mg/d)	VPA (µg/ml)	Free VPA (µg/ml)
−28	300	9.0	5000	55	6
−24	200	<2.5	5000	87	13
−7	100	<2.5	5000	110	19
+7	—	—	5000	110	20
+22	—	—	5000	130	37

−day refers to the period during PHT co-treatment. +day refers to the period of VPA monotherapy.

of PHT at which the inductive effect was still seen varied among patients. The absence of an increase in VPA was observed in only one patient. The effect on VPA levels caused by discontinuing CBZ was less than when PHT was stopped: VPA levels rose only an average of 21%. This greater inductive effect of PHT was confirmed in three patients needing to resume two-drug therapy. Each patient had experienced a doubling of VPA levels after discontinuation of PHT. Monotherapy provided insufficient seizure control so CBZ was added to VPA. However, little inductive effect by CBZ was seen because VPA levels did not decline. Table 1 lists means and standard deviations of changes in VPA serum concentrations indicating the magnitude of change.

Timing of disinduction

The timing of disinduction was variable. A rise in VPA levels (on constant dose) typically began when PHT dose dropped below 200 mg/day, or with PHT levels below 5 µg/ml. Four of 11 patients showed evidence of disinduction and increased VPA levels before PHT was discontinued. In three patients, changes were seen a week after discontinuation, and in two others the rise in VPA blood levels was not seen until two weeks after PHT discontinuation. In two patients, disinduction did not appear until PHT was totally discontinued. One patient had PHT rapidly tapered over three days in a hospital setting. VPA level was unchanged at 56 µg/ml two days after discontinuation. Six days later, on constant dose, VPA had risen to 99 µg/ml and subsequent samples remained in this range (105 µg/ml) until VPA dosage was reduced. Thus, disinduction occurred between day 2 and day 8, or within the week. Table 2 describes an example with disinduction of VPA during tapering of PHT doses. The timing of CBZ disinduction was similar to PHT but less easily defined due to the modest changes.

DISCUSSION

Interactions between VPA and the co-medications CBZ or PHT were observed before, during, and after crossover to VPA monotherapy. The effects of enzyme induction from co-administration of PHT can be inferred from the marked rise of VPA (average 74%) during monotherapy. This potent effect is consistent with findings by Perucca et al. (20), and Shaw et al. (21) showing a marked increase in antipyrine or glucaric acid clearance in subjects given PHT compared to controls. Patsalos et al. (22) studied antipyrine clearance in patients following removal of a variety of antiepileptic drugs and found that PHT was a potent inducer. CBZ has been identified as possessing enzyme inducing properties in the same studies cited above, although changes in valproate clearance were modest in two or three children taken off CBZ in the study of Cloyd *et al.* (23). Our experience in this group of patients also showed surprisingly modest change in valproate levels in six patients after CBZ discontinuation. Further observation was possible in the three patients who had breakthrough tonic-clonic seizures on VPA monotherapy after PHT was discontinued. All had shown marked increase in VPA levels on constant dose after stopping PHT. However, the later addition of CBZ to VPA caused little change in VPA levels. The opportunity to observe the lack of inductive effect of CBZ was important because it was documented in patients known to have had a marked response to PHT. The dosages of CBZ were low to moderate prior to crossover and CBZ levels were in the low range after addition in the monotherapy failures. Possibly, CBZ induction would have been more evident at high dose with corresponding levels. The effect of dose and blood levels appeared to be important for PHT induction. VPA levels had begun to rise in several patients well before PHT had been totally discontinued, when PHT levels were 5 μg/ml or less.

Our studies did not afford an opportunity to evaluate the time required for enzyme induction or increased valproate clearance in the presence of other antiepileptic drugs, but we were able to look at the approximate time for disinduction. Although the process of disinduction appeared to occur over a variable span of approximately four weeks among these patients, timing of increased valproate levels may well have resulted from varying effects of the quantity of enzyme inducing drug present during the gradual tapering process. Indeed, once evidence of disinduction was detected, the short VPA half life required only about three days to reach the new steady state. Once begun, the overall disinduction was fairly rapid and took place within a week or less. Others have reported more long-term inductive effects. PB, a potent enzyme inducer with a long half life, was found to have a continuing induction effect for a lengthy period after discontinuation (24). Kater (25) reported that increased clearance of PHT caused by co-administration of alcohol, another potent inducer, persisted for up to two months after ETOH was discontinued.

The clinical implications of the timing of new steady state serum concentrations when going to VPA monotherapy are important. If valproate levels are high before elimination of an enzyme inducing drug, readjustment of dose likely will be necessary to avoid toxicity, such as tremor. Evidence from our studies suggests that these changes occur rather quickly, within two weeks after discontinuing drug. With other drugs, the timing will depend on the elimination half life of the particular drug. If a drug is abruptly discontinued, the disinduction can be expected to occur rapidly and probably within the first week. The time to determine blood levels and any dose change will be based on the elimination half life of the drug being maintained in monotherapy. The issue becomes more complex in circumstances in which there is a tapering of medication over a period of time during the crossover process (26). Specifically, the co-administered drug causing the enzyme induction will exert significant effects at some dosage. In our study a number of patients showed evidence of disinduction when dose of PHT had decreased to about 2 mg/kg, whereas in others some effect continued until drug had been totally withdrawn. This pilot study is being expanded to more patients to clarify the timing and dose relationship of the disinduction process.

CONCLUSIONS

The use of valproate is associated with frequent drug interactions that are clinically significant. The mechanisms include alterations of protein binding and enzyme inhibition by valproate, as well as enzyme induction and increased clearance of valproate by concomitant enzyme inducing antiepileptic drugs. Our studies suggest that PHT has a much more marked enzyme inducing effect than CBZ, so that doubling of valproate levels following discontinuation of PHT and conversion to monotherapy is common. During the tapering process, the loss of enzyme inducing properties by PHT was quite variable. Initial dose reduction had an effect in some patients but disinduction did not begin in others until PHT levels were very sub-therapeutic. CBZ had more modest enzyme inducing effect. The timing and magnitude of disinduction have clinical significance in everyday management of patients both during polytherapy and monotherapy, particularly during a crossover period.

ACKNOWLEDGMENT

Supported by the Veterans Administration Medical Research Service and USPHS Grant No. NS 06208-23.

REFERENCES

(1) Mattson RH, Cramer JA. Valproate: Interactions with other drugs. In: Levy RH, Mattson RH, Meldrum BS, Penry JD, Dreifuss FE, eds. *Antiepileptic drugs*, 3rd Ed. New York: Raven Press, 1989.

(2) Mattson RH, Cramer JA. Antiepileptic drug interactions in clinical use. In: Pitlick W, ed. *Drug interactions*. New York: Demos Press, 1989: 75–85.

(3) Mattson RH, Cramer JA, Williamson PD, Novelly R. Valproic acid in epilepsy: Clinical and pharmacological effects. *Ann Neurol* 1978; **3**: 20–25.

(4) Kissin B. Interaction of ethyl alcohol and other drugs. In: Kissin B, Begleiter H, eds. *The biology of alcoholism. Clinical pathology*. New York: Plenum Press, 1971; **3**: 119.

(5) Cramer JA, Mattson RH. Valproic acid: In vitro plasma protein binding and interactions with phenytoin. *Ther Drug Monit* 1979; **1**: 105–16.

(6) Cramer JA, Mattson RH, Bennett DM, Swick CT. Variable free and total valproic acid concentrations in sole and multi drug-therapy. In: Levy RH *et al.*, eds. *Metabolism of antiepileptic drugs*. New York: Raven Press, 1984; 105–14.

(7) Mattson RH, Cramer JA. Valproic acid. In: Browne TR, Feldman RG, eds. *Epilepsy, diagnosis and management*. Boston: Little Browne & Co, 1983: 225–34.

(8) Kapetanovic I, Kupferberg HJ, Porter RJ, Penry JK. Valproic acid-phenobarbital interaction: A systematic study using stable isotopically labeled phenobarbital in an epileptic patient. In: Morselli PL, Pippenger CE, Richens A, *et al.*, eds. *Antiepileptic drug therapy: Advances in drug monitoring*. New York: Raven Press, 1980: 373–80.

(9) Wilder BJ, Willmore LJ, Bruni J, Villareal HJ. Valproic acid: Interaction with other anticonvulsants drugs. *Neurology* 1978; **28**: 892–6.

(10) Bruni J, Gallo JM, Lee CS, Perchalski RJ, Wilder BJ. Interactions of valproic acid with phenytoin. *Neurology* 1980; **30**: 1233–6.

(11) Windorfer A, Sauer W, Gadeke R. Elevation of diphenylhdantoin and primidone serum concentration by addition of dipropylacetate, a new anticonvulsant drug. *Acta Paediatr Scand* 1972; **64**: 771–2.

(12) Mattson RH, Cramer JA. Valproic acid and ethosuximide interaction. *Ann Neurol* 1980; **7**: 583–4.

(13) Pisani F, Narbone MC, Trunfio C, *et al.* Valproic acid-ethosuximide interaction: a pharmacokinetic study. *Epilepsia* 1984; **25**: 229–33.

(14) Bowdle TA, Levy RH, Cutler RE. Effect of carbamazepine on valproic acid kinetics in normal subjects. *Clin Pharmacol Ther* 1979; **26**: 627–34.

(15) Cramer JA, Mattson RH, Bennett DM, Swick CT. Variable free and total valproic acid concentrations in sole and multi drug therapy. *Therapy Drug Monit* 1986; **8**: 411–6.

(16) Sackellares JC, Sato S, Dreifuss FE, Penry JK. Reductions of steady state valproate levels by other antiepileptic drugs. *Epilepsia* 1981; **22**: 437–41.

(17) Cramer JA, Mattson RH, Prevey ML, Ouellette V. How often is medication taken as prescribed? A novel assessment technique. *JAMA* 1989; **261**: 3273–7.

(18) Dreifuss FE, Santilli N, Langer DH, Sweeney KP, Moline KA, Menander KB. Valproic acid hepatic fatalities: A retrospective review. *Neurology* 1987; **37**: 379–85.

(19) Scheffner D, Konig ST, Rauterberg-Ruland I, Kochem W, Hofmann WJ, Unkelbach ST. Fatal liver failure in 16 children with valproate therapy. *Epilepsia* 1988; **29**: 530–42.

(20) Perucca E, Hedges A, Makki KA, Ruprah M, Wilson JF, Richens, A. A comparative study of the relative enzyme inducing properties of anticonvulsant drugs in epileptic patients. *Br J Clin Pharmacol* 1984; **18**: 401–10.

(21) Shaw PN, Houston JB, Rowland M, Hopkins K, Thiercelin JF, Morselli PL. Antipyrine metabolite kinetics in healthy human volunteers during multiple dosing of phenytoin and carbamazepine. *Br J Clin Pharmacol* 1985; **20**: 611–18.

(22) Patsalos PN, Duncan JS, Shorvon SD. Effect of the removal of individual antiepileptic drugs on antipyrine kinetics, in patients taking polytherapy. *Br J Clin Pharmacol* 1988; **26**: 253–9.

(23) Cloyd JC, Kriel RL, Fischer JH. Valproic acid pharmacokinetics in children. II. Discontinuation of concomitant antiepileptic drug therapy. *Neurology* 1985; **35**: 1623–7.

(24) Breckenridge A, Orme ML, Davies L, Thurgiersson SS, Davies DS. Dose dependent enzyme induction. *Clin Pharmacol Ther* 1973; **14**: 514–20.

(25) Kater RMH, Roggin G, Tobon F, Zieve P, Iber FL. Increased rate of clearance of drugs from the circulation of alcoholics. *Am J Med Sci* 1969; **258**: 35–9.

(26) Mattson RH, Cramer JA. Crossover from polytherapy to monotherapy in primary generalized epilepsy. *Am J Med* 1988; **84**: 23–8.

DISCUSSION

Professor Mattson *(Connecticut, USA):* I would like to ask the audience the following:

Do you think the effect on valproate level was greatest	Response
1 Following removal of carbamazepine	17%
2 Following removal of phenytoin	53%
3 Similar for both drugs	20%
4 Don't know	10%

I am pleased to say that the majority you were correct. Of the nine patients taking phenytoin six of them had a doubling of the valproate level after it was discontinued, two of them had a 2.5-fold increase, and only one of them showed no change. In the five who were on carbamazepine when the drug was eliminated there was only a very modest increase of about 20% in the level of valproate. So although we think of carbamazepine as a significant inducer, in our experience it is much less problematic to deal with it, rather than phenytoin in combination with valproate.

Dr Duncan *(Chalfont St Peter, UK):* We performed a double blind study of the withdrawal of phenytoin, carbamazepine and valproate, in patients on polytherapy. We looked at the time course of drug interactions fairly carefully and the most important finding with the deinduction was that the changes were complete within one week after the end of the withdrawal of the drug. The only exception was patients taking phenobarbitone who took a lot longer; that obviously reflects the long half life of phenobarbitone.

Professor Mattson *(Connecticut, USA):* That is quite consistent with our observations. We only had one phenobarbitone patient, so we could not comment on that.

Professor Orme *(Liverpool, UK):* Studies that we performed about 10 years ago showed that one of the most important things in deinduction was the length of time on therapy. With regard to protein binding, my view is that protein binding interactions are almost absent in clinical medicine unless you have an inhibitor as well. The rise in free concentrations are not important unless you have got an inhibitor. Valproate, unfortunately, is also an inhibitor and that is why problems arise, but protein binding interactions in general I think can be excluded from most of the pharmacology textbooks.

Professor Mattson: When patients are taking high doses of drug in an effort to get them controlled and are close to the toxic range then the rises and falls in free levels may have a greater effect than you might suspect, but most of the time this is not clinically important.

Overview of the incidence of unwanted effects of antiepileptic drugs

H. Meinardi

Instituut voor Epilepsiebestrijding, Heemstede, The Netherlands

Of the side-effects caused by antiepileptic drugs the following four have probably received most attention in the past decade.

SPINA BIFIDA

The first indication that the association of spina bifida in the child with use of valproate by the mother during pregnancy might be a bigger problem than revealed by different prospective studies on teratogenicity of antiepileptic drugs, came from Robert and Guibaud (1).

Though the information from a case register like the one in Lyon provides an important indication that valproate is associated with the occurrence of spina bifida it is not an absolute indication of the true risks as the size of the cohort of 'pregnant users of valproate' is not known. The causal link is presumed to be a metabolite of valproate or valproate itself (2). Proof that any particular metabolite is responsible is so far lacking. In fact the actual mechanism of interference with proper closure of the spinal column and neural tube is completely unknown. Several authors have suggested that a lack of folic acid might be part of the mechanism (3,4). If so, the likelihood of spina bifida would be greater in the case of mothers using phenytoin. Yet in the Lyon register this association was present less often. There should be more efforts to analyse the mechanism of this malformation. This will not be an easy task. In studying the effect of serum from persons using carbamazepine on cultured rat embryos, Lindhout et al. (5) found a positive association between neural tube closure defects and hyponatraemia while no correlation with either the level of carbamazepine or carbamazepine-epoxide could be demonstrated, though a positive but weaker association with the ratio of epoxide metabolite to carbamazepine was found.

VALPROATE HEPATOXICITY

Another side-effect in the limelight was the occurrence of fatal hepatitis in some patients using valproate. At first reports seemed to derive mainly from Anglo-Saxon countries, suggesting a possible pharmacogenetic aspect. Recently, Scheffner published a series of 16 fatal liver failures in German children on valproate therapy (6). Dreifuss's data (7) suggest that, in particular, children less than two years old on polypharmacy are at risk, with an incidence of 1/1500: this is contested by Scheffner (6).

Several studies have been performed to determine the mechanism of action of valproate hepatotoxicity. Scheffner et al. have suggested that enhanced levels of the 4-ene metabolite of valproate might be associated with fatal liver failure. This, however, has been challenged by Tennison et al. (8). In rats, microvesicular steatosis and mitochondrial swelling in liver cells can be demonstrated on treatment with valproate, particularly if valproate is administered together with an oxidase-inducing drug like phenobarbitone (9). This, however, is contrary to the situation in man, where it seems an idiosyncratic and not a toxic phenomenon.

Fourth international symposium on sodium valproate and epilepsy, edited by David Chadwick, 1989; Royal Society of Medicine Services International Congress and Symposium Series No. 152, published by Royal Society of Medicine Services Limited.

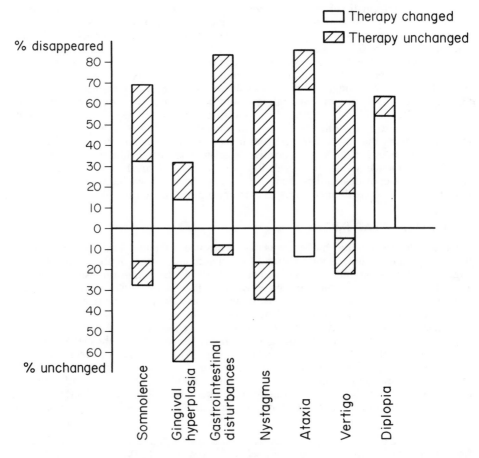

Effects on cognition, I, during treatment; II, after 25% reduction, III, after 50% reduction; IV, after 100% reduction. CBZ=carbamazepine, PHT=phenytoin.

Figure 1   *Cognition: drug effects. (These data were originally published in* Arch Neurol *1988; **45**: 893 (12). Copyright ©1988, American Medical Association. Reprinted by kind permission.)*

Figure 2   *Outcome of common drug reactions. (This figure was originally published in* Epilepsia *1988; **29**: 787–93 (15). Reprinted by kind permission.)*

Perhaps after this meeting new information will permit a clearer view of the risk and appropriate indicators.

COGNITIVE FUNCTION

Emphasis on the social aspects of living with epilepsy has increased concern about cognitive side-effects of antiepileptic drugs. In England, Trimble and co-workers (11) have provided greater insight into the impairment of cognitive function caused by antiepileptic drugs. Gallassi and co-workers (12) recently published the results of neuropsychological testing before and after drug withdrawal in 13 patients on carbamazepine monotherapy and 12 patients on phenytoin monotherapy, both groups being seizure-free for at least two years. To summarize all test results in a single value for each subject, they calculated the mean of all T-scores. This value, called global performance score, was considered to be an indicator of global level of performance. As can be seen from Fig. 1, phenytoin users performed worse than carbamazepine users and only after complete withdrawal did this group perform equal or better than the 26 normal controls matched for age, sex, educational and social level.

Few studies have been performed with respect to the influence of valproate on cognitive function. The pharmacokinetic-pharmacodynamic relationship of valproate makes it difficult to interpret results. Trimble and Thompson (11) found few significant impairments, though volunteers exposed to valproate for two weeks did show a reduced speed on decision-making tasks.

In patients on monotherapy with valproate in whom doses were either increased or decreased, minimal adverse effects were detected and those that are seen (increased decision-making time for the more complex decisions, impairment of immediate recall of pictures, increased visual scanning time and impaired auditory detection) are probably dose related (13).

TOLERANCE

Development of tolerance giving rise to loss of seizure control can also be considered an adverse effect. Benzodiazepines particularly show this phenomenon. However, it is often difficult to distinguish between the development of tolerance and the occurrence of escape. Valproate is not considered a drug to which tolerance develops; relapse after a hitherto unknown period of freedom from seizures in a patient with intractable epilepsy has therefore been classified as escape (14).

Though much attention is paid to the development of tolerance to beneficial effects, tolerance to adverse effects is rarely studied, at least not with respect to the mechanism of action of the drug. In a recent paper the Collaborative Group for Epidemiology of Epilepsy in Milan (15) gave a graphic representation of the outcome of most common adverse drug reactions. As can be seen, an important percentage of adverse drug reactions disappeared though the therapy remained unchanged (Fig. 2).

Side-effects are part and parcel of handling antiepileptic drugs. A drug that is designed to control excessive neuronal discharges apparently is not capable of doing only that. There are always other, dose-dependent, less desirable actions on the CNS.

The importance of side-effects has recently been stressed by Arafeh and Wallace (16). In an important percentage of cases signs of intoxication were reported. However, these data for children include temporary side-effects and also side-effects while first introducing the drug.

In children Herranz et al. (17) have looked at the percentage of users of particular drugs that required cessation of treatment or changes in the treatment regimen and those that could readily tolerate or did not experience adverse effects (Fig. 3). In the case of behavioural changes both positive and negative side-effects were observed. While nearly 61% of phenobarbitone users experienced some untoward effect on behaviour, part of the behavioural changes seen in children taking carbamazepine was due to children with an apparent 'mood elevation' (Fig. 4).

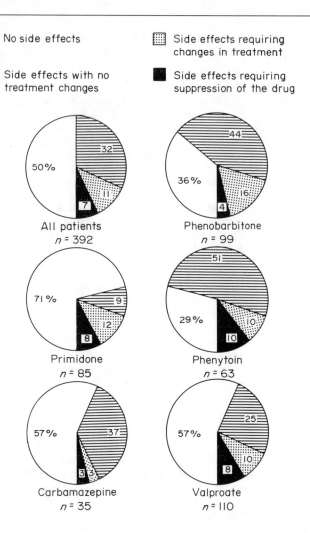

Figure 3 *Changes in treatment required because of drug reactions. (This figure was originally published in* Epilepsia *1988; **29**: 794–804 (17). Reprinted by kind permission.)*

IDIOSYNCRATIC ADVERSE EFFECTS

Toxic side-effects are partly avoidable. Before the general use of drug level determinations it was common practice to increase drug dosages either to an appropriate level to suppress all seizures, or until side-effects became apparent. At present many physicians try to prevent occurrence of side-effects by switching to a second drug when levels approach the toxic range without sufficient effect on seizure control. Also the number of side-effects can be reduced by monitoring the development of metabolic tolerance when introducing a drug for the first time.

Idiosyncratic reactions are by definition dosage-independent. In our Institute, 6.4% of 2649 patients suffered idiosyncratic reactions; 80% of these were allergic skin reactions. Hyponatraemia and gingival hyperplasia were registered as idiosyncratic reactions. Carbamazepine was the drug most often implicated in the allergic skin reactions, but this has to be considered against the frequency with which drugs are prescribed by epileptologists at the Institute. Fig. 5 shows the situation in 1986.

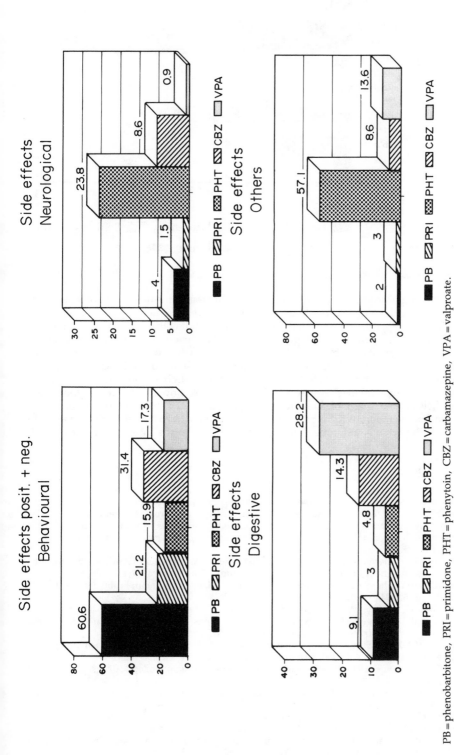

PB = phenobarbitone, PRI = primidone, PHT = phenytoin, CBZ = carbamazepine, VPA = valproate.

Figure 4 *Behavioural and neurological side-effects of anticonvulsant drugs. (These data were originally published in Epilepsia 1988; 29: 794–804 (17). Reprinted by kind permission.)*

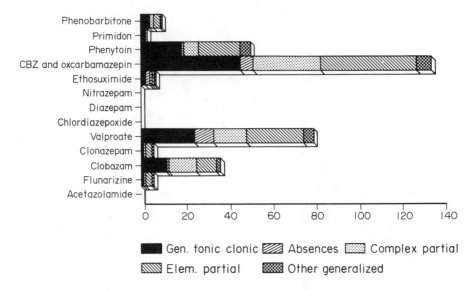

Figure 5   *Drug use 1986 (at the author's Institute, The Netherlands).*

It is surprising how little research is reported on the mechanism of action of side-effects. While studies are ongoing in order to understand the development of tolerance to efficacy of drugs, little work appears to be directed towards understanding the development of tolerance to adverse effects. In particular, complaints about sedation and drowsiness often disappear within weeks after initiation of medication. We neither know why we feel drowsy or sedated, nor why this feeling disappears. Electroencephalographers claim that drowsiness is accompanied by increased synchronization of electroencephalographic (EEG) activity, but our knowledge ends there, because the mechanisms of EEG synchronization are still very hypothetical.

Nevertheless, the mass of knowledge is gradually expanding with an occasional paroxysmal acceleration. No doubt when we have assimilated all the information available at this meeting we will again be better equipped to serve the interests of our patients.

REFERENCES

(1) Robert E, Guibaud P. Maternal valproic acid and congenital neural tube defects. *Lancet* 1982; **ii**: 937.
(2) Lindhout D, Meinardi H, Meijer JWA, Nau H. Antiepileptic drugs and teratogenesis in two consecutive cohorts: changes in prescription policy paralleled by change in pattern of malformations. In: Lindhout D, ed. *Teratogenesis in maternal epilepsy; new aspects of prevention.* Thesis. 1985; 81–105.
(3) Dansky LV, Andermann E, Rosenblatt D, Sherwin AL, Andermann F. Anticonvulsants, folate levels, and pregnancy outcome: a prospective study. *Ann Neurol* 1987; **21**: 176–82.
(4) Smithells RW, Sheppard S, Schorah CJ. Vitamin deficiencies and neural tube defects. *Arch Dis Child* 1976; **51**: 944–50.
(5) Lindhout D, Meijer JWA, Verhoef A, Peters PWJ. Metabolic interactions in clinical and experimental teratogenesis. In: Nau H, Scott WJ Jr, eds. *Interspecies comparison and maternal/ embryonic-fetal drug transfer.* Boca Raton, Florida: CRC Press, 1987; 233–50
(6) Scheffner D, König St, Rauterberg-Ruland I, Kochen W, Hofmann WJ, Unkelbach St. Fatal liver failure in 16 children with valproate therapy. *Epilepsia* 1988; **29**: 530–42.
(7) Dreifuss FE, Langer DH. Hepatic considerations in the use of antiepileptic drugs. *Epilepsia* 1987; **28**: S23–9.
(8) Tennison MB, Miles MV, Pollack GM, Thorn MD, Dupuis RE. Valproate metabolites and hepatotoxicity in an epileptic population. *Epilepsia* 1988; **29**: 543–7.
(9) Sugimoto T, Woo M, Nishida N, Takeguchi T, Sakane Y, Kobayashi Y. Hepatotoxicity in rat following administration of valproic acid. *Epilepsia* 1987; **28**: 142–6.
(10) Shields WD, Saslow E. Myoclonic, atonic, and absence seizures following institution of carbamazepine therapy in children. *Neurology* 1983; **33**: 1487–9.

(11) Trimble MR, Thompson PJ. Anticonvulsant drugs, cognitive function and behavior. *Epilepsia* 1983; **24**: S55–63.
(12) Gallassi R, Morreale A, Lorusso S, Procaccianti G, Lugaresi E, Baruzzi A. Carbamazepine and phenytoin. *Arch Neurol* 1988; **45**: 892–4.
(13) Trimble MR, Thompson PJ. Sodium valproate and cognitive function. *Epilepsia* 1984; **25** (Suppl): S60–4.
(14) Meinardi H, Smits H, Bakhuizen van den Brink R. Clinical significance of tolerance. In: Frey HH, Fröscher W, Koella WP, Meinardi H. *Tolerance to beneficial and adverse effects of antiepileptic drugs*. New York: Raven Press, 1986: 101–8
(15) Collaborative Group for Epidemiology of Epilepsy. Adverse reactions to antiepileptic drugs: a follow-up study of 355 patients with chronic antiepileptic drug treatment. *Epilepsia* 1988; **29**: 787–93.
(16) Abu-Arafeh IA, Wallace SJ. Unwanted effects of antiepileptic drugs. *Dev Med Child Neurol* 1988; **30**: 117–20.
(17) Herranz JL, Armijo JA, Arteaga R. Clinical side effects of phenobarbital, primidone, phenytoin, carbamazepine and valproate during monotherapy in children. *Epilepsia* 1988; **29**: 794–804.

FURTHER READING

Oxley J, Janz D, Meinardi H, eds. *Chronic toxicity of antiepileptic drugs*. New York: Raven Press, 1983; 300 pp.
Schmidt D, ed. *Adverse effects of antiepileptic drugs*. New York: Raven Press, 1982; 240 pp.

Hepatic side effects of valproate

F. E. Dreifuss

Department of Neurology, School of Medicine, University of Virginia Health Sciences Center, Charlottesville, USA

Since valproate (VPA) was introduced as an antiepileptic drug an increasing number of cases of fatal hepatotoxicity coincident with its use have been reported in the medical literature (1–6). At the same time VPA has proved effective as both the sole and adjunct therapy for simple and complex absence seizures and as adjunctive for patients with multiple seizure types that include absence seizures (7–10). Moreover, it is generally regarded as the drug of choice in the management of patients suffering from a primary generalized epilepsy including myoclonic and generalized tonic-clonic seizure types (11–12).

The tendency for VPA to produce various metabolic abnormalities has been described since it was first introduced. However, the clinical significance of effects of mitochondrial dysfunction and its various biochemical alterations have not been clarified. These include hyperammonaemia which may be consequent on increased renal production of ammonia or inhibition of nitrogen elimination secondary to inhibition to urea synthesis. It may be enhanced in the presence of multiple drugs and may be secondary to increased glycine and propionic acid concentrations similar to the mechanism postulated in propionyl CoA carboxylase deficiency (13). Carnitine deficiency may be a contributing factor and frequently accompanies valproate therapy though is rarely of any clinical significance (14). Hyperglycinaemia and hyperglycinuria may occur, again asymptomatically. It is not felt that any of these abnormalities of mitochondrial function are clinical indicators of impending hepatic failure. This complication, however, has been postulated to result from the idiosyncratic transformation of metabolic activity into a pathway resulting in a toxic metabolite. Rettie et al. (15) showed that 2-n-propyl-4-pentenoic acid, a metabolite which is formed via the omega oxidation pathway may be associated with hepatic toxicity. The 4-ene metabolite inhibits both cytochrome P-450 and fatty acid beta oxidation and induces microvesicular steatosis. The 4-ene metabolite production is increased by cytochrome P-450 induction and this in turn occurs with phenobarbital and other enzyme-inducing drugs. It is not generally believed that the detection of the 4-ene metabolite is necessarily a good biochemical indicator of impending hepatic toxicity though it has been found in patients suffering this complication by Scheffner et al. (16) and others.

Dose-related elevations in liver enzymes may occur in over 40% of persons receiving valproate (17). Such elevations are not generally accompanied by clinical symptoms and, in most, the elevations occur in the absence of abnormalities of liver synthetic function such as the production of fibrinogen and of abnormalities in the prothrombin time. They may represent transient enzyme induction.

Hepatic reactions to antiepileptic drugs may occur with drugs other than valproate but probably by a different mechanism. Thus the abnormalities seen with phenytoin and carbamazepine which may also be fatal in more than 10% of persons affected, are usually associated with fever, rash, eosinophilia and a history of a relatively short exposure prior to the onset of symptoms. The liver histology suggests an allergic rather than a toxic phenomenon (18). Hepatic injury in association with valproate may not become clinically apparent early in the course of treatment and the liver

Fourth international symposium on sodium valproate and epilepsy, edited by David Chadwick, 1989; Royal Society of Medicine Services International Congress and Symposium Series No. 152, published by Royal Society of Medicine Services Limited.

histology suggests microvesicular steatosis rather than the consequence of an allergic phenomenon (19).

Because the reported literature up to 1986 did not identify either a biochemical or a clinical risk factor and because of a clinical impression that smaller children appeared to be at higher risk, a study was undertaken to evaluate this and to try to identify which patients were at particular risk of developing fatal hepatotoxicity (17). The first reports from this study identified 37 cases of fatal hepatotoxicity in the United States. There were 47 cases originally reported to the manufacturer. Some of these had not received valproate, others had no relationship between hepatic disease and the valproate and yet others had identifiable familial hepatic problems. Thirty-seven patients revealed a profile of high risk versus low risk of developing fatal hepatic illness coincident with valproate use. It was found that the highest risk existed in children between the ages of 0–2 years who were receiving multiple antiepileptic drugs and who had other medical diseases including mental retardation, congenital abnormalities and other neurological dysfunction. The risk of hepatic fatality in the 0–2 year group on polytherapy was 1 in 500 which was 20 times the overall incidence of fatal hepatic toxicity (1 in 10 000). The overall incidence in patients above the age of two treated with polytherapy was 1 in 12 000 and those over age two treated with monotherapy had a 1 in 45 000 risk. Both the monotherapy and polytherapy patients in the older age group were at considerably less risk than the younger age group and no person over age 10 on monotherapy was reported in the fatality category.

Because enzyme elevations are seen in up to 40% of patients receiving valproate, this was not regarded as a reliable indicator. The initial clinical manifestations of hepatic failure, namely nausea, vomiting, anorexia and lethary and the findings of oedema and jaundice were sinister events as was a sudden loss of seizure control, particularly status epilepticus. Serum elevations more than three times the baseline and the finding of low fibrinogen or an elevated prothrombin time were regarded as important indicators of serious hepatic dysfunction.

The importance of this study was enhanced by the use of a market survey which calculated the denominator for incidence figures by establishing the number of patients receiving anticonvulsant treatment with VPA in a specific period of time and identified monotherapy versus polytherapy groups in age-stratified data. This set the study apart from those which used incidence and prevalence data estimates based on epidemiological data from other contexts.

Following this report, prescribing patterns changed and a decline in the overall number of hepatic fatalities occurred when the survey was repeated for the two years subsequent to the identification of the previously identified high risk group (20). In the follow-up two-year study, four cases were reported in the United States and, though it is conceivable that an occasional death may have occurred and not have come to the attention of the manufacturer, an analysis of the data was consonant with that previously found in terms of identifying a relatively high risk group of children under the age of two years on

Table 1 *Rate of hepatic fatality by age group in patients receiving valproate as monotherapy or polytherapy (1978–1984)*

Age group	Monotherapy			Polytherapy[a]		
	Total patients	Deaths	Rate per 10 M	Total patients	Deaths	Rate per 10 M
0–2	7025	1	1.42	7889	15	19.01
3–10	35 593	4	1.12	39 975	7	1.75
11–20	51 951	0	0	58 348	5	0.86
21–40	59 107	0	0	66 386	4	0.60
41+	34 145	0	0	38 351	1	0.26
Monotherapy total	187 821	5	0.27			
Polytherapy total				210 949	32	1.52
Combined total				398 770	37	0.93

[a]*Other anticonvulsants taken with valproate: phenytoin (17 patients); phenobarbital (16); clonazepam (10); carbamazepine (8); primidone (3); diamox, diazepam, and paraldehyde (2 each); ethosuximide and mesantoin (1 each). (from Neurology **37**: 383 with permission)*

Table 2 *Rate of hepatic fatality by age group in patients receiving valproate as monotherapy or polytherapy,*
(1985–1986)

Age group	Monotherapy			Polytherapy[a]		
	Total patients	Deaths	Rate per 10 M[a]	Total patients	Deaths	Rate per 10 M[a]
0–2	<1188[b]	0	0	<792[b]	1	12.62
3–10	20 702	1[c]	0.48	13 802	2	1.45
11–20	30 226	0	0	20 150	0	0
21–40	33 977	0	0	22 651	0	0
41+	33 848	0	0	22 566	0	0
Total	118 753	1	0.08	79 169	3	0.38
Combined total				197 922	4	0.20

[a]*Number of deaths per 10 000 new and continuing patients.* [b]*Number of treated patients in the 0–2 year old range not perceptible in patient database; to calculate the rate, an estimate of 1% of the total was utilized (estimated total, 1986: monotherapy <1188; polytherapy, <792).* [c]*+Fatality that occurred in 1985 but not reported until 1988.*
(from Neurology 39: 203 with permission)

with a decreasing polytherapy event incidence with increasing age and an absence of monotherapy deaths over the age of 10 years. The accompanying table illustrates this concordance.

Greater use of monotherapy and decreased use of the drug in small children with severe neurological disease may have influenced the fatality rate leading to a nearly three-fold decrease. The occurrence of only one hepatic fatality among the monotherapy patients in the second survey confirms the greater safety of valproate monotherapy over polytherapy though the hepatic fatality rate for the latter has also decreased.

The increased risk of fatal hepatotoxicity in patients receiving valproate with other anticonvulsant drugs may be due to the aberrant cytochrome P-450-dependent metabolism previously referred to. This enzyme activity can be induced by other anticonvulsant drugs such as phenytoin, phenobarbital and carbamazepine.

Some of the familial cases of reported hepatotoxicity with valproate may be cases of familial liver disease and several instances were seen in populations where siblings of affected patients died of fatal hepatotoxicity without ever having been treated with valproate. Such events are exemplified by Alper's disease or progressive hepato-cerebral degeneration (21).

Out of our experience have come several recommendations to minimize the risk of serious reactions: (22)
(1) Avoid the administration of valproate as part of anticonvulsant polytherapy in children under the age of three years unless monotherapy has failed or the potential for benefits of polypharmacy outweigh the risks.
(2) Avoid the administration of valproate to patients with existing liver disease or a family history of childhood hepatic disease.
(3) Administer valproate in the lowest possible dose consistent with seizure control or avoid concomitant administration of valproate and salicylates and avoid fasting in children with intercurrent illnesses.
(4) Monitor clinically for such symptoms as nausea, vomiting, headache, lethargy, oedema, jaundice or seizure breakthrough especially after febrile illness.
If any of these symptoms develop, valproate therapy should be discontinued until a definitive diagnosis is obtained.

It is recommended that enzyme tests of liver function, though proving less predictive of hepatic complications, should continue but should not replace good clinical judgement. Substantial elevations of enzyme values appearing early in the course of treatment might be clinically significant given the predominance of fatalities within the first three months of therapy. It is our recommendation that should the enzyme levels be elevated to three times the baseline level, tests of liver synthetic function such as the prothrombin time of fibrinogen levels should be carried out.

The identification of a high-risk group is of clinical usefulness. On the other hand it should not lead to a false sense of security. The concept of a high risk group is challenged by the findings of Scheffner *et al.* (16) who have presented retrospective data on 16 West German children who died of liver failure while on valproate therapy and reviewed 95 previously reported world-wide cases. However, all of the 16 cases from Germany and more than 90% of the previously reported 95 cases were under 20 years of age and none of the hepatic fatalities in the 16 children in the reported series occurred in patients over the age of 10 years receiving valproate as monotherapy. The majority also had associated mental retardation and/or underlying neurological disease.

While the overall incidence of fatal hepatotoxicity with valproate therapy is rare, the ideal high-risk detection by means of a biochemical marker has so far proved elusive but continues to represent the best chance of achieving the goal which is to keep the risk/benefit ratio to a minimum in the application of one of the most useful available antiepileptic drugs.

REFERENCES

(1) Zimmerman H, Ishak K. Valproate-induced hepatic injury: analysis of 23 fatal cases. *Hepatology* 1982; **2**: 591–7.
(2) Zafrani E, Berthelot P. Sodium valproate in the induction of unusual hepatotoxicity. *Hepatology* 1982; **2**: 648–9.
(3) Jeavons PM. Non-dose-related side effects of valproate. *Epilepsia* 1984; **25**: S50–S55.
(4) Fenichel GM, Greene HL. Valproate hepatotoxicity: two new cases, a summary of others, and recommendations. *Pediat Neurol* 1985; **1**: 109–13.
(5) Rothner AD. Valproic acid: a review of 23 fatal cases. *Ann Neurol* 1985; **10**: 287.
(6) Berkovic SF, Bladin PF, Jones DB, Smallwood RA, Vajda FJ. Hepatotoxicity of sodium valproate. *Clin Exp Neurol* 1983; **19**: 192–7.
(7) Sato S, White B, Penry JK, Dreifuss FE, Sackellares JC, Kupferberg H. Valproic acid versus ethosuximide in the treatment of absence seizures. *Neurology* 1982; **32**: 157–63.
(8) Callaghan N. O'Hare J, O'Driscoll D, O'Neill B, Daly M. Comparative study of ethosuximide and sodium valproate in the treatment of typical absence seizures (petit mal). *Dev Med Child Neurol* 1982; **24**: 830–6.
(9) Covanis A, Gupta AK, Jeavons PM. Sodium valproate: monotherapy and polytherapy. *Epilepsia* 1982; **23**: 693–720.
(10) Ramsay RE. Controlled and comparative trials with valproate: United States. *Epilepsia* 1984; **25** (Suppl): S40–S43.
(11) Chadwick D. Comparison of monotherapy with valproate and other antiepileptic drugs in the treatment of seizure disorders. *Am J Med* 1988; **84** (Suppl 1A): 3–6.
(12) Wilder BJ, Rangel RJ. Review of valproate monotherapy in the treatment of generalized tonic-clonic seizures. *Am J Med* 1988; **84** (Suppl 1A): 7–13.
(13) Wolf B, Paulsen EP, Dreifuss FE. Valproate in the treatment of seizures associated with propionic acidemia. *Pediatrics* 1981; **67**: 162–3.
(14) Ohtani Y, Eudo F, Matsudo J. Carnitine deficiency and hyperammonemia associated with valproic acid therapy. *J Pediatr* 1982; **101**: 782–5.
(15) Rettie AE, Rettenmeier AW, Howard WN, Baillie TA. Cytochrome P450-catalyzed formation of VPA, a toxic metabolite of valproic acid. *Science* 1987; **235**: 890–3.
(16) Scheffner D, König ST, Rauterberg-Ruland I, Kochen W, Hoffmann WJ, Unkelbach ST. Fatal liver failure in 16 children with valproate therapy. *Epilepsia* 1988; **29**: 530–42.
(17) Dreifuss FE, Santilli N, Langer DH, Sweeney KP, Moline KA, Menander KB. Valproic acid hepatic fatalities: a retrospective review. *Neurology* 1987; **37**: 379–85.
(18) Gram L, Bentsen KD. Hepatic toxicity of anti-epileptic drugs: a review. In: Iivanainen MV, ed. Current therapy in epilepsy. *Acta Neurol Scand* 1983; **68** (Suppl 97): 81–90.
(19) Gram L, Bentsen KD. Hepatic toxicity of antiepileptic drugs: a review. *Acta Neurol Scand* 1983; **68** (Suppl 97): 81–90.
(20) Dreifuss FE, Langer DH, Moline KA, Maxwell JE. Valproic acid hepatic fatalities. II. U.S. experience since 1984. *Neurology* 1989; **39**: 201–7.
(21) Egger J, Harding BN, Boyd SG, *et al.* Progressive neuronal degeneration of childhood with liver disease. *Clin Pediat* 1987; **26**: 167–73.
(22) Dreifuss FE. Fatal liver failure in children on valproate. *Lancet* 1987; **i**: 47–8.

Management of the pregnant patient with epilepsy

Part 1: An obstetrician's view

I. G. Robertson

Department of Obstetrics and Gynaecology, Sharoe Green Hospital, Preston, UK

When a woman with epilepsy is referred to the Obstetric Ante-Natal Clinic for booking in early pregnancy, the Obstetrician is faced with the problems of providing adequate control of the seizures by way of appropriate anticonvulsant therapy, and yet minimizing the risk to the foetus. This risk to the foetus may come from either the anticonvulsant drugs or the seizures themselves. This presentation will concentrate on the aspects of maternal care and foetal well-being with regard to the use of anticonvulsant drugs in pregnancy. Pre-pregnancy counselling of epileptic women and the use of anticonvulsant drugs in pregnancy-induced hypertension/eclampsia will not be discussed.

MATERNAL CARE

The principle of good maternal care of epileptic women is to provide adequate control of the seizures with anticonvulsant drugs. The recent 'Confidential Enquiry into Maternal Deaths in England & Wales, 1982–84' (1) highlighted the importance of epilepsy as a contribution to maternal mortality in England & Wales. In order to understand the current importance of epilepsy it is necessary for the reader to look at the maternal mortality figures for the last 150 years. This has been very well reviewed in Chapter 19 of the above mentioned report. Since 1937 there has been a sharp and constant fall in maternal mortality which is due to a multitude of different factors but it remains interesting that maternal mortality continues to halve every 10 years. In the 'Maternal Mortality' report for 1982–84 there were seven women who developed status epilepticus during or immediately after pregnancy. All the women were young (18–32 years) and multiparous. Three deaths occurred during pregnancy and four within four weeks of delivery. All the deaths were attributed to acute asphyxia due to convulsions. All the women were known to have epilepsy at the time of their initial visit to the Ante-Natal Clinic for booking. They were all on anticonvulsant drugs throughout pregnancy. Only one, however, had blood taken for anticonvulsant drug monitoring. The drug concentrations were below the therapeutic range and no action was taken. In two other women the drug concentration was measured at autopsy and found to be below the therapeutic range.

  The histories of the epileptic women who died suggest that most obstetricians and physicians are content to allow pregnant women with epilepsy to continue on the same anticonvulsant therapy prescribed before pregnancy. It is now well known and established that drug concentrations will change during pregnancy despite maintaining the same daily dose and, therefore, it seems unavoidable for doctors involved in the care of epileptic women in pregnancy to carry out regular therapeutic drug monitoring. The measure of the seizure frequency as a prognostic factor does not seem to be satisfactory as two of the women who died from convulsions had had no seizure for more than one year. The number of pregnant women with epilepsy who have died due to convulsions has remained

Fourth international symposium on sodium valproate and epilepsy, edited by David Chadwick, 1989; Royal Society of Medicine Services International Congress and Symposium Series No. 152, published by Royal Society of Medicine Services Limited.

unchanged since 1970 when the figures were first recorded. Major advances have been made in reducing the other causes of maternal death (e.g. hypertension, pulmonary embolism, haemorrhage and anaesthesia). Epilepsy has now emerged as a possible avoidable cause of death in pregnancy and, therefore, general practitioners, obstetricians and physicians/neurologists need to co-operate in providing optimum management for their patients. This will undoubtedly involve monitoring drug concentrations both in the Ante-Natal Clinic and in the puerperium. The cause of death of two of the epileptic women was attributed to having drowned in the bath. Appropriate advice should be given to the patients and their attendants to try and avoid this unnecessary loss of life.

FOETAL WELL-BEING

The principle of management is to minimize the risk to the foetus. The foetus is at risk from both the epileptic convulsions and also the anticonvulsant drug. The affect of the seizures on the foetus can cause hypoxia due to decreased placental blood flow or post-ictal apnoeia.

In Fig. 1 this pregnant woman at term, who was in early labour, suffered a generalized tonic-clonic seizure treated with an oxygen face mask and intravenous diazepam. The seizure was relatively short-lived but the foetal bradycardia persisted for 14 minutes. It is likely that the foetal bradycardia was an indication of foetal hypoxia. This foetal hypoxia may be sufficient to cause significant mental retardation.

It is well documented that there is a 2–3 times risk of physical malformation in children born to epileptic women. These structural abnormalities must be due to an effect during the time of organogenesis in the first trimester of pregnancy (e.g. heart defect, facial clefts, and neural tube defects) and may be due to a number of factors one of which could be the anticonvulsant drug. There is no study which clearly links a specific drug to a particular defect although all drugs have been implicated in the literature in some way or another. It is now 25 years since the first report of abnormal children born to epileptic mothers and no doubt there will be many more in the future. However, until we can establish monotherapy in female epileptic patients and measure the drug concentration in the first trimester we will not be in a position to give definite advice to our patients.

With regard to sodium valproate, this is a popular and effective anticonvulsant drug. It is widely used in the United Kingdom but over the last decade reports have appeared with regard to the association with neural tube defects (spina bifida). It is recommended that in current obstetric practice an epileptic woman attending the Ante-Natal Booking Clinic in early pregnancy is offered screening to check the foetus for possible defects.

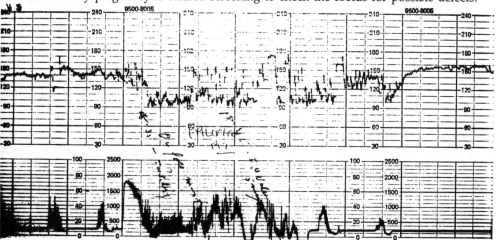

Figure 1 *Intrapartum cardiotocograph of a patient, showing foetal heart deceleration for 14 min following the onset of a grand mal seizure. (Figure originally published in* Clin Obstet Gynecol North Am *1986; 13: 365–84. Reprinted by kind permission.)*

In practice this is done by carrying out an anomaly ultra-sound scan and a maternal serum alpha feto protein. If either of these tests suggest a foetal abnormality then amniocentesis is offered to establish a diagnosis. This will allow, under the present Abortion Act of 1967, for a therapeutic termination of pregnancy to be performed if that is the wish of the parents.

CONCLUSION

In conclusion I wish to alert this Conference to the risks of the seizure to the mother and the baby rather than the previously well published and discussed risk of the anticonvulsant drugs to the foetus. In no way do I underestimate the potential teratogenic effect of any drug taken during pregnancy. However, to establish a well-balanced approach it seems essential to bear in mind the risk to mother and baby of the potentially hazardous effects of a convulsion.

REFERENCES

(1) *Report on confidential enquiries into maternal deaths in England & Wales, 1982–84*. London: HMSO, 1989.

Management of the pregnant patient with epilepsy

Part 2: A neurologist's view

P. Loiseau

Department of Neurology, University Hospital, Pellegrin, Bordeaux, France

The aims of neurologists who look after patients with epilepsy are first, to put an end to seizures, second to render the patient's life as normal as possible.

A prescription of antiepileptic drugs is usually the best way to make a patient seizure free, but in the pregnant patient it is not so simple. Many young women consider that having a child is an important part of normal life, but unfortunately in epileptic patients pregnancy should always be considered a high-risk situation. Friis (1) pointed out that three factors must be taken into consideration:

the desire of the patient to have a child;

the risk of the foetus and the mother being exposed to seizures during pregnancy;

a 2–3 fold increased risk of malformations among the offspring of women with epilepsy One must weigh these three factors differently in different patients.

Neurologists try to control seizures under any circumstances—seizures are not a problem particular to pregnancy. However, all anticonvulsants must be viewed as teratogenic agents.

Before pregnancy there are two possible situations: the patient is either seizure free or not. If a patient has been seizure free for a long time (at least two years) then a cautious interruption of antiepileptic therapy should be considered. In more cases the patient still suffers from seizures or is at risk of relapse during pregnancy and anticonvulsant treatment is necessary.

Neurologists greatly fear the occurrence of seizures in the pregnant patient because of the danger to the mother and to the baby. The risks are obvious for the mother—falling or loss of consciousness may be the cause of domestic or road traffic accidents. Maternal seizures may cause foetal hypoxia with severe effects on the foetus (2). We do not want to stop therapy but it must be adjusted to achieve control or to maintain a low frequency of seizures with a minimal dose of drugs.

Some patients are controlled by unnecessarily high doses of anticonvulsants, either because of overprescribing or because of resistant seizures. Dosage should be reduced to the lowest effective dose. Polytherapy is usually unnecessary and should also be reduced since the more antiepileptic drugs taken by the patient, the higher the risks of malformation in the foetus. Blood levels should be checked regularly, but a decrease in level does not *per se* justify an increase of dosage. It is often a sign of poor compliance because many pregnant women are afraid of taking drugs. This is one of the reasons why prepregnancy and pregnancy counselling is most important.

The role of the neurologist in counselling includes informing the patient on the possible course of epilepsy during pregnancy, although in fact this course is often variable and unpredictable. According to Schmidt (3) the frequency of seizures is reduced in 25%, increased in 25% and unchanged in 50% of cases, and different figures have been published elsewhere.

Counselling should include information on the risk of major malformations, minor anomalies and developmental disturbances. The risk is multifactorial, with genetic, environmental and therapeutic components. As all antiepileptic drugs are weak teratogenic

Fourth international symposium on sodium valproate and epilepsy, edited by David Chadwick, 1989; Royal Society of Medicine Services International Congress and Symposium Series No. 152, published by Royal Society of Medicine Services Limited.

agents, it is not necessary to change a beneficial therapy, and indeed most epileptic women are reluctant to change their medication.

Primary prevention of malformations is by administering a single drug in divided doses, and where possible, as sustained release preparations. For secondary prevention, women should have regular ultrasound examinations and, where sodium valproate is used, amniocentesis is advisable.

In many cases, most of the first trimester, the period of organogenesis, has elapsed when the patient first consults for advice. At that stage one can only reconsider the daily dosages of drugs, with a view to avoiding sedation and drug withdrawal effects during the neonatal period.

It must be stressed, however, that in most cases there is no problem for an epileptic pregnant patient or her child.

REFERENCES

(1) Friis ML. Antiepileptic drugs and teratogenesis. How should patients, doctors and health authorities be counselled? *Acta Neurol Scand* 1984; **Suppl 94**: 39–43.
(2) Teramo K, Hiilesmaa VK. Pregnancy and fetal complications in epileptic pregnancies: review of the literature. In: Janz D, Dam M, Richens A, Bossi L, Helge H, Schmidt D. *Epilepsy, pregnancy and the child*. New York: Raven Press, 1982: 53–59.
(3) Schmidt D. The effect of pregnancy on the natural history of epilepsy: review of the literature. In: Janz D, Dam M, Richens A, Bossi L, Helge H, Schmidt D. *Epilepsy, pregnancy and the child*. New York: Raven Press, 1982: 3–14.

Discussion after Professors Meinardi and Dreifuss, Mr Robertson and Professor Loiseau

Interactive question from Professor Richens

In terms of adverse reactions, monotherapy is better than polytherapy	**Response**
1 Yes	95%
2 No	2%
3 Don't know	3%

Professor Richens *(Chairman)*: An overwhelming majority of people say that mono-therapy is better than polytherapy. I wonder if we will be saying the same in 10 years time in the next epilepsy meeting. Would you like to comment on that Professor Meinardi?

Professor Meinardi (Heemstede, The Netherlands): I quite agree. Recently, Joan Lockhart published a paper on an experimental drug stiripentol which combined well with carbama-zepine, so some people are again looking at polytherapy, but it is too early to comment.

Interactive question from Professor Meinardi

When you administer an antiepileptic drug do you feel you should check haematology, liver and kidney functions on at least a 3-monthly basis?	**Response**
1 During the first year	38%
2 As long as the drug is used	15%
3 Only once after starting the drug	28%
4 Never	19%

Professor Meinardi: I was interested to know what my colleagues thought about that because to catch the adverse reactions by these type of tests is rather difficult. On the other hand never to do these tests is probably the other extreme.

Professor Dreifuss *(Virginia, USA)*: That response is what one might expect among the medico-legally naïve. Those of us who are constantly exposed to litigation continue these blood tests for as long as drugs are used.

Interactive question from Professor Dreifuss

The patient on valproate has an elevation of ALT and AST twice the normal range, what would you do?	**Response**
1 Stop treatment immediately because of the risk of liver failure	16%
2 Undertake a liver biopsy	2%
3 Do nothing but monitor and do clotting studies because it is likely to be transient	82%

Note: ALT = SGOT. AST = SGPT.

Dr Hall *(London, UK)*: Could Professor Dreifuss comment on the various isolated reports of children with other specific inborn errors of metabolism who showed evidence of valproate toxicity.

Professor Dreifuss: The easiest answer is that it is itself an inborn error of metabolism or it is an aberration of normal metabolism with what appears to be an excessive production of the 4-ene metabolite which is the result of cytochrome P450 enzyme induction; on the other hand, there are some reports of ornithine transcarbamylase deficiency which is another potentially fatal hepatic abnormality, and the two may be interacting here, one is precipitating the other.

Dr Pearce *(Hull, UK)*: Following the last two questions, the vast majority of us seem to think that we should check haematology and biochemistry at three-monthly intervals. What are the most common idiosyncratic drug reactions which may be missed by such monitoring?

Professor Meinardi: If there are idiosyncratic reactions, most of them occur during the first month, but some occur many years later. Patients should be warned, and also the general practitioners, that when someone takes antiepileptic drugs certain clinical signs become important, and should be acted upon while in case of a non-drug user it would be appropriate to wait.

Dr Duncan *(London, UK)*: Professor Dreifuss, we know that in some people there is an increase in ammonia levels when they are treated with valproate. Would it be worth measuring ammonia before and shortly after starting valproate as a predictive test for who may be at increased risk of developing severe hepatotoxic reactions to the drug?

Professor Dreifuss: The majority of patients on valproate show an increase in their ammonia levels and a decrease in their carnitine levels that are not predictive of anything in particular.

Interactive question from Professor Richens

In a young woman with juvenile myoclonic epilepsy what would be your drug of first choice?	**Response**
1 Phenytoin	1%
2 Carbamazepine	3%
3 Sodium valproate	92%
4 None of these	4%

Most of us seem to agree that sodium valproate is the drug of choice.

Interactive question from Professor Richens

A woman says that she wishes to become pregnant, she wants to have a family during the next year. Would you like to choose a drug.	**Response**
1 Phenytoin	1%
2 Carbamazepine	9%
3 Sodium valproate	65%
4 None of these	24%

The pattern has changed slightly; the number of people who would prescribe valproate has reduced and the number who would prescribe none has gone up. Professor Loiseau would you like to comment on that. Should we or shouldn't we be using Epilim in young women who want to become pregnant?

Mr Robertson *(Preston, UK):* When a patient comes to my antenatal clinic I counsel her about the potential teratogenic effects of valproate, I arrange a scan checking the anterior abdominal wall and the neural tube, I arrange a maternal serum α-feto protein to ensure that is within normal range. If there is any problem with either of those investigations I arrange a diagnostic amniocentesis. If that is abnormal I explain it to the patient and if she wishes, I offer her a prostaglandin termination of pregnancy.

Professor Richens *(Chairman):* Will your investigations pick up all patients at risk?

Mr Robertson: The ultrasound scan nowadays will pick up 90–95% simply on a single 16-week ultrasound carried out by a well-trained radiographer. In the hands of people slightly more expert, that might rise to 98%. It is very rare for a neural tube defect to be missed.

Professor Jeavons *(Birmingham, UK):* In my experience a great number of patients with juvenile myoclonic epilepsy cease to have their myoclonic attacks when they become pregnant. I think one has to consider the type of seizure when you are advising. In a number of patients who are on sodium valproate I advise them, if they wish to become pregnant, to stop the sodium valproate beforehand in order to avoid spina bifida, because by the time they know they are pregnant it is too late. I give this advice to a number of specific patients, depending on the type of seizure.

Professor Richens *(Chairman):* When does the therapeutic effect of pregnancy begin?

Professor Jeavons *(Birmingham, UK):* I can not answer that, but I think it is reasonable risk, particularly if patients have been absolutely free from seizures for a long period of time. However, I tell all these patients that they must restart their Epilim prior to delivery because of the higher risk at that point.

Dr van Oorschot *(The Netherlands):* I would suggest that Mr Robertson advise his pregnant epileptic patients not only to unlock the bathroom door, but to take a shower because more epileptic patients drown in the bath than in the swimming pool, and if someone has a seizure during a bath, even when the door is unlocked it is very hard to get them out of the tub without aspiration.

Mr Robertson: This is a difficult area because many ladies like to have a bath after childbirth and would not take my advice to have a shower, some Health Authorities do not have showers in their lying-in wards because women sometimes trip over getting in there. I know of one case where the woman was advised not to go in the bath, she was advised to have a shower and that if she did go into any room at all to leave it unlocked. She decided not to take the advice of any of her attendants and regrettably she died, so advice does not always work.

Dr Kyllerman *(Sweden):* Dr Jeavons comment on the risk of treatment is well taken. I am presently caring for two children with a meningomyclocoele secondary to the mother having had valproate treatment during pregnancy in ordinary dosages and serum levels. These patients are severely affected with mental retardation, upper extremity malformations, they are hypotonic and of low intelligence. Furthermore, there is probably a spectrum of disorder. There are three more patients born to the same mother, one of them with a spastic one-sided monoparethesis and the other two, twins, with definite signs of a fetal valproate syndrome and psychomotor retardation. This is much larger problem than has been appreciated and has to be considered in the risk benefit ratio for treatment during pregnancy.

Mr Robertson: Would those lesions not have been picked up by the obstetrician antenatally?

Dr Kyllerman: Yes they would, but sometimes parents choose to have their children born, and sometimes the damage is done in the first six to eight weeks of gestation when the women do not realize that they are pregnant. This information must be given to fertile women before pregnancy.

Mr Robertson: You are advocating prepregnancy counselling and I fully agree with you.

Dr Kyllerman: That is right, and especially necessary when the pregnancy is planned rather than accidental.

Professor Loiseau *(Bordeaux, France):* In such cases the pregnancy may be compared to a clinical trial, and as in a clinical trial there must be fully informed consent from the mother.

Dr Fenwick *(London, UK):* It is not uncommon for those of us who work in epilepsy clinics occasionally to have a sudden death. Is the rate of sudden death that you have given for pregnant women higher or lower than the overall rate for sudden death among women who are not pregnant?

Mr Robertson: I cannot answer that. The point I am trying to make is that as other maternal causes of death decline, suddenly epilepsy has arrived at the point where it is very important. And we need to look at this more carefully than we have done in the past.

Hyperammonaemia and the use
of antiepileptic drugs, including valproate

J. Hulsman

Epilepsy Centre, Kempenhaeghe, Heeze, The Netherlands

INTRODUCTION

The choice of an antiepileptic drug (AED) is based mainly on its efficacy against a certain seizure type. This is not the only criterion, however, since a definitive selection for an individual patient has to be based on the balance between efficacy and side-effects occurring with the drug, as side-effects may significantly affect the quality of life for the patient.

The more patients treated with AED, the more side effects are reported. Care should be taken, however, in interpretation of the reported adverse effects, as in many cases it may not be clear whether and to what extent the relationship with drug treatment is causal.

With this background in mind it is of interest to look into the phenomenon of hyperammonaemia (1,2,3) connected with the use of valproate (VPA). Since hyperammonaemia is observed in certain hepatic disorders, hyperammonaemia occurring simultaneously with the use of VPA is often considered as an indication of hepatotoxicity of the drug.

Careful review of the literature indicates that hyperammonaemia is most commonly found when concomitant AEDs are used together with VPA.

METHODS

Patients (aged 7–68 years) attending our epilepsy clinic were randomly selected, and were divided into subgroups based on therapy as described in Table 1. There was an almost equal number of men and women in each group. There were no clinical signs or laboratory indications of liver disease. All patients were on a stable dosage for at least three months prior to the investigation. Blood samples were obtained by venepuncture before food or medication intake. After venepuncture patients received a standard meal containing 30 g milk protein (Meritene, Wander, Brussels) followed by blood sampling at 60 min and 90 min. Serum ammonium values and concentration(s) of AED were estimated according to procedures described in laboratory methods.

Besides the patients a control group of 52 healthy volunteers, not on medication, was studied following the same protocol.

Table 1 *Description of the patient group: Age, VPA dose per 24 h. Percentage of patients having a serum value above the norm of SGOT, SGPT, gamma-GT and AP*

Medication	Age (y) Mean	Age (y) Range	VPA dose (mg) Mean	VPA dose (mg) Range	SGOT	SGPT	γ-GT	AP
					% above reference value			
VPA mono	30.2	(7–68)	1365	(600–2000)	5	9	27	9
AED–VPA	27.8	(13–56)	—	—	0	0	48	10
VPA+AED	29.6	(15–57)	1950	(900–3600)	2	2	55	5

Fourth international symposium on sodium valproate and epilepsy, edited by David Chadwick, 1989; Royal Society of Medicine Services International Congress and Symposium Series No. 152, published by Royal Society of Medicine Services Limited.

Laboratory methods

Ammonia (NH_3) is in equilibrium with ammonium ions (NH_4+)

$$NH_3 + H_3O^+ \leftrightharpoons NH_4^+ + H_2O$$

The amount of free ammonia depends on the concentration of protons (H^+) in the environment. The pH of this equilibrium is 7.24, which means that at physiological pH of 7.40 the concentration of free NH_3 is 2% of the concentration of NH_4^+. Ammonia passes across the cell membrane causing toxic side effects, which NH_4^+ does not.

In the laboratory, however, NH_4^+ is estimated, which means that the literature data correlating ammonium levels with side-effects only can be interpreted when the pH is measured simultaneously. In this study hyperammonaemia indicates the sum of NH_3 and NH_4^+. For this reason no attempt is made to correlate ammonium values with observed side-effects.

Ammonium values were assessed by an enzymatic method (4) using glutamate dehydrogenase and alpha-ketoglutarate as substrate (Boehringer, Mannheim, Germany).

After venepuncture, samples were centrifuged and frozen immediately in order to eliminate falsely elevated values. Concentration of VPA was assessed by gas-liquid chromatography (4% FFAP–140 °C) after extracting the serum with tetrachloromethane, using cyclohexane carboxylic acid as an internal standard.

RESULTS

Ammonium values are presented in Table 2 and Figs 1 and 2.

Fasting ammonium concentrations

There is no significant difference in ammonium levels between the VPA monotherapy and the group on AED without VPA. The group on VPA and concomitant AED has a significantly elevated mean ammonium value compared to volunteers and patients on VPA monotherapy and patients receiving AEDs other than valproate. There is a significant different between volunteers and patients receiving valproate.

Twenty-one per cent of patients on VPA monotherapy had elevated NH_4^+ values (>35 μmol/l) compared with 22% of patients on AED without VPA. Forty-six per cent of patients on polypharmacy including VPA show a percentage of elevated ammonium levels.

Table 2 *Ammonium values (mean $\pm$ SE) in fasting patients and after standard protein meal*

Medication		Ammonium (fasting) mean		Ammonium (after protein) mean	
		μmol/l	SE	μmol/l	SE
Controls	($n=$ 52)	17.9	8.5	23.9	11.2
CBZ	($n=$ 20)	21.2	6.1	25.7	10.6
PHT	($n=$ 6)	19.8	13.1	17.5	14.3
CBZ+PHT	($n=$ 17)	23.2	8.9	31.3	11.3
CBZ+PHB	($n=$ 4)	16.5	7.7	30.3	12.0
Polypharmacy excl. VPA	($n=$ 23)	23.9	12.0	28.3	13.0
AED—therapy without VPA	($n=$ 70)	22.2	9.8	27.5	12.0
VPA	($n=$102)	24.1	12.8	39.3	19.8
VPA+CBZ	($n=$ 93)	36.2	21.7	67.1	40.4
VPA+CBZ+PHT	($n=$ 67)	39.3	23.6	78.3	48.2
VPA+ >3 AED	($n=$114)	37.0	21.1	71.1	46.4
VPA+1 or more AED	($n=$274)	37.3	21.9	71.5	44.9

Groups are specified in numbers of patients and type of medication. VPA = valproate, CBZ = carbamazepine, PHT = phenytoin, PHB = phenobarbitone.

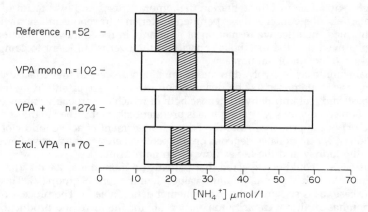

Figure 1 *Comparison of ammonium values in four groups: Healthy volunteers (reference). Patients on monotherapy VPA (VPA mono). Patients on VPA and one or more other AED (VPA+). Patients on one or more AED without VPA (VPA−). The solid lines represent values of the mean ± SE. The striped area represent the confidence limits of the group mean (<0.05).*

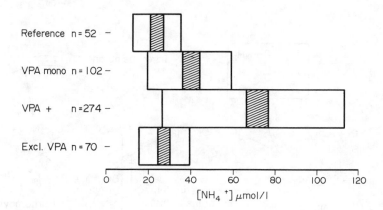

Figure 2 *Comparison of ammonium values after standard protein load. Identification of patient groups as in Fig. 1.*

Ammonium concentrations after a protein load

Volunteers and patients received a protein-rich meal under standard conditions. It was found that approximately 90 min after intake ammonium values reached a maximum. The control group showed a small increase in the mean ammonium value results compared to fasting values (Table 2). The VPA-monotherapy group had higher values than the reference group, and the polypharmacy group without VPA showed similar ammonium values to the control group. The VPA and comedication group however, had ammonium values far higher than the controls (Fig. 2).

DISCUSSION

Elevated serum ammonium values may be explained by increased formation of ammonia or decreased metabolism. The main source of production is deamination of amino acids taking place in different tissues (kidney, skeletal muscle and the colon (5)). Warter *et al.* (6) demonstrated that an important source of ammonia production is located in the renal tubule cells. Selective catheterization showed the ammonium concentration in the vena renalis to be higher by a factor of three than in the femoral artery, and by a factor of 10 than in the hepatic vein. Repetition of the experiments after an intravenous infusion with 1500 mg VPA confirmed the selective formation of ammonia in the kidney, stimulated by VPA. It further proved that the metabolic capacity of the liver is sufficient to compensate for the excess production of ammonia.

The main amino acids involved in the deamination process in the renal tubule cells are glutamine and glutamic acid. The deamination reactions are catalyzed by the enzymes glutaminase and glutamic dehydrogenase both of which are probably enhanced by VPA. The question still remains why ammonia is preferentially reabsorbed in the venous blood, since the pH of the primary urine, the other compartment of active inflow of ammonia, is much lower. Much probably depends on competition between the relative flows of venous blood in the kidney and the lesser flow of primary urine.

On this basis it could be expected that patients on monotherapy with VPA (Group B) would present much higher ammonium values than the control group (V). This, however, is not the case, as is shown in the experimental data (Table 2). The process of ammonia elimination has sufficient capacity to compensate for the increased production. Only in approximately 20% of cases was the metabolic rate smaller than the production of ammonia.

We stimulated the production of ammonia by giving a standardized protein load. Healthy volunteers receiving a standard protein meal show increased ammonium values ($p < 0.01$)

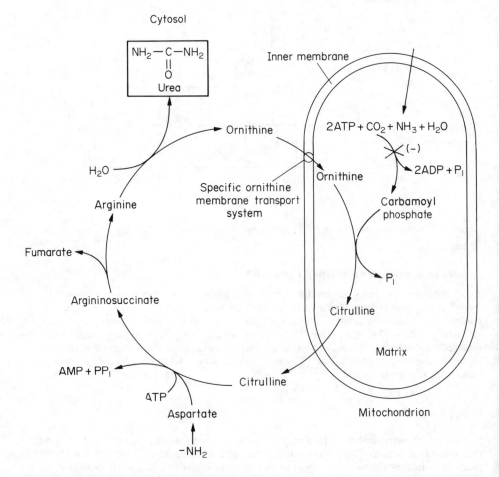

Figure 3 *Ornithine cycle, with special interest of the first step taking place in the mitochondrion. The first step is inhibited by propionate ($-$).*

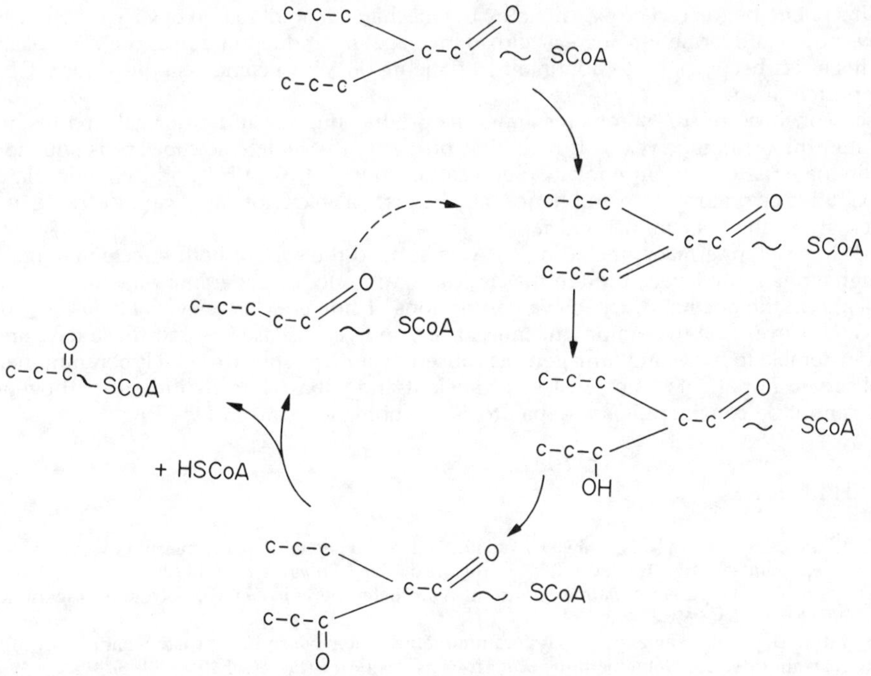

Figure 4 *Pathway of β-oxidative degradation of VPA. The process is iterated as indicated by the dotted arrow finally resulting in two moles prionyl-S CoA and one mole acetyl-S CoA.*

as compared to their fasting values (Table 2). These values are considered to be reference values after protein load, with an upper limit of 46 μmol/l. Patients in Group B show an increase in ammonium levels after protein load, compared to the mean value of the reference group (V) after protein load ($p<0.01$). It therefore seems that VPA elevates ammonia production, for which the metabolic capacity can only partly compensate, especially when there is a higher protein intake.

In order to explain this it is necessary to discuss the elimination process.

Ammonia is metabolized in the ornithine cycle, beginning in the liver mitochondria (Fig. 3). The first reaction step $NH_3 + CO_2 + ATP$ is complex and is catalysed by carbamoyl-phosphate transferase (CPT). When this enzyme (CPT) is partly deficient, hyper-ammonaemia occurs (7,8). Furthermore, CPT may be inhibited by several compounds, among which is propionate, a degradation compound of VPA. The metabolism of VPA is interesting, with regard to the influence of concomitant antiepileptic drugs. VPA is metabolized by beta- and omega-oxidation. Beta-oxidation leads to a meta-bolic pathway as demonstrated in Fig. 4. Since VPA is a branched-chain fatty acid this pathway finally yields two molecules propionate and one molecule acetate per mole VPA. The acetate is introduced into the citric acid cycle in the form of acetyl-thionyl-CoA and is thus completely eliminated. The propionate molecules are eliminated slowly by renal clearance. All types of (co)-medication that induce beta-oxidation of VPA, such as carbamazepine, phenytoin and phenobarbitone may cause accumulation of propionate and hence inhibition of CPT, leading to decreased rate of ammonia elimination. In this respect it is interesting to study patient data concerning concomitant AED.

From these data it is clear that in fasting patients using AEDs without VPA (Group A) the ammonium levels are only slightly higher than in the control group of healthy volunteers (V). When the patients in Group A receive a protein load the mean value of ammonium in the group stays almost constant. The group of patients receiving VPA and comedication (Group C) show significantly higher fasting ammonium values than the control group (V) or the monotherapy VPA (Group B).

This phenomenon can be explained by the mechanism of inhibition of CPT activity caused by propionate formed by increased oxidative enzyme induction due to the comedication. This effect becomes quite dominant in patients on VPA+comedication (Group C) after a protein load.

In conclusion, VPA stimulates ammonia production, but under normal circumstances, when the ornithine cycle is functioning properly, the metabolic capacity is sufficient to eliminate the excess ammonia. Comedication such as CBZ, PHT and PHB stimulate the oxidative enzyme system and hence may be responsible for a significant decrease in CPT activity in the liver mitochondria.

When polypharmacy, including VPA, is applied the sum of both effects may result in high ammonium levels, though the clinical significance of hyperammonaemia is far from clear. On the one hand, extensive descriptions of side-effects are available in cases of so-called irreversible hyperammonaemia in certain liver diseases (9) but these data are not transferable to hyperammoniagenesis caused by antiepileptic drugs. Hyperammonaemia observed in patients using AEDs is transient and is based on a different pathogenesis. It cannot be considered as a hepatotoxic phenomenon caused by VPA.

REFERENCES

(1) Iinuma K, Hayasaka K, Narisawa K, Tada K, Hori K. Hyperamino-acidaemia and hyperammonemia in epileptic children treated with valproic acid. *Eur J Pediatr* 1988; **148**: 267–9.
(2) Laub MC. Hyperammonämie Während Valproate-Therapie bei Kindern und Jugendlichen. *Nervenartz* 1986; **57**: 314–8.
(3) Ettlin Th, Scollo-Lavizarri G. Hyperammonämie unter Natriumvalproatebehandlung: klinisch relevant oder ein Nebenbefund. *Schweiz Rundschau Med (PRAXIS)* 1986; **29**: 881–5.
(4) Da Fonveca-Wollheim F. Bedeutung von Wasserstoffionen Konzentration und ADP-Zusatz bei der Ammoniak-bestimmung mit Glutamatdehydrogenase. *Z Klin Chem Klin Biochem* 1973; **11**: 421–6.
(5) Kvamme E. Ammonia metabolism in the CNS. *Prog Neurobiol* 1983; **20**: 109–32.
(6) Warter JM, Brandt C, Marescaux C, *et al.* The renal origin of sodium valproate-induced hyperammonemia in fasting humans. *Neurology* 1983; **33**: 1136–40.
(7) Hjelm M, Oberholzer V, Seakins J, Thomas S, Kay TDS. Valproate-induced inhibition of urea synthesis and hyperammonemia in healthy subjects. *Lancet* 1986; **ii**: 859.
(8) Tripp JH, Hargreaves T, *et al.* Sodium valproate and ornithine carbamoyltransferase deficiency. *Lancet* 1981; **i**: 1165–6.
(9) Conn HO, Lieberthal MM. *The hepatic coma syndromes and lactulose*. Baltimore: Williams and Wilkins, 1979.

Anticonvulsants, thyroid and other endocrine functions

R. T. Jung

Ninewells Hospital and Medical School, Dundee, UK

Long-term administration of anticonvulsant drugs is well known to affect blood thyroid hormone levels (1–6). Both phenytoin and carbamazepine reduce the serum levels of total thyroxine (T_4), triiodothyronine (T_3), free T_4, free T_3 and, in some, reverse triiodothyronine (rT_3). Thyroid binding globulin (TBG), prealbumin and thyroid stimulating hormone (TSH) are usually unaltered. Sodium valproate depresses thyroid hormone levels to a lesser degree. In a recent study of 71 adults on various anticonvulsant monotherapies, total T_4 was within the normal range in 85% of patients on sodium valproate but in only 40% on carbamazepine or phenytoin (7). Free T_4 was within the normal reference range in more patients, namely, in 95% of those on sodium valproate, in 70% on carbamazepine and in 65% on phenytoin. There was no significant difference in the distribution of normal TSH results between anticonvulsants; 90% on sodium valproate or on carbamazepine, 94% on phenytoin.

It is well known that a free T_4 level below the normal reference range is usually not associated with an elevated basal serum TSH level and that the patient appears euthyroid. Nevertheless, symptoms due to the side-effects of the anticonvulsant drug such as weakness, fatigue, lack of motivation, constipation and sedation may be difficult to discriminate from those due to hypothyroidism. There is also a small number of patients in whom abnormalities of TSH do occur (8) and cases of reversible hypothyroidism induced by phenytoin and carbamazepine have been reported (9). Therefore, two questions arise, namely, why serum free T_4 can be below normal but the patient remains euthyroid and why do anticonvulsants differ in their ability to reduce free T_4?

Although the above three anticonvulsants can displace T_4 from TBG this does not appear to be the major reason for the depressed thyroid hormone levels seen in patients on therapeutic dosages. This is illustrated by the work of Franklyn et al. (10). Phenytoin added to normal serum in vitro to reproduce a therapeutic phenytoin concentration of 12.5 μg/ml, increased free T_4 by only 6.5% from 21.7 to 23.1 pmol/l. If the phenytoin added was increased to reproduce a toxic level of 50 μg/ml then displacement increased by 41% to 30.7 pmol/l. This contrasted with the situation in 31 euthyroid patients with therapeutic phenytoin levels (7 to 17 μg/ml) where total T_4 was reduced by 40%. Larsen et al. (11) has calculated that phenytoin given to man in therapeutic dosages is about 10-fold more effective in lowering T_4 than would be predicted from its in vitro potency for displacing T_4 from its serum protein binding sites. This lack of any significant displacement as a cause of the reduced serum T_4 would explain why both T_4 and T_3 thyroid uptakes are unaltered and why tests of T_4 binding capacity to TBG are also unchanged (or only just slightly decreased) at therapeutic anticonvulsant levels of sodium valproate, carbamazepine or phenytoin.

If T_4 displacement from TBG happened to be the only reason for the reduced serum total T_4 then one would have difficulties in explaining why free T_4 levels are also reduced. The reason for the latter is that the anticonvulsants accelerate hormone clearance by hepatic enzyme induction at therapeutic anticonvulsant levels. This has been demonstrated by

Fourth international symposium on sodium valproate and epilepsy, edited by David Chadwick, 1989; Royal Society of Medicine Services International Congress and Symposium Series No. 152, published by Royal Society of Medicine Services Limited.

measuring two indirect indices of hepatic enzyme induction, namely antipyrine clearance and the urinary excretion of D-glucaric acid both of which are increased with enzyme induction (12). Patients treated with carbamazepine, phenytoin, primidone and phenobarbitone show increased values for the above two indices. The relative potency at average dose levels for antipyrine clearance is phenobarbitone 1, phenytoin 0.92, carbamazepine 0.84 and primidone 0.82. D-glucaric acid excretion is also significantly higher in patients on carbamazepine compared with phenytoin.

Whether sodium valproate causes hepatic enzyme induction has been argued for some time. Certainly, in the above work, sodium valproate (see Table 1) increased mean antipyrine clearance by an insignificant 19% but D-glucaric acid excretion was elevated 94% on average, although even this failed to reach statistical significance. These indices are limited in their capacity to predict accurately enzyme induction. Although sodium valproate does not appear to increase cytochrome P450 content, aniline hydroxylase or aminopyrine-N-demethylase activity in rodents, it is an effective inducer of hepatic 8-aminolaevulinic acid synthetase in the rat and chick embryo and can also markedly increase porphyrin and cytochrome P450 concentration in chick embryo's hepatocytes (12,13). There are also anecdotal reports of sodium valproate precipitating acute attacks of porphyria (14) and markedly elevating both antipyrine clearance and D-glucaric acid excretion in individual patients (12). Nevertheless, it is clear that any enzyme-stimulating effect of sodium valproate is appreciably less than with other anticonvulsants and this possibly accounts for the differences in serum thyroid hormone levels observed.

Serum T_3 is decreased less than serum T_4 by anticonvulsants. The available evidence suggests that this is not due solely to preferential enhanced monoiodination of T_4 to T_3 in the liver (15). Whereas Hufner and Knopfle (16) reported a twofold increase in T_3 production from T_4 in rat liver homogenates, Kaplan et al. (17) did not detect any significant changes in T_4 to T_3 conversion rate in both liver and anterior pituitary homogenates of phenytoin treated rats. The unaltered or slightly reduced serum rT_3 levels in patients on anticonvulsant therapy is also unlikely to be due to any preferential monodeiodination to rT_3 but due to enhanced degradation of rT_3. This decremental difference of T_3 compared to T_4 is also unlikely to be due to a relative increased thyroidal T_3 secretion, for carbamazepine treated hypothyroid subjects on T_4 replacement have unaltered T_4 to T_3 ratios (18). The most likely explanation is that the anticonvulsants nonspecifically enhance the metabolism of T_4, T_3 and rT_3, with T_3 metabolism being enhanced less than T_4 (15).

The paradox of a reduced serum total T_4 and T_3 in patients who are euthyroid is understandable if free T_4 and free T_3 remained unaltered. However, this is often not the case. So why are patients with a low free T_4 and/or low free T_3 not hypothyroid—or are they? A diagnostic index such as that of Crooks Wayne suggests that the patients are euthyroid clinically (7). This is supported by unaltered 4 and 25 h thyroidal I^{131} uptakes and unaltered resting metabolic rate measurements (15,19). Serum cholesterol and triglyceride have been reported elevated in patients on phenytoin (20) but this does not necessarily indicate hypothyroidism since phenytoin can affect hepatic metabolism and may inhibit insulin secretion, both of which would increase lipid levels (21). Basal serum TSH is often reported unchanged by anticonvulsant therapy, again suggesting a euthyroid state. Nevertheless, a rise in serum TSH has been reported in the initial stages

Table 1   *Mean indices of drug metabolizing capacity on various anticonvulsants (from data of Perucca et al. (12))*

| Anticonvulsant | Antipyrine kinetics | | D-glucaric acid excretion nmol/kg/24 h |
	Clearance ml/h/kg	Half-life h	
Controls (nil)	47	11.2	90
Sodium valproate	56	9.7	175
Carbamazepine	83	5.9	1030
Phenytoin	92	5.5	565
Phenobarbitone	98	4.8	1020

of anticonvulsant medication with carbamazepine, phenytoin or phenobarbitone (6). In one such report, the serum TSH rose by day 4 of therapy, peaked by day 20 and then fell to pre-treatment levels (5). A marked rise in TSH (from 5 to 21 μU/mol) has been reported in anecdotal cases of under-replaced thyroxine treated hypothyroid patients (8) but not in those on adequate or more than adequate thyroxine replacement (18).

The reason why those patients with a low free T_4 and low free T_3 are not hypothyroid has yet to be adequately explained. One explanation is that the anticonvulsant may have a slight thyroid agonistic effect (15). This has been suggested for phenytoin although there is a fine dividing line between phenytoin's action as a thyroid agonist at low concentrations and as a potent antagonist at higher concentrations. The agonist action is suggested by experiments in the induction of the liver cytosolic malic enzyme (22). If phenytoin is injected into athyreotic rats, malic enzyme activity is increased 2.2-fold within 48 h; this compares to a 31.5-fold increase induced by T_3 in the same studies. Hence phenytoin has about 4% of the effect of T_3 on the induction of malic enzyme. However, increasing phenytoin concentration antagonises the action of T_3 as shown by using the model of cultured GC cells wherein growth hormone (GH) production is regulated by T_3; increasing concentrations of phenytoin inhibit and eventually abolish GH production induced by T_3 possibly by inhibiting T_3 entry into the cells (15,23,24).

The anticonvulsants phenytoin and carbamazepine have also been reported to have a marked influence at the hypothalamus-pituitary level. Thyrotrophin releasing hormone (TRH) is suppressed at the hypothalamic level as is TRH-stimulated TSH in the pituitary. These drugs have also been reported to induce a hypothalamic type TSH response to TRH in some and hence may blunt the usual hyperdynamic rise in TSH to TRH observed if hypothyroidism ensued with anticonvulsant therapy. Sodium valproate, an inhibitor of gamma aminobutyric acid (GABA) transaminase, does not appear to affect significantly the prolactin and TSH dynamics to TRH (200 μg) or metoclopramide when given chronically for 6 months (26). Likewise, acute administration of sodium valproate does not affect the usual rise of TSH to TRH although variable prolactin responses have been reported (26,27,28). One does wonder if the stereochemical similarity of carbamazepine and phenytoin to each other and in the linked diphenyl groups with T_4 may explain the differences between these anticonvulsants and sodium valproate on the TSH responsiveness of the hypothalamic-pituitary axis (5). Nevertheless, sodium valproate can have a marked effect on the secretion of other hypothalamic-pituitary hormones, especially growth hormone (GH) and corticotrophin (ACTH).

The effect of sodium valproate on GH shows marked differences between acute and chronic administration. Acute sodium valproate administration does not affect the GH response to TRH (29), levodopa or insulin-induced hypoglycaemia (30,31). Short-term administration (3 to 7 days) attenuates the GH response to diazepam, insulin, hypoglycaemia and physical exercise but not to levodopa (30,32,33,34). Chronic administration for 6 months significantly reduces the GH response to levodopa and attenuates, but not to a statistically significant extent, the GH rise to growth hormone releasing hormone (GHRH) (26). Nevertheless, Invitti et al. (26) have reported reversible growth arrest in one patient on sodium valproate which was associated with abolition of the GH response to levodopa and GHRH which were both normal before treatment, indicating that the above observations may have profound clinical relevance in growing children. This effect on GH of sodium valproate is in contrast to that observed with other anticonvulsants. Chronic phenytoin administration has no effect on the GH response to clonidine but actually increases the GH response to diazepam, glucagon or levodopa (32,36). On the other hand, chronic carbamazepine therapy does not alter the GH responsiveness to glucagon, diazepam or clonidine (36).

Abraham et al. (31) reported no effect of sodium valproate on ACTH and cortisol responses to insulin induced hypoglycaemia in normal subjects treated with sodium valproate for three weeks. However, recently, Invitti et al. (26) have reported a progressive attenuation of the ACTH and cortisol responses to metyrapone and corticotrophin releasing hormone (CRH) with chronic sodium valproate therapy over six months, although urinary free cortisol and morning cortisol levels were not significantly altered, hence the clinical importance in chronic epileptic patients is, as yet, not fully apparent. Recent research, however, suggests that sodium valproate does not alter the hypothalamic-pituitary-gonadal axis in males in contrast to that observed with phenytoin and carbamazepine. Both the latter anticonvulsants reduce blood dehydro-epiandrosterone sulphate levels and increase sex hormone binding globulin whereas carbamazepine has been reported by some but not others to reduce free testosterone and increase basal luteinizing hormone levels (37,38). This may be clinically relevant for epileptic men often report reduced libido and impairment of sexual function (37).

In *conclusion*, one has to be cautious in assessing hypothyroidism in patients receiving anticonvulsant therapy, especially if on phenytoin and carbamazepine, but less so on sodium valproate. In monitoring one should measure free T_4 and not total T_4. TSH measured alone would also give a certain degree of discrimination but in the light of the known suppressant action of carbamazepine and phenytoin on the hypothalamic and pituitary TSH release possibly free T_4 should always be measured and if below the reference range then basal TSH and the possibility of a TRH test may be indicated. Until we have a reliable method of assessing peripheral intracellular thyroid maintenance, the question of whether some degree of hypothyroidism, albeit mild, is present in patients on anticonvulsant therapy must remain an open and tantalizing question. Finally, the apparent minimal effect of sodium valproate on thyroid function compared with the other anticonvulsants should be tempered with the realisation that sodium valproate may cause other hypothalamic-pituitary alterations, the significance of which is only now being investigated and understood.

REFERENCES

(1) Liewendahl K, Majuri H. Thyroxine, triiodothyronine and thyrotropin in serum during long term diphenyl hydantoin therapy. *Scand J Clin Lab Invest* 1976; **36**: 141–4.
(2) Liewendahl K, Majuri H, Helenius T. Thyroid function tests in patients on long term treatment with various anticonvulsant drugs. *Clin Endocr* 1978; **8**: 185–91.
(3) Fichsel H, Knopfle G. Effects of anticonvulsant drugs on thyroid hormones in epileptic children. *Epilepsia* 1978; **19**: 323–36.
(4) Yeo PPB, Bates D, Howe JG, *et al*. Anticonvulsants and thyroid function. *Br Med J* 1978; **1**: 1581–3.
(5) Rootwelt K, Ganes T, Johannessen SI. Effect of carbamazepine, phenytoin and phenobarbitone on serum levels of thyroid hormones and thyrotropin in humans. *Scand J Clin Lab Invest* 1978; **38**: 731–6.
(6) Bentsen KD, Gram L, Veje A. Serum thyroid hormones and blood folic acid during monotherapy with carbamazepine or valproate. *Acta Neurol Scand* 1983; **67**: 235–41.
(7) Connacher AA, Borsey DQ, Browning MCK, Davidson DLW, Jung RT. The effective evaluation of thyroid status in patients on phenytoin, carbamazepine or sodium valproate attending an epilepsy clinic. *Postgrad Med J* 1987; **63**: 841–5.
(8) Blackshear JL, Schultz LA, Napier JS, Stuart DD. Thyroxine replacement requirements in hypothyroid patients receiving phenytoin. *Ann Intern Med* 1983; **99**: 341–2.
(9) Aanderud S, Strandjord RE. Hypothyroidism induced by anti-epileptic therapy. *Acta Neurol Scandinav* 1980; **61**: 330–2.
(10) Franklyn JA, Sheppard MC, Ramsden DB. Measurement of free thyroid hormones in patients on long term phenytoin therapy. *Eur J Clin Pharmac* 1984; **26**: 633–4.
(11) Larsen PR, Atkinson AJ, Wellman HN, Goldsmith RE. The effect of diphenyl hydantoin on thyroxine metabolism in man. *J Clin Invest* 1970; **49**: 1266–79.
(12) Perucca E, Hedges A, Makki KA, *et al*. A comparative study of the relative enzyme inducing properties of anticonvulsant drugs in epileptic patients. *Br J Clin Pharmac* 1984; **18**: 401–10.
(13) Bonkowsky HL, Sinclair PR, Emery S, Sinclair JF. Seizure management in acute hepatic porphyria: Risks of valproate and clonazepam. *Neurology* 1980; **30**: 588–92.
(14) Garcio Merino JA, Lopez-Lozaro JJ. Risks of valproate in porphyria. *Lancet* 1980; **ii**: 856 (letter).
(15) Smith PJ, Surks MI. Multiple effects of diphenyl hydantoin on the thyroid hormone system. *Endoc Rev* 1984; **5**: 514–24.
(16) Hufner M, Knopfle M. Pharmacological influences in T_4 to T_3 conversion in rat liver. *Clin Chim Acta* 1976; **72**: 337.
(17) Kaplan MM, Brietbart R, Larsen PR, Tatro JB, Appiah A. Effects of phenytoin on thyroxine 5′ deiodinase in rat liver and anterior pituitary. *Clin Res* 1980; **28**: 261A.
(18) Aanderud S, Myking OL, Strandjord RE. Influence of carbamazepine on thyroid hormones and thyroxine binding globulin in hypothyroid patients substituted with thyroxine. *Clin Endoc* 1981; **15**: 247–52.

(19) Oppenheimer JM, Fisher LV, Nelson KM, Jailer JW. Depression of the serum protein bound iodine level by diphenylhydantoin. *J Clin Endocrinol Metab* 1961; **21**: 252–62.

(20) Pelkonen R, Fogelholm R, Nikkila EA. Increase in serum cholesterol during phenytoin treatment. *Br Med J* 1975; **4**: 85.

(21) Malherbe C, Burrill KC, Levin SR. Karam JM, Forsham PM. Effect of diphenyl hydantoin on insulin secretion in man. *N Engl J Med* 1972; **286**: 339–42.

(22) Mann DN, Kumara-Siri MK, Surks MI. Response of hepatic enzymes to L triiodothyronine and diphenyl hydantoin. *Endocrinology* 1983. **112**: 1732–8.

(23) Gingrich SA, Smith PS, Shapiro LE, *et al.* Diphenyl hydantoin (phenytoin) attenuates the action of 3,5,3' triiodothyronine in cultured GC cells. *Endocrinology* 1985; **116**: 2306–13.

(24) Zemel LR, Biezunski DR, Shapiro LE, Surks MI. Diphenyl hydantoin decreases the entry of 3,5,3 L triiodo-L-thyronine but not L thyroxine in cultured GH producing cells. *Acta Endocrinol (Copenh)* 1988; **117**: 392–8.

(25) Surks MI, Ordene KW, Kumara-Siri MH, Mann DN. Effect of diphenylhydantoin on TSH secretion in man and in the rat. *J Clin Endocrinol Metab* 1983; **56**: 940–5.

(26) Invitti C, Danesi L, Dubini A, Cavagnini F. Neuroendocrine effects of chronic administration of sodium valproate in epileptic patients. *Acta Endocrinol (Copenh)* 1988; **118**: 381–8.

(27) Elias AN, Szekeres AV, Stone SC, Valenta LJ, How T, Ascher MS. GABAergic and dopaminergic mechanisms in gonadotrophin secretion in males—effects of baclofen and metoclopramide. *Acta Endocrinol (Copenh)* 1983; **103**: 451–6.

(28) Melis GB, Mais V, Paoletti AM, Antenori D, de Ruggiero A, Fioretti P. GABAergic control of anterior pituitary function in humans. In: Racagni G, Danoso AO, eds. *GABA and endocrine function.* New York: Raven Press, 1986: 219–42.

(29) Personal observation.

(30) Koulu M, Lammentousta R, Dahlstrom S. Effects of some GABAergic drugs on the dopaminergic control of human growth hormone secretion. *J Clin Endocrinol Metab* 1980; **51**: 124–9.

(31) Abraham RR, Darnhorst A, Wynn V, *et al.* Corticotrophin, cortisol, prolactin and growth hormone responses to insulin induced hypoglycaemia in normal subjects given sodium valproate. *Clin Endocrinol* 1985; **22**: 639–44.

(32) Koulu M, Lammintausta R, Kangas L, Dahlstrom S. Effect of methysergide, pimozide and sodium valproate on the diazepam stimulated growth hormone secretion in man. *J Clin Endocrinol Metab* 1979; **48**: 119–22.

(33) Steardo L, Iovino M, Monteleone P, Agrusta M, Orio F. Pharmacological evidence for a dual GABAergic regulation of growth hormone release in humans. *Life Sci* 1986; **39**: 979–85.

(34) London DR, Loizou LA, Butt WR, Rovei V, Bianchetti G, Marselli PL. Effects of anticonvulsant drugs on hormonal responses in normal volunteers. In: Johannessen SI, ed. *Antiepileptic therapy: Advances in drug monitoring.* New York: Raven Press, 1980: 405–10.

(35) Dornhorst A, Jenkins JS, Lamberts SWJ, *et al.* The evaluation of sodium valproate in the treatment of Nelson's syndrome. *J Clin Endocrinol Metab* 1983; **56**: 985–91.

(36) Crawford PM, Belchetz P, Davies C, Chadwick D. Growth hormone response to diazepam, clonidine and glucagon in patients with epilepsy. *Epilepsy Res* 1989; **3**: 63–9.

(37) Macphee GJA, Larkin JG, Butler E, Beastall GH, Brodie MJ. Circulating hormones and pituitary responsiveness in young epileptic men receiving long term antiepileptic medication. *Epilepsia* 1988; **29**: 468–75.

(38) Isojarvi JIT, Myllyla VV, Pakarinan AJ. Effects of carbamazepine on pituitary responsiveness to luteinising hormone-releasing hormone, thyrotropin releasing hormone and metoclopramide in epileptic patients. *Epilepsia* 1989; **30**: 50–6.

Discussion after Drs Hulsman and Jung

Interactive questions from Dr Hulsman

1. Do you agree that valproate may originate or cause hyperammonaemia mainly in patients using polypharmacy with antiepileptic drugs? **Response**
   1 Yes 95%
   2 No 5%

2. If you found a blood ammonia level twice that of the upper limit of the normal range in a child who had just started on sodium valproate what would you do? **Response**
   1 Stop the drug 15%
   2 Continue but observe 65%
   3 Don't know 19%

Professor Richens *(Chairman):* So there you are Dr Hulsman, most people would continue, but observe. Is that right?

Dr Hulsman *(Heeze, The Netherlands):* I agree with that. We have to decide whether we use arterial or venous values and we have to know at what time and in what position the blood sample was taken because there is a normal range, of say, an increase by a factor of two or three after food intake, mainly caused by protein. So even when you find increased values you need not necessarily consider this as a hepatotoxic phenomenon.

Professor Richens: So that is a predictable adverse effect which occurs very commonly, but there is severe hyperammonaemia which may be associated with a deficiency of enzymes in the liver.

Dr Hulsman: Patients on valproate plus antiepileptic drugs may have values of approximately five to ten times the normal range, which can be correlated with side effects, but it does not indicate hepatoxicity as I have shown in my paper.

Dr Sundqvist *(Sweden):* As we know valproate is the first drug of choice in atonic, tonic-clonic seizures and myoclonic seizures. We have become increasingly aware during recent years of the mitochondrial cytopathy and its disorders. What would Dr Hulsman advise us to do about the use of valproate in these disorders?

Dr Hulsman: With a metabolic disorder at this level I would prefer not to use a branched chain fatty acid with an odd number of carbon atoms like valproate. However, there is a small percentage of branched chain fatty acids in food also, so even when you do not use valproate you can run into hepatic troubles.

Interactive questions from Dr Jung

1.	When monitoring for hypothyroidism in epilepsy would you	**Response**
	1 Consider it sufficient to measure total serum thyroxine	2%
	2 Pick up most cases by measuring free T_4 and TSH	90%
	3 T_4	8%

2.	Do you monitor thyroid function in your patients after starting drug therapy, in the absence of possible clinical signs of thyroid dysfunction?	**Response**
	1 Always	5%
	2 Sometimes	25%
	3 Never	70%

Professor Richens: Apparently most of us never measure thyroid function in our epileptic patient starting on drug therapy. Is that right, or should we be doing it?

Dr Jung *(Dundee, UK):* I would certainly measure thyroid function if a patient was complaining of symptoms such as weakness, fatigue, constipation, sedation, but of course these are not exclusive to hypothyroidism for antiepileptic therapy may also produce such symptoms. May I suggest that all new cases referred, thyroid function is checked and that is probably quite sufficient during long-term surveillance unless something happens which changes your clinical decision.

Professor Richens: Now that we know a little more about the mechanisms we may be more inclined to do so. I have found low T_4s on many occasions in euthyroid patients and therefore I have stopped measuring them as a routine. But obviously there are some patients we should look at very specifically.

Dr Price *(Swindon, UK):* Can Dr Jung explain why he found a discrepancy between the TRH tests and the sensitive TSH in isolation in those patients who had low free T_4s on anticonvulsants, as you would expect them to measure the same thing.

I think it has been shown that the effects of sodium valproate in improving the features of Nelson's Syndrome are not due to specific effect of the valproate itself, but simply to the fact that the drug increases cortisol levels and a group in London has shown that when cortisol replacement is given, cortisol levels are higher on valproate than when the patient is not on valproate, and this is the reason that ACTH levels and the features of Nelson's syndrome are improved. A similar effect probably occurs in patients with Cushing's syndrome taking metyrapone since another study has shown that levels of 11-deoxycortisol are increased when sodium valproate is added in to metyrapone at the same time as their cortisol levels fall. It is probably inhibition of hepatic metabolism leading to increased metyrapone levels that causes the improvement.

Dr Jung: I quite agree you might expect to see the TSH baseline up in 6 or 7 mU/l range when you find a hyperdynamic response; we do not always find that.

The second question is most interesting. I too have read those papers but I have seen morning ACTH values falling from over 1000 down to about 60 on sodium valproate, and when I have measured the hydrocortisone levels in the blood stream there are not elevated unduly and I therefore wonder whether the above is a true reflection of its action. There are also patients in whom sodium valproate has no effect on the elevated ACTH level. I think one has to leave that as an open question.

SESSION V

RECENT DEVELOPMENTS WITH VALPROATE

Chairman: L. Gram

Pharmacokinetics of a newly developed sustained release form of sodium valproate

J. Barre[1] and Y. Berger[2]

[1]Laboratoire Hospitalo-Universitaire de Pharmacologie, Centre Hospitalier Intercommunal de Créteil, France and [2]Sanofi-Recherche, Montpellier, France

INTRODUCTION

The activity of sodium valproate and valproic acid in the treatment of different forms of epilepsy is now well established (1). In order to obtain an optimal therapeutic index (efficacy versus side effects), a good stability of valproic acid levels in the body is required within dosing intervals. Two to three daily intakes of the dosage forms currently available on the market throughout the world are mandatory to achieve this goal.

A sustained release dosage form (LA 40220 SRF) has been developed by Sanofi in order to reduce the number of daily doses, to improve patient compliance and to maintain the concentration within the optimum range over a 24 h period with minimum fluctuations. The purpose of this article is to review the pharmacokinetic properties of this sustained release form in comparison with the enteric-coated Depakine® tablet currently marketed in France.

SINGLE DOSE STUDY

The aim of this investigation was to compare the pharmacokinetic properties as well as the relative bioavailability of LA 40220 SRF versus Depakine at three dose levels.

The study was carried out with 18 healthy volunteers divided into three groups containing six subjects each. Group I, II and III received a single dose of 0.5, 1 and 2 g of sodium valproate respectively, administered with each form (LA 40220 SRF and Depakine). In each group, the two forms were administered in a randomized cross-over design with a wash-out interval of one week. All subjects fasted overnight and for an additional 4 h after drug dosing. Blood samples were collected until 72 h post-administration.

Total and free concentrations were assayed with the EMIT System® (homogeneous enzyme immunoassays) (Syva Co, Palo Alto). Free levels could be measured after isolation by ultrafiltration using the EMIT Free Level® System.

The pharmacokinetic profiles are given in Figure 1. The pharmacokinetic parameters are summarized in Table 1. The values of Tmax of LA 40220 SRF are twice as great as those observed with Depakine. On the contrary, LA 40220 SRF exhibits significantly lower Cmax as compared with Depakine, whatever the dose. No lag time was observed with the sustained release form unlike the results with Depakine. LA 40220 SRF shows an increase of AUCo-∞ and plasma concentrations proportional to the dose whereas this is not the case for Depakine (Fig. 2). LA 40220 SRF exhibits a profile of total valproic acid concentration vs time which is much more regular than that of Depakine. In addition LA 40220 SRF does not yield high peaks of free valproic acid level unlike Depakine (Fig.3).

Fourth international symposium on sodium valproate and epilepsy, edited by David Chadwick, 1989; Royal Society of Medicine Services International Congress and Symposium Series No. 152, published by Royal Society of Medicine Services Limited.

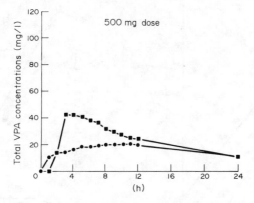

Figure 1a *Mean plasma levels of total VPA after administration of LA 40220 SRF (●) and enteric coated Depakine (■).*

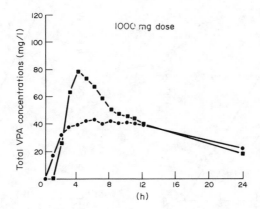

Figure 1b *Mean plasma levels of total VPA after administration of LA 40220 SRF (●) and enteric coated Depakine (■).*

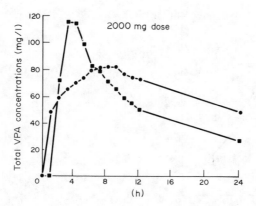

Figure 1c *Mean plasma levels of total VPA after administration of LA 40220 SRF (●) and enteric coated Depakine (■).*

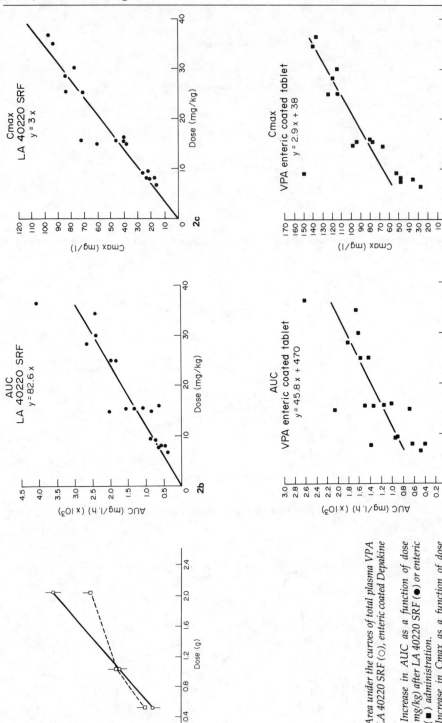

Figure 2a *Area under the curves of total plasma VPA versus dose. LA 40220 SRF (○), enteric coated Depakine (□).*

Figure 2b *Increase in AUC as a function of dose (expressed in mg/kg) after LA 40220 SRF (●) or enteric coated VPA (■) administration.*

Figure 2c *Increase in Cmax as a function of dose (expressed in mg/kg) after LA 40220 SRF (●) or enteric coated VPA (■).*

Table 1 *Pharmacokinetic parameters measured after single administration of three doses: 500, 1000 and 2000 mg of Depakine and LA 40220 SRF*

	Tmax (h)		
Dose (mg)	500	1000	2000
Depakine	4.3 ± 0.7	3.7 ± 0.4	3.2 ± 0.2
LA 40220 SRF	9.8 ± 0.7	8.0 ± 1.3	7.7 ± 0.4
Wilcoxon's Test	$p < 0.01$	$p < 0.01$	$p < 0.01$
	Cmax (mg/l)		
Dose (mg)	500	1000	2000
Depakine	45.2 ± 3.9	82.0 ± 4.4	124.8 ± 4.6
LA 40220 SRF	21.7 ± 1.7	50.3 ± 5.6	86.2 ± 4.1
ANOVA	$p < 0.005$	$p < 0.005$	$p < 0.005$
	AUCo-∞ (mg/l)		
Dose (mg)	500	1000	2000
Depakine	788.4 ± 151.6	1283 ± 190	1784 ± 173
LA 40220 SRF	614.5 ± 67.7	1238 ± 205	2554 ± 328
ANOVA	NS	NS	$p < 0.005$

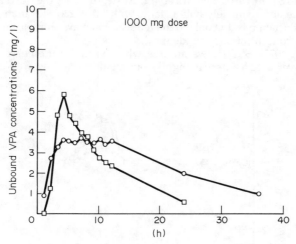

Figure 3a *Time course of unbound VPA levels after administration of LA 40220 SRF (○) and enteric coated Depakine (□).*

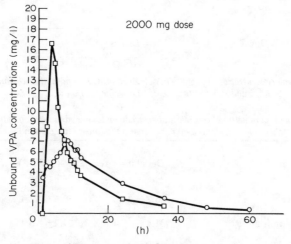

Figure 3b *Time course of unbound VPA levels after administration of LA 40220 SRF (○) and enteric coated Depakine (□).*

This first study showed that the sustained-release form has some potential advantage over the enteric-coated Depakine tablet owing to AUCo-∞ of total drug proportional to the dose and regular distributions of total and free drug levels as well as the cut-down peaks of free concentrations of valproic acid.

MULTIPLE DOSE STUDIES

The pharmacokinetic profile of valproic acid was investigated after multiple dosing of sodium valproate administered as LA 40220 SRF (0.5 g twice a day), in comparison with Depakine (0.5 g twice a day).

Sixteen healthy subjects received daily over an 8 day period either LA 40220 SRF or Depakine twice a day (0.5 g at 8 a.m. and 0.5 g at 8 p.m.) in a cross-over study design. After the morning intake on days 7 and 8, blood samples were withdrawn and valproic acid levels were determined by gas-liquid chromatography with a flame ionisation detector.

Figure 4 shows the time course of valproic acid levels observed on days 7 and 8 after the morning intake of the two forms. Pharmacokinetic parameters calculated 12 h after the dose (8 a.m. to 8 p.m.) are listed in Table 2. At steady state, the fluctuations of plasma concentrations are approximately half as large with LA 40220 SRF than with Depakine. This decrease in fluctuation is due only to the reduction in maximum plasma concentrations since the trough concentrations are identical.

In addition LA 40220 SRF shows an area which is under the curve of total plasma concentrations over a 12 h interval slightly but significantly lower ($p < 0.01$) than that

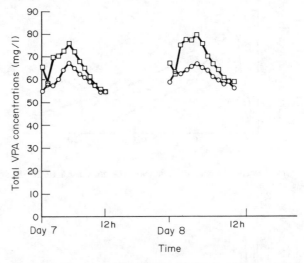

Figure 4 *Mean plasma concentrations of total VPA obtained at day 7 and 8 after chronic administration of 0.5 g LA 40220 SRF (○) b.i.d and 0.5 g enteric-coated Depakine (□) b.i.d.*

Table 2 *Pharmacokinetic parameters of valproic acid at steady-state after administration for 8 days of LA 40220 SRF and Depakine (500 mg of sodium valproate twice a day)*

	Depakine	LA 40220 SRF	Statistical significance
Css,max mg/l	88.2± 15.2	69.6± 12.8	ANOVA $p < 0.001$
Css,min mg/l	56.7± 16.6	55.5± 12.4	ANOVA N.S.
Css,max – Css,min mg/l	31.4± 8.4	14.2± 6.4	ANOVA $p < 0.001$
AUC12h mg/l	832 ±182	746 ±162	ANOVA $p < 0.01$

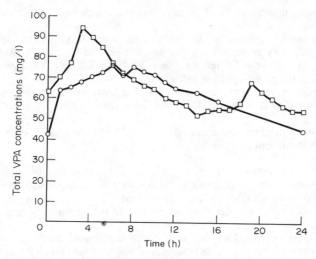

Figure 5   *Mean plasma levels of total VPA after 10 days of administration of 1 g LA 40220 SRF (○) once a day and 0.5 g enteric coated Depakine (□) b.i.d.*

Table 3   *Pharmacokinetic parameters of valproic acid after administration for 10 days of 1 g LA 40220 SRF once a day versus Depakine 500 mg twice a day.*

	Depakine	LA 40220 SRF	Statistical significance
Css,max mg/l	95.2± 15.8	81.6± 15.8	ANOVA $p < 0.005$
Css,min mg/l	54.3± 16	44.7± 9.6	ANOVA $p = 0.05$
Css,max – Css,min mg/l	40.9± 11.4	36.9± 13.7	ANOVA N.S.
AUC 24 h mg/l	1572 ±285	1486 ±249	ANOVA N.S. Westlake confidence intervals : 14%

of Depakine. The oral bioavailability of valproic acid is slightly lower after LA 40220 SRF administration than after Depakine intake, but this slight decrease is acceptable for a sustained release form.

In the light of these results, another investigation was conducted in order to evaluate the time course of valproic acid plasma levels after a once a day administration of LA 40220 SRF (1 g of sodium valproate), in comparison with a twice a day administration of Depakine 500 mg tablet.

Twelve healthy subjects received for 10 days either 1 g LA 40220 SRF at 8.00 a.m. or 500 mg Depakine twice a day (8 a.m. and 8 p.m.) in a cross-over study. On day 10, plasma levels of valproic acid were determined by gas liquid chromatography.

The plasma levels obtained after both regimens are depicted in Fig. 5. As shown in Table 3, LA 40220 SRF yielded lower Css,max ($p < 0.005$) and Css,min ($p = 0.05$), whereas no significant differences were found with plasma level flucations (Css,max–Css,min) and with AUC over 24 h.

DISCUSSION

LA 40220 SRF tablets exhibited pharmacokinetic behaviour meeting the requirement of a sustained release form since the comparison with the regular-release enteric-coated form Depakine showed:

— a comparable bioavailability at steady-state during chronic administration,
— no lag time,
— a 50% decrease in Cssmax/Cssmin fluctuations owing to a lowered Cssmax when 0.5 g LA 40220 SRF was given twice a day as compared to 0.5 g of Depakine twice a day,
— similar Cssmax/Cssmin fluctations when 1 g LA 40220 SRF was given once a day as compared to 0.5 g of Depakine twice a day,
— plasma drug levels at a steady state swinging between 40 and 80 mg/ml over a 24 h dosing interval after a once a day administration of 1 g of LA 40220 SRF.

The pharmacokinetic characteristics of LA 40220 SRF may offer several advantages in the long-term treatment of epilepsy:

— single daily dose administration in common epilepsies, improving compliance,
— easier management of treatment owing to the proportional dose-concentration relationship that facilitates dosing adjustment,
— easier monitoring of plasma drug levels due to the greater stability of valproic acid concentrations,
— and because peaks of total and free drug concentrations are cut down, a better protection against concentration-related side-effects of valproic acid (such as tremors) (2) and/or side-effects of commonly associated drugs such as phenytoin (3) may be expected.

NOTE

The studies reviewed in this article were conducted under the responsibility of Drs A. Brachet Liermain (Bordeaux, France), H. Jaeger (Neu Ulm, West Germany) and J. P. Tillement (Paris-Créteil, France).

REFERENCES

(1) Chadwick D. Comparison of monotherapy with valproate and other antiepileptic drugs in the treatment of seizure disorders. Am J Med 1988; 84 (Suppl 1A): 3–6.
(2) Dreifuss FE, Langer DH. Side effects of valproate. Am J Med 1988; 84 (Suppl 1A): 34–41.
(3) Bourgeois BF. Pharmacologic interactions between valproate and others drugs. Am J Med 1988; 84 (Suppl 1A): 29–33.

Sustained release valproate versus conventional formulation valproate. A study of the tolerance and efficacy of LA 40220

Th. Rentmeester and J. Hulsman

Epilepsy Centre, Kempenhaeghe, Heeze, The Netherlands

INTRODUCTION

Valproate is an effective drug in the treatment of patients suffering from primary generalized epilepsy, while it is also effective in other epileptic syndromes (1–5). In general, valproate is well tolerated, yet a considerable number of patients complain of side-effects (6). There are indications that the side-effects are caused by the degree of serum level fluctuations (7). The pharmacokinetic properties of valproate and the comparatively short half-life can result in considerable inter-individual variations in plasma concentrations.

With the enteric-coated form of valproate, the resorption peak occurs between 0 and 5 h (8). As a result of competitive protein binding interactions with comedication may occur and the fluctuating serum-level results in fluctuation of the comedication. Although treatment with monotherapy is to be preferred, an estimated 20% of the patients with epilepsy are treated with polytherapy (9). This study investigates efficacy and tolerance of the sustained release form of valproate (LA 40220 = Depakine Chrono) in patients treated with monotherapy and polypharmacy.

MATERIALS AND METHODS

Thirty patients suffering from epilepsy were treated with valproate (Fig. 1); 10 patients received valproate monotherapy, six patients received a combination of valproate and

VPA mono	7 female, 3 male	:	M1–M10
	Age range	:	25–55 years
	Age mean	:	35.4 years
	Height range	:	156–194 cm
	Weight range	:	49–90 kg
	Seizure type	:	9 PG, 1 PSG.
VPA + PHT	2 female, 3 male	:	P1–P5
	Age range	:	24–36 years
	Age mean	:	28.6 years
	Height range	:	172–184 cm
	Weight range	:	61–99 kg
	Seizure type	:	1 PG, 4 CP, 1 SG
VPA + CBZ	5 female, 7 male	:	C1–C12
	Age range	:	24–36 years
	Age mean	:	36.1 years
	Height range	:	156–181 cm
	Weight range	:	53–87 kg
	Seizure type	:	3 PG, 7 CP, 2 SG

Figure 1 *Patient characteristics. PG = Primary generalized seizures. CP = complex partial seizures. SG = Secondary generalized seizures.*

Fourth international symposium on sodium valproate and epilepsy, edited by David Chadwick, 1989; Royal Society of Medicine Services International Congress and Symposium Series No. 152, published by Royal Society of Medicine Services Limited.

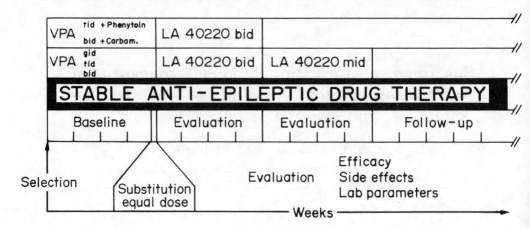

Figure 2 *Flow chart.*

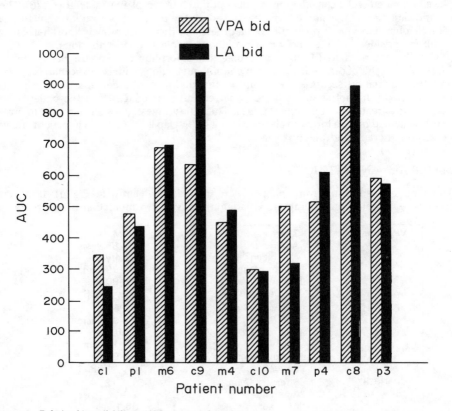

Figure 3 *Relative bioavailability. AUC = area under curve.*

carbamazepine. Twelve patients suffered from primary generalized epilepsy, four from secondary generalized epilepsy, and 12 from partial epilepsy. One patient had a combination of primary generalized and complex partial epilepsy.

After a baseline period of four weeks in which the doses of valproate were administered 1–4 times a day, the conventional formulation of valproate was replaced by LA 40220 twice daily for four weeks. During this period any comedication was unchanged. Most of the patients were subsequently admitted to a follow-up study of one year. After each period

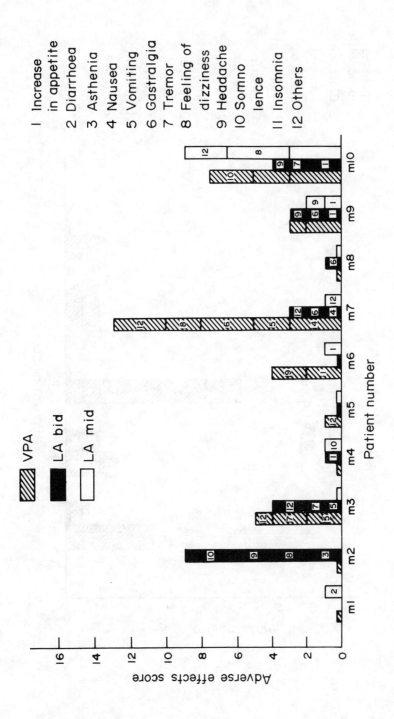

Figure 4 *Adverse effects in valproate monotherapy.*

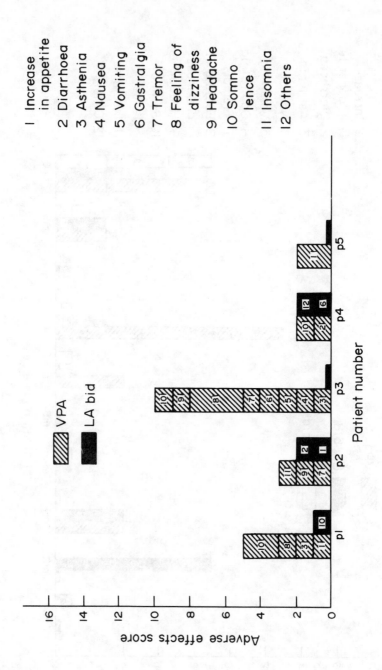

1 Increase
  in appetite
2 Diarrhoea
3 Asthenia
4 Nausea
5 Vomiting
6 Gastralgia
7 Tremor
8 Feeling of
  dizziness
9 Headache
10 Somno
   lence
11 Insomnia
12 Others

Figure 5 *Adverse effects in valproate and phenytoin therapy: Patients' subjective assessment.*

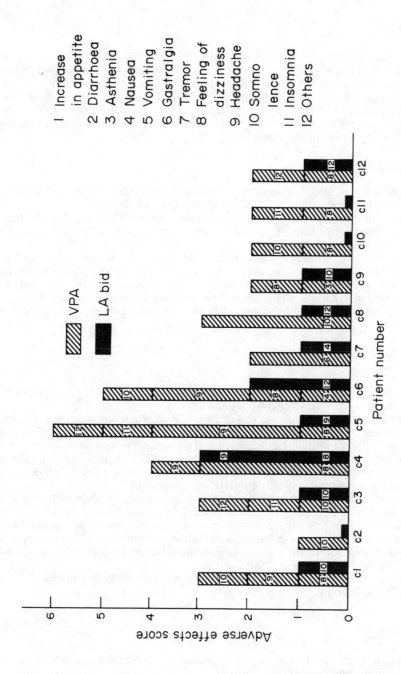

Figure 6 *Adverse effects in valproate and carbamazepine therapy: Patients' subjective assessment.*

of four weeks serum levels of the drug were measured every 2 h over a 12 h period (Fig. 2). Patients were asked in consultation to assess subjective symptoms and side-effects.

RESULTS

It appeared from the pharmacokinetic studies that the relative bioavailability of LA 40220 did not differ substantially in comparison with the conventional formulation (Fig. 3). This did not depend on whether the conventional dose was administered 1, 2, 3 or 4 times a day, compared with twice daily LA 40220. With the long-acting formulation the peak level islower than with the conventional formulation, while the trough levels are identical. The appearance of the peak level is predictable with LA 40220 and usually occurs within 2 h of administration of the medication.

Side effects

Most patients using VPA monotherapy tolerated the medication well. No change was observed after substitution of LA 40220 once or twice a day (Fig. 4).

Patients receiving phenytoin or carbamazepine in addition to valproate frequently reported side-effects. These side-effects were partially avoided by increasing the daily number of doses of all drugs.

After switching from valproate to LA 40220 a considerable reduction of side-effects occurred, especially those indicating intermittent intoxication (dizziness, drowsiness, ataxia and accommodation disturbances). These appeared to be less frequent and less severe, and in a number of patients the side-effects disappeared completely (Figs. 5, 6). These effects remained the same after a follow-up period of one year (to be published).

CONCLUSION

We studied 30 patients suffering from primary generalized epilepsy and partial seizures and some with secondary generalization. All patients were treated with valproate. In the latter two types of case valproate was often administered in combination with phenytoin or carbamazepine. We studied the pharmacokinetic effects, efficacy and tolerance of valproate in the conventional formulation and a sustained release formulation (LA 40220).

From this study it appears that the efficacy of LA 40220 is comparable with the efficacy of the conventional formulation of VPA, and this study revealed that a high peak in serum levels is not necessary to obtain effective seizure control.

Side-effects, even in frequent daily dosages, occur regularly when valproate is used in combination with phenytoin or carbamazepine. After switching to the sustained release formulation side effects appeared to be less frequent and less severe, particularly those side effects that can be an expression of the influence of the central nervous system. The sustained release formulation also appears to have far less influence on comedication, as judged by the fluctuations in serum levels.

As a result, the quality of life can be improved substantially in patients with epilepsy receiving polytherapy.

REFERENCES

(1) Meinardi H, Magnus O. Drug therapy. In: Vinken PJ, Bruyn GW. *Handbook of clinical neurology.* Amsterdam: North-Holland, 1977: 664–73.
(2) Sonnen AEH. De medicamenteuze behandeling van epilepsie. *Ned Tijdschr Geneeskd* 1979; **123**: 485.
(3) Reynolds EH. Drug treatment of epilepsy. *Lancet* 1978; ii: 721.
(4) Heycop ten Ham MW van. *Epilepsie.* Leiden: Stafleu, 1974.
(5) Roger J. *et al. Epileptic syndromes in infancy, childhood and adolescence.* London: John Libbey, 1985.

(6) Schmidt D. *Adverse effects of antiepileptic drugs*. New York: Raven Press, 1982.
(7) Schobben AFAM. *Pharmacokinetics and therapeutics in epilepsy*. Nijmegen: Stichting Studentenpers, 1979.
(8) Rowan AJ, Binnie CD, de Beer-Pawlikowski NKB. *et al*. Serial twenty-four-hour serum level monitoring in the study of sodium valproate. In: Parsonage MJ, Caldwell ADS, eds. *The place of sodium valproate in the treatment of epilepsy*. RSM International Congress and Symposium Series No. 30. London: The Royal Society of Medicine, 1980.
(9) Schmidt D. Withdrawal of antiepileptic drugs. *16th Epilepsy International Congress*. Hamburg, 1985.

Pharmacokinetic aspects of
sodium valproate suppositories

J. Issakainen

University Children's Hospital, Zürich, Switzerland

INTRODUCTION

Since the description of successful treatment of status epilepticus by rectal administration of valproic acid (1) there have been few reports about the clinical use of this drug by the rectal route. In six adult patients with status epilepticus refractory to parenteral treatment with diazepam, amytal or both, seizure control could be achieved in five patients and a 75% reduction in seizure frequency in one patient with the use of sodium valproate (NaVPA) suppositories (2). Rectally administered NaVPA has been used successfully in some further cases, both children and adults (3–6).

Occasionally, the oral route of drug administration may be impossible, for example because of an intermittent gastrointestinal infection, in an unconscious patient, during convulsive or non-convulsive status epilepticus, prior to and during surgery, prior to radiological examinations in fasting condition or occasionally because of drug refusal in psychiatric and mentally retarded patients. Administration of valproate by a rectal route might be clinically useful in such instances.

BIOAVAILABILITY

The extent of absorption or absolute bioavailability has been determined by comparison of the areas under the plasma concentration-time curves following single oral and intravenous bolus administration. Despite differences in population and formulation (oral solution, immediate release tablet, and enteric coated tablet), the absolute bioavailability of valproate (VPA) was consistently found close to unity (7). The absorption of VPA in the form of sodium salt is essentially complete.

The bioavailability of oral preparations is dependent on the extraction rate and metabolization during the first pass in the liver. However, the loss of drug by first-pass metabolism is not of consequence among antiepileptic drugs, since they have low extraction ratios (VPA 0.03). Cloyd & Kriel (4) could show that the bioavailability of VPA syrup given rectally was comparable to that following oral administration.

We have studied the bioavailability of NaVPA suppositories during repeated administration at steady state in epileptic children (8). The relative bioavailability of fatty suppositories (100 and 300 mg) was measured in comparison to oral solution (300 mg/ml) and enteric coated tablets (150, 300, 500 mg). Eight patients were treated with the oral solution (Group A, mean age 10.6 years) and five patients with enteric coated tablets (Group B, mean age 16.4 years). In every patient five serum levels of VPA over a 24 h period were measured. Thereafter, suppositories were administered for 2–7 days and serum levels were again determined (under identical dosing and sampling times). The bioavailability

Fourth international symposium on sodium valproate and epilepsy, edited by David Chadwick, 1989; Royal Society of Medicine Services International Congress and Symposium Series No. 152, published by Royal Society of Medicine Services Limited.

of NaVPA was calculated on the basis of the area under concentration vs time curve over 24 h.

Five concentrations were used for the determination of the area under the serum concentration curve because a preliminary investigation indicated that these five points adequately represented the concentration profile over 24 h. Although NaVPA enteric coated tablets have different absorption kinetics and different concentration profiles than suppositories the preliminary study in one patient with three additional blood samples during the night showed only a difference of 2.8% in the relative bioavailability.

The average bioavailability for suppositories compared with the oral form was 112.4% in Group A (solution) and 99.5% in Group B (enteric coated tablets) (Table 1). Fluctuations of serum VPA levels were very similar with suppositories and oral solution (Fig. 1), and more pronounced than with the enteric coated tablets (Fig. 2).

LOCAL EFFECTS

Stool frequency was not increased by repeated administration of suppositories, except for a three-fold increase in one patient. There was no evidence of local irritation from the suppositories. However, the older patients showed an increasing tendency to refuse the rectal application. We had to administer up to four suppositories per dose or up to 11 suppositories in one day. Therefore, suppositories with a higher drug content than 100 and 300 mg would be desirable.

Table 1 *Relative bioavailability of sodium valproate suppositories compared with sodium valproate solution (Group A) and enteric coated tablets (Group B)*

Group A		Group B	
Patient	Bioavailability (%)	Patient	Bioavailability (%)
1	103.5	1	86.2
2	110.0	2	116.2
3	121.6	3	96.3
4	109.75	4	73.9
5	137.8	5	124.7
6	109.2		
7	119.5		
8	88.0		
Mean	112.4%	Mean	99.5%
±SD	±14.5	±SD	±21.0

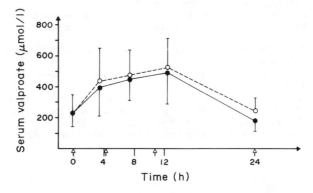

Figure 1 *Mean serum concentration of sodium valproate in μmol/l (with SD) in Group A during treatment with suppositories and with solution (Suppositories: open circles, dashed lines; solution: full circles, solid lines. Arrows indicate time of drug administration. Time 0 corresponds to 08:00 a.m.).*

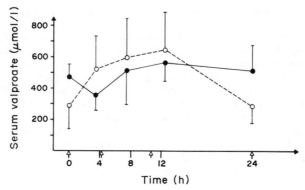

Figure 2   *Mean serum concentration of sodium valproate in μmol/l (with SD) in Group B during treatment with suppositories and with enteric coated tablets (Suppositories: open circles, dashed lines; tablets: full circles, solid lines. Arrows indicate time of drug administration. Time 0 corresponds to 08:00 a.m.).*

CLINICAL EFFICACY

In the whole group of 13 children, only one had more seizures during the therapy with NaVPA suppositories. This increase was probably due to spontaneous fluctuation of seizure frequency, because this patient tends to have periodic clusters of seizures, which also occurred during treatment with enteric coated tablets.

CONCLUSION

There are few reports in the literature about successful treatment with VPA by rectal application. The results of our study show that a short period of treatment with rectal NaVPA suppositories at steady-state as a substitute for the oral solution or enteric coated tablets is a safe alternative with regard to bioavailability, clinical efficacy and tolerability in epileptic children in whom the oral route is temporarily not available.

REFERENCES

(1) Vajda FJE, Symington GR, Bladin PF. Rectal valproate in intractable status epilepticus. *Lancet* 1977; i: 359–60.
(2) Vajda FJE, Mihaly GW, Miles JL, Donnan GA, Bladin PF. Rectal administration of sodium valproate in status epilepticus. *Neurology* 1978; **28**: 897–9.
(3) Thorpy MJ. Rectal valproate syrup and status epilepticus. *Neurology* 1980; **30**: 1113–4.
(4) Cloyd JC, Kriel RR. Bioavailability of rectally administered valproic acid syrup. *Neurology* 1981; **31**: 1348–52.
(5) Scanabissi E, Dal Pozzo D, Franzoni E, Galloni C, Mengoli G, Caliva R. Rectal administration of sodium valproate in children. *Ital J Neurol Sci* 1984; **5**: 189–93.
(6) Kanazawa O, Sengoku A, Kawai I. Treatment of childhood epilepsy with rectal valproate. *Brain Dev* 1987; **9**: 615–20.
(7) Levy RH, Lai AA. Valproate: absorption, distribution and excretion. In: Woodbury DM, Penry JK, Pippenger CE, eds. *Antiepileptic drugs*. New York: Raven Press, 1982: 555–65.
(8) Issakainen J, Bourgeois BFD. Bioavailability of sodium valproate suppositories during repeated administration at steady state in epileptic children. *Eur J Pediatr* 1987; **146**: 404–7.

Discussion after Drs Barre, Rentmeester, and Issakainen

Professor Dam *(Copenhagen, Denmark):* Was your study blinded any way? It is very important, when we look for the effect and the side effect of drugs, that it is a controlled trial.

Dr Rentmeester *(Heeze, The Netherlands):* We compared the pharmacokinetic values of the sustained release formulation and we also asked the patient about side effects in the trial period. Nearly all patients asked us to continue with the long acting formulation. We were surprised by the good reduction of side effects. I agree it is desirable to perform a double blind study but we did not do so [but see comment by Dr Brodie]. Perhaps we can do this in the future. Nevertheless, if we see remarkable reduction of side effects for a long period we think that is a clinically reliable effect.

Dr Kyllerman *(Sweden):* I have a question for Dr Barre. Is it correct that there is not a great difference in serum concentrations at 12 h with slow release preparation compared to the enteric coated variety? The major difference is the peak at one and a half hours.

Dr Barre *(Creteil, France):* There are two advantages of the sustained release form. First, the same bioavailability over the 24 h period, so when it is given once a day you have the same bioavailability as compared to twice a day for the enteric coated form. Second, with the sustained release form you reduce the two peak levels that you have with enteric coated form.

Dr Brodie *(Glasgow, UK):* We are doing a double dummy comparison of the new slow release carbamazepine with conventional carbamazepine. We have built in some objective measures of psychomotor function, and are also looking at the kinetics as well. The only time I see the patients is when they complete the study and the vast majority of them have picked the controlled release formulation. I would therefore, echo the previous questioner.

Dr Fenwick *(London, UK):* I would be grateful for the speakers' comments on the usefulness of measuring serum levels is not helpful because of the wide fluctuations in serum levels after dosing, although trough levels are probably worth measuring first thing in the morning. Has this changed with the sustained release formulation? And what would you say now is the advantage of measuring serum levels?

Dr Rentmeester: Before there was a sustained release formulation I measured blood levels of valproate, but only when I took blood for liver function tests etc. and to control the plasma levels of co-mediation phenytoin and carbamazepine. Levels above 100 mg/l nearly always correlate with side effects like dizziness and drowsiness. Under 40 mg/l it seems less effective, so we have a wide window in which we can treat a patient. Now we have valproate in the long acting formulation in the Netherlands we can check the blood level even in the middle of the day when the patient is in a poly-clinic situation.

Dr Barre: When the sustained release form is given once a day the blood levels are less affected by diurnal fluctuations and in terms of monitoring this can be an advantage.

1. Is there an indication to prescribe sustained release valproate instead of **Response**
   conventional valproate?
   1 Yes 83%
   2 No 17%
   PREVIOUS VOTE TAKEN BEFORE THE SESSION
   1 Yes 70%
   2 No 30%

2. Would you prescribe valproate sustained release because **Response**
   1 It has a better clinical effect 8%
   2 Fewer side effects 50%
   3 Less frequent dosage 42%

Dr Issakainen *(Zurich, Switzerland):* If you plot the serum concentration curve showed for valproate enteric coated tablets you see that the serum concentration falls at first and then rises. This is not because absorption is slower with this formulation, but it is delayed.

Interactive question from Dr Issakainen

If available to use would you consider the use of valproate suppositories? **Response**
1 When oral therapy is temporarily impossible 60%
2 In the treatment of status epilepticus 5%
3 Both situations 35%

Dr Gram *(Dianalund, Denmark):* It seems not many people would use it for the treatment of status epilepticus and I think that is due to the fact that the acute effect of this drug has not yet been established. There are a number of publications where status has been stopped, with this treatment, but that has only been within 24 h. We do not know if the drug has an acute effect.

Interactive question from Dr Barre

If you switch from the enteric coated VPA to the sustained release form what **Response**
would you do to get the same bioavailability?
1 You would increase the dose of the sustained release form 12%
2 You would give the same dose of sustained release form 80%
3 You would give a smaller dose of sustained release form 9%

Dr Oxley *(Chalfont St Peter, UK):* Does anybody have experience or can you guess whether rectal valproate would be of use in the intermittent prophylaxis of febrile convulsions?

Dr Knudsen *(Copenhagen, Denmark):* We have just completed a study of about 200 patients in which we investigated that problem. Patients were treated after the first febrile seizure. One group was given intermittent valproate as suppositories and the other group received diazepam solution. The response rate was the same and it was the only outcome which was inconclusive. I cannot be sure but I think that the lack of effect in the diazepam group was due to lack in compliance, and the lack of effect in the valproate group is probably an acute effect.

Intravenous valproate: Experience in neurosurgery

D. J. Price

Leeds General Infirmary, Yorkshire, UK

Anticonvulsants are the most widely prescribed group of drugs in a neurosurgical service. Seizures in neurosurgical practice may be due to evolving underlying pathology, the operative intervention or to head injury. They may contribute significantly to peri-operative morbidity and mortality. When patients at risk of developing epilepsy are recovering from a general anaesthetic or are in coma with or without ventilatory support, an oral preparation of an anticonvulsant is usually inappropriate and intravenous or rectal preparations are necessary alternatives.

Intravenous therapy is useful for the following three groups of patients:

1. *Low risk prophylaxis*
Patients who have had seizures in the past, are taking oral anticonvulsant medication and now require an anaesthetic for an operation when gastrointestinal absorption is inhibited for a period of 12 h or more.
2. *High risk prophylaxis*
Those who have had recent seizures due to the pathology requiring neurosurgery, during the peri-operative period.
3. *Status epilepticus*
For rapid seizure control when two or three boluses of an intravenous benzodiazepine have failed to abort this life-threatening condition. By this stage, airway protection and ventilatory support are mandatory.

MANAGEMENT OF STATUS EPILEPTICUS IN BRITAIN

In Britain, the selection of the definitive drug for control of benzodiazepine-resistant status is usually made in the Accident and Emergency Department or the neurosurgical ward by relatively junior doctors. As no one doctor is likely to see more than one patient a year with this medical emergency, the choice of the second line drug and its dosage is often inappropriate. Failure to respond to a second anticonvulsant often given at sub-optimal doses may lead to further administration of a series of other alternatives from a choice of nine that are currently available in intravenous form. A polypharmaceutical approach often leads to as many as four or five drugs being given concurrently and status may continue until one of them is given at the necessary high dose-rate. Apart from phenytoin, they all depress cerebral function sufficiently to induce and maintain clouding of consciousness. Dosage titration to achieve control by steadily increasing the dose rate of anticonvulsants with sedating side effects inevitably causes delays. Although it is reasonable to recommend initiation of treatment with the rapid bolus administration of a fast-acting CNS depressant such as diazepam, longer term control requires an agent with minimal sedative properties. The 'perfect' anticonvulsant for this purpose should be relatively non-toxic, particularly as high initial doses are required to develop the necessary plasma/brain gradient needed for rapid brain loading.

Fourth international symposium on sodium valproate and epilepsy, edited by David Chadwick, 1989; Royal Society of Medicine Services International Congress and Symposium Series No. 152, published by Royal Society of Medicine Services Limited.

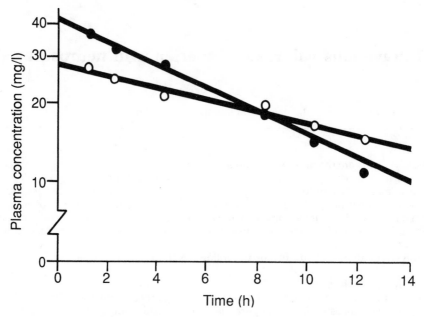

Figure 1 *Plasma concentrations of sodium valproate in two patients following bolus intravenous injections of 400 mg.*

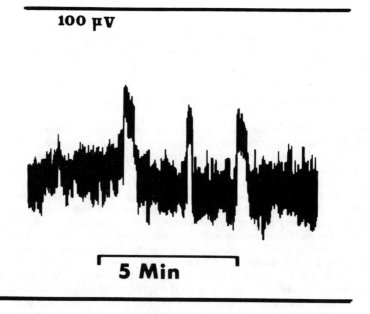

Figure 2 *A typical recording of status epilepticus on a cerebral function monitor.*

Until recently, phenytoin was the only non-sedative drug available as an intravenous preparation. Although effective, it may be necessary to limit the rate of administration of the initial loading dose to avoid cardiac irregularities (1). Any leakage around the intravenous cannula causes tissue reactions (2). Fifteen years ago, I abandoned its use as an oral prophylactic anticonvulsant in neurosurgical practice as blood-level optimization

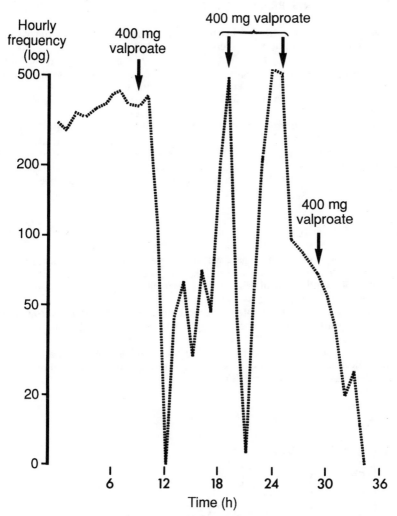

Figure 3 *The influence of bolus doses of valproate on the frequency of seizure discharges in a patient with status epilepticus.*

required regular monitoring. In principle, I was reluctant to change from one drug for the management of status to another more suitable for long term protection and welcomed the opportunity to assess the usefulness of sodium valproate in an intravenous formulation. It had already proven moderately effective for status by nasogastric administration (3). When this agent was introduced in Europe in 1968 and in Britain in 1974, many neurologists suggested that it was most useful for generalized seizures and would be of less value for the management of partial seizures with focal features (4,5).

When it was first used for the partial epilepsies in neurosurgical patients, it proved capable of completely controlling 50% of patients with repeated partial seizures provided doses of up to 5 g/day were given (6). If a maximum of 3 g/day were given, only 35% were controlled and if the initial recommended maximum of 1.6 g/day was given only 20% were controlled for at least a year. The relationship of the dosage with probability of control convinced me that this was an important addition to the pharmaco-logical armamentarium for the partial seizures so commonly seen in neurosurgical practice and encouraged me to use high doses of intravenous valproate for the control of status epilepticus.

VALPROATE ADMINISTERED BY BOLUS

When the intravenous formulation became available in 1978, the pharmacokinetics were studied in neurosurgical patients given a single bolus of 400 mg (7).

It was initially used for the treatment of status epilepticus which had already proved resistant to diazepam boluses and then continuous infusions of phenytoin at high doses. The patients were paralysed and ventilated and seizure activity was detected from the modified EEG signal derived from a cerebral function monitor (8).

The seizure discharge frequency was generated by on-line analysis on a PDP11 minicomputer using Trigg's tracking function. In the first patient, the response of the seizure frequency to single 400 mg bolus doses of valproate appeared very dramatic. Subsequent patients proved less responsive and it soon became apparent that control in most patients would usually not be achieved until at least 2 g had been administered in bolus dose.

CONTINUOUS INFUSION

After a loading dose of 400 mg was given over a period of 5 min, a continuous infusion of 100 mg/h was then set up. If the seizure frequency did not respond, the rate was increased to 200 or even 300 mg/h until all seizures had been abolished. This technique also resulted in delays in control for as long as 12 h.

Although the higher infusion rate procured blood levels of over 200 µg/ml I considered it necessary to start the infusion at 300 mg/h and only reduce it when control became evident.

This resulted in a more rapid control and formed the basis of a closed-loop application with the sodium valproate infusion rate being automatically controlled according to the response of the seizure frequency (9).

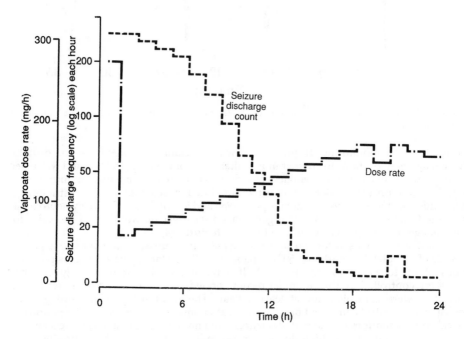

Figure 4 *The slow response of seizure discharge counts to gradually increasing valproate dose rates.*

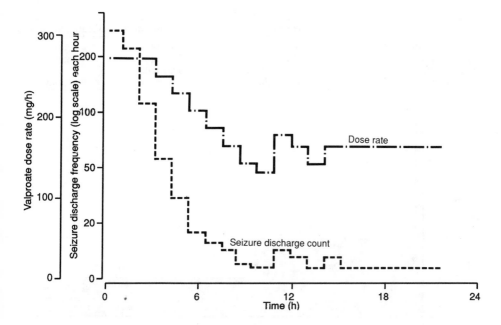

Figure 5 *The more rapid response of seizure discharge counts to initial high valproate loading and gradual reduction of the dose rates as soon as control is established.*

PRELIMINARY RETROSPECTIVE SERIES

Over a period of seven years, intravenous valproate was administered to 36 patients. Fifteen of these had diazepam resistant status epilepticus, 11 had recent seizures ('high risk prophylaxis') and 10 had lower chances of developing epilepsy ('low risk prophylaxis'). When this series was retrospectively analysed, a wide range of maintenance doses (expressed as milligrams/kilograms/hour) became evident (Table 1). This reflected the increasing confidence over the years in starting with higher dose rates of up to 400 mg/h. Of the 15 patients in status, only six had abolishment of seizure discharges at 2 h but 14 were controlled at 4 h. One patient remained resistant despite administration of a total dose of 50 g given over a period of eight days.

Table 1

Seizure abortion (15 patients)	1–16 mg/kg/h
High risk prophylaxis (11 patients)	1–12 mg/kg/h
Low risk prophylaxis (10 patients)	1–2 mg/kg/h

After experience of the previous seven years, it was considered that higher loading doses were required for status epilepticus particularly as all the patients had already received diazepam. Cross tolerance of valproate with diazepam has been reported in experimental animals (10) and may account for the need for the use of higher doses in these patients to create steep plasma/brain gradients to achieve higher brain levels as soon as possible.

PROSPECTIVE SERIES

Over a period of two years, nine patients with diazepam resistant status and six patients at high risk of developing epilepsy were treated according to the following protocol (Table 2).

Table 2

	Hourly rate	Hourly adult dose	Total daily dose
Low risk prophylaxis	1.5 mg/kg/h	100 mg/h	2.4 g/day
High risk prophylaxis	3.0 mg/kg/h	200 mg/h	4.8 g/day
Status loading	15.0 mg/kg/h	1000 mg/h	—
Status maintenance	6.0 mg/kg/h	400 mg/h	9.6 g/day

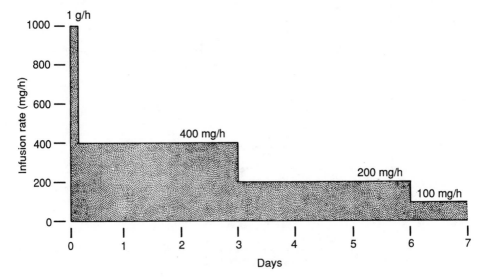

Figure 6 *An example of valproate dosage rates used for a patient to control status epilepticus.*

Table 3 *Results—seizure control*

	Preliminary series	Definitive series
Seizure control at 1 h	—	7/9
Seizure control at 2 h	6/15	7/9
Seizure control at 4 h	14/15	7/9

For status (Fig. 6) it did prove inconvenient, tedious and time consuming to open 24 ampoules each containing only 400 mg of valproate to fill two 50 ml syringes for the syringe pump to be set up for the first 18 h of treatment and the drug cost of *c.* £180 for that first day had to be considered. It is perhaps fortunate that only a few patients with status epilepticus do require management such as this as the majority have responded to initial bolus doses of diazepam. The results of the series as shown in Table 3.

SIDE EFFECTS

In both series, no localized reactions were encountered at the intravenous catheter insertion site. On two occasions, concentrated valproate was allowed to leak into the tissue accidentally but this caused no erythema and only swelling. In one patient with status epilepticus, thrombocytopenia did develop but other factors may have contributed to this.

CONCLUSION

The intravenous formulation of sodium valproate provides a convenient alternative to the oral preparation for prophylaxis of epilepsy. It is also a useful alternative to phenytoin as a second-line non-sedative anticonvulsant for status epilepticus which has failed to respond to bolus doses of diazepam. High doses, however, are required for initial loading in order to achieve urgent seizure abortion. No local side effects have been seen but one patient did develop thrombocytopenia.

REFERENCES

(1) Zoneraich S, Zoneraich O, Siegel J. Sudden death following intravenous sodium diphenylhydantoin. *Am Heart J* **91**: 375–7.
(2) Rao VK, Feldman PD, Dibbell DG. Extravasation injury to the hand by intravenous phenytoin. *J Neurosurg* 1988; **68**: 967–9.
(3) Manhire AR, Espir M. Treatment of status epilepticus with sodium valproate. *Br Med J* 1974; **3**: 808.
(4) Kerfriden P, Kerfriden M, Albe-Fessard D. The Toul-ar-c'Hoate experience in the treatment of epileptic children with Depakine. *Presse Méd* 1978; **78**: 1943–6.
(5) Jeavons PM, Clark JE. Sodium valproate in the treatment of epilepsy. *Br Med J* 1974; **2**: 584–6.
(6) Price DJ. The efficiency of sodium valproate as the only anticonvulsant administered to neurosurgical patients. In: Parsonage MJ, Caldwell ADS, eds. *The place of sodium valproate in the treatment of epilepsy.* London, Toronto, Sydney: Academic Press, 1980: 23–34.
(7) Mehta AC, Calvert RT, Rigby J, Price DJE. Pharmocokinetics of sodium valproate in epileptic patients after an intravenous bolus administration. *J Clin Hosp Pharm* 1980; **5**: 329–31.
(8) Prior PF. *Monitoring cerebral function.* Amsterdam: Elsevier, 1979.
(9) Mason J, Price DJ, Dugdale RE. Automated control of status epilepticus by closed loop techniques. *Int Care Med* 1979; **5**: 159–60.
(10) Gent JP, Bentley M, Feely M, Heigh JRM. Benzodiazepine cross-tolerance in mice extends to sodium valproate. *Eur J Pharmacol* 1986; **128**: 9–15.

Intravenous sodium valproate in neurosurgery: Repeat dose pharmacokinetic study and safety assessment in neurosurgical patients

A. J. Moore[1], B. A. Bell[1] and D. J. Berry[2]

[1]Atkinson Morley's Hospital, Wimbledon, London, UK
and [2]Poisons Unit, New Cross Hospital, London, UK

INTRODUCTION

The development of epilepsy may abruptly blight the process of recovery from intracranial surgery or head injury. Estimates of the risk of this complication vary widely (1), being as high as 20% or more post-craniotomy (1,2) and around 10% after serious head trauma (3). Opinions differ as to the efficacy of anti-convulsants in the prevention of post-craniotomy and post-traumatic seizures (2,4,5,6,7). Recent studies have suggested that phenytoin, commonly used in neurosurgical units, has little effect on the development of epilepsy after craniotomy or head injury (5,7).

In view of the far-reaching effects that seizures may have on a patient's work and eligibility to drive, and the controversy over currently used anticonvulsant prophylaxis, a trial is in progress at Atkinson Morley's Hospital, Wimbledon to test the efficacy of sodium valproate when used prophylactically.

REPEAT DOSE PHARMACOKINETIC STUDY

Sodium valproate has a low volume of distribution, being apparently restricted to the bloodstream and the rapidly exchangeable extracellular water. It is 90% protein bound at therapeutic levels, and only the unbound fraction is cleared. Its half-life is quoted as between 8 and 20 h (8), but is reduced in patients on enzyme inducing anti-convulsants (9) and may be increased in old age (10) and in various pathological conditions.

A number of investigators have studied the pharmacokinetic parameters of sodium valproate in human volunteers or epileptic patients using a single intravenous dose (11), notably Perucca *et al.* in 1978 (9,12), Mehta and co-workers in 1980 (13) and Nitsche and Mascher in 1982 (14). Results are essentially in agreement, and show that the plasma concentration decay curve after a bolus intravenous dose fits a two-compartment open model, with first order elimination.

In a study performed by Loiseau and co-workers in 1980 (15), patients received an intravenous (i.v.) bolus dose of 800 mg sodium valproate, and plasma levels were measured over the ensuing 37 h. A plasma concentration decay curve was produced for each patient, and was used to calculate the size of a second intravenous dose and constant infusion, according to each patient's individual parameters, to maintain a specified plasma level, as follows:

Fourth international symposium on sodium valproate and epilepsy, edited by David Chadwick, 1989; Royal Society of Medicine Services International Congress and Symposium Series No. 152, published by Royal Society of Medicine Services Limited.

Total body clearance (l/h) = i.v. dose/area under curve (l/h)
Bolus dose (mg)   = ([Vc.SVP] + [Vd.SVP])/2
Infusion rate (mg(h)   = Clearance × SVP

Where: SVP is required plasma level (in mg(l), Vc = volume central compartment (in litres) and Vd = apparent distribution volume (litres: calculated from the area under the curve of the plasma valproate profile). The infusion rate was calculated as recommended by Gibaldi & Perrier (1975 (16) (2-compartment open model)

Sanofi Recherche in Montpellier used Loiseau's results to derive a theoretical protocol for the present trial (17).

METHOD

The trial is randomized, double-blind and placebo-controlled. It includes patients over the age of 12 years, without previous fits, who are at risk of developing epilepsy after head injury or craniotomy. Those on drugs with known anticonvulsant effects are excluded, as are those with renal or hepatic dysfunction.

A bolus dose (10 mg/kg bodyweight) of sodium valproate i.v., or placebo is given on entry (usually at induction of anaesthesia for craniotomy patients) and this is followed by an infusion (0.6 mg/kg/h), which is continued until 12 h after the first oral dose is tolerated. Except in unusual circumstances, oral liquid is started 12 h after entry, and enteric coated tablets the day after surgery. The tablets, equivalent to 500 mg sodium valproate, are taken three times a day for one year, then discontinued. Assessments are made every three months for the first year, then at two years. Patients are withdrawn if they suffer a fit or serious side-effect. So far, 125 patients have been recruited to the trial.

In the main trial only limited data were available regarding plasma levels of valproate—a single reading is taken at 24 h, and then every three months in the clinic. So, a more detailed study was undertaken on 10 patients who formed part of the main trial. Their ages ranged between 21 and 76 years, and their weights between 60 and 80 kg. Five underwent craniotomy for aneurysm surgery, four for tumour and one for trauma. Blood samples were taken at increasing intervals over the 48 h following the i.v. bolus dose, and plasma valproate levels were determined by a specific gas-liquid chromatographic assay (18).

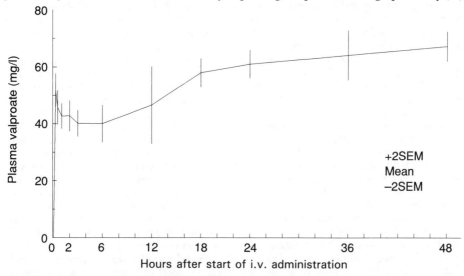

Figure 1 *Plasma valproate levels after i.v. administration regime: 10 mg/kg bolus + 0.6 mg/kg/h infusion*

RESULTS

No reactions were noted at sites of bolus injection or infusion, and there were no complaints of pain or discomfort. During the period of administration of the i.v. infusion no systemic ill-effects were recorded whatsoever. None of the 10 patients in the pharmacokinetic study suffered a fit during the 48-h period after entry. The plasma concentration curve of valproate is shown in Fig. 1. The valproate level remains within the therapeutic range throughout the 48-h study period.

DISCUSSION

The plasma levels of sodium valproate observed in the first 12 h are slightly lower than would have been expected from theoretical considerations. In the study by Loiseau where a bolus dose was followed by an infusion (15), plasma concentrations of sodium valproate fluctuated by as much as 33% during a constant delivery rate of the drug. It was hypothesized that this variability was due to oscillations in the amount of plasma-protein binding. A reduction in protein binding capacity would be expected to result in enhanced elimination leading to a decrease in total drug levels. Sodium valproate is mainly bound to albumin, which has been shown to fall after surgery. In addition, free fatty acids compete with the drug for protein binding, and serum levels of free fatty acids would be elevated in the body's response to surgical stress. As all the patients studied were post-perative, these factors may account for the lower plasma levels of sodium valproate, which nevertheless remained within the therapeutic range throughout the 48 h of the study.

SAFETY ASSESSMENT

Since the mid-1970s, published and unpublished reports (9,12,15,19,20) on the use of intravenous valproate detail more than 200 patients and volunteers who have received the drug. Studies have been carried out using bolus injections given over 30 s to 5 min periods, followed by infusions delivering widely differing total doses in a 24 h period. Not all workers have commented on the occurrence of side-effects, but the majority did. Tartara *et al.* (19), recorded one child who complained of nausea during administration of the drug, and vomited afterwards. In an unpublished report, Waltregny (Belgium) noted one patient who also suffered transient nausea. All workers reported good local tolerance of intravenous valproate, and apart from the nausea, there were no reports of any adverse gastrointestinal, cardiovascular or respiratory effects.

In our small pharmacokinetic study, no reactions were noted at sites of bolus injection or infusion, and there were no complaints of pain or discomfort (with the proviso that the patients were anaesthetized for surgery during the initial infusion period). During the period of administration of the i.v. infusion no systemic ill effects were recorded whatsoever.

The same can be said for the patients so far entered into the main trial who were randomized to receive active treatment. In over 60 such patients, even the long-term side-effects have been few. One patient developed disturbed liver function tests and was withdrawn without any further adverse effects (21). There have been several patients who noticed a tremor, which disappeared on discontinuing treatment at the end of the trial period, and several more who complained of weight gain. The latter complaint is difficult to assess because of the number of contributory factors. This is also true of alopecia—one lady who asked to be withdrawn because of hair loss was in fact receiving placebo. Interestingly, the three other patients with alopecia had serum levels in excess of 100 mg/l despite a total dosage of only 1500 mg/day. This effect could hardly be attributed to the intravenous drug, however, occurring as it did several months after entering the trial.

Intravenous valproate is easy to use, has excellent local tolerance and seemingly no adverse systemic effects.

ACKNOWLEDGMENT

The authors would like to express their thanks to Dr Derrick Easter and the anaesthetic registrars and senior registrars at Atkinson Morley's Hospital for their assistance in this study.

REFERENCES

(1) Jennett B, Ward P, Murray L. Risk of epilepsy after head injury and intracranial surgery. Implications for driving. *J Neurol Neurosurg Psychiat* 1984; **47**: 104.
(2) Deutschman CS, Haines SJ. Anticonvulsant prophylaxis in neurological surgery. *Neurosurgery* 1985; **17**: 510–17.
(3) McQueen JK, Blackwood DHQ, Harris P, Kalbag RM, Johnson AL. Low risk of late post-traumatic seizures following severe head injury: implications for clinical trials of prophylaxis. *J Neurol Neurosurg Psychiatry* 1983; **46**: 899–904.
(4) North JB, Penhall RK, Hanieh A, Frewin DB, Taylor WB. Phenytoin and post-operative epilepsy. A double-blind study. *J Neurosurg* 1983; **58**: 672–7.
(5) Young B, Rapp RP, Norton JA, Haack D, Tibbs PA, Bean JR. Failure of prophylactically administered phenytoin to prevent late post-traumatic seizures. *J Neurosurg* 1983; **58**: 236–41.
(6) Price DJ. The efficacy of sodium valproate as the only anticonvulsant administered to neurosurgical patients. In: Parsonage MJ, Caldwell ADS, eds. *The place of sodium valproate in the treatment of epilepsy*. RSM International Congress and Symposium Series 30, 1980; London: Royal Society of Medicine, 23–30.
(7) Shaw MDM, Foy P, Chadwick D. The effectiveness of prophylactic anticonvulsants following neurosurgery. *Acta Neurochir* 1983; **5**: 495–9.
(8) Epilim Technical Brochure, December 1988.
(9) Perucca E, Gatti G, Frigo GM, Crema A, Calzetti S, Visintini D. Disposition of sodium valproate in epileptic patients. *Br J Clin Pharmacol* 1978; **5**: 495–9.
(10) Bryson SM, Verma N, Scott RJW, Rubin PC. Pharmacokinetics of valproic acid in young and elderly subjects. *Br J Clin Pharmacol* 1983; **16**: 104–5.
(11) Gugler R, van Unruh GE. Clinical pharmacokinetics of valproic acid. *Clin Pharmacokinet* 1980; **1**: 67–83.
(12) Perucca E, Gatti G, Frigo GM, Crema A. Pharmacokinetics of valproic acid after oral and intravenous administration. *Br J Clin Pharmacol* 1978; **5**: 313–18.
(13) Mehta AC, Calvert RT, Rigby J, Price DJE. Pharmacokinetics of sodium valproate in epileptic patients after an intravenous bolus administration. *J Clin Hosp Pharmacy* 1980; **5**: 329–31.
(14) Nitsche V, Mascher H. The pharmacokinetics of valproic acid after oral and parenteral administration in healthy volunteers. *Epilepsia* 1982; **23**: 153–62.
(15) Loiseau P, Cenrand B, Levy RH, *et al*. Diurnal variations in steady-state plasma concentrations of valproic acid in epileptic patients. *Clin Pharmacokinet* 1980; **7**: 544–52.
(16) Gibaldi M, Perrier D. *Multicompartment models in pharmacokinetics*. New York: Marcel Dekker, 1975: 45–95.
(17) Cautreds W. Sanofi Direction des Recherches. Montpellier Internal Report, 1983.
(18) Berry DJ, Clarke LA. The determination of valproic acid (dipropyl acetic acid) in plasma by gas-liquid chromatography. *J Chromatogr* 1978; **156**: 301–310.
(19) Tartara A, Moglia A, Verri AP, Savoldi F, Bo P. Effects of sodium valproate administered acutely I.V. on human and experimental epileptic foci. *Farmaco (Prat)* 1980; **35**: 623–31.
(20) Clinical evidence on the administration, safety and tolerability of sodium valproate by the intravenous route. *Internal Report, Labaz* 32–41.
(21) Turnbull DM, Dick DJ, Wilson L, Sherratt HSA, Albert KGMM. Valproate causes metabolic disturbance in normal man. *J Neurol Neurosurg Psych* 1986; **49**: 405–10.

Intravenous sodium valproate in the neonatal intensive care unit

N. Marlow[1] and R. W. I. Cooke

Department of Child Health, Liverpool Maternity Hospital, Liverpool, UK
[1]Present address: Bristol Maternity Hospital, Bristol, UK

INTRODUCTION

Seizures are a common occurrence during neonatal intensive care and generally carry a poor prognosis. Commonly used drugs are only partially effective and many children rapidly progress to multiple drug regimes because of continuing seizures. In a recent presentation it was suggested that sodium valproate may be more effective than phenobarbitone, phenytoin or clonazepam in the rapid control of seizures monitored by continuous EEG (1), but study numbers were small. We present preliminary findings from an ongoing randomized trial of sodium valproate versus phenobarbitone for the rapid control of clinically monitored neonatal seizures.

METHODS

This study was designed to test the hypothesis that sodium valproate therapy achieves rapid control of seizures more frequently than phenobarbitone. All children admitted to the Mersey Regional Neonatal Intensive Care Unit and who were deemed to require anticonvulsants were randomly assigned to receive either phenobarbitone or sodium valproate using prerandomized proforma in sealed envelopes. Assuming that pheno-barbitone will fail to control seizures in 75% of children, 26 children would be required in each treatment group to achieve 50% improvement in control, significant at the 5% level with a power of 80%. Randomization was stratified by gestational age (above and below 36 weeks) as seizures in term infants tend to be associated with perinatal asphyxia in contrast to preterm infants in whom seizures are associated with periventricular haemorrhage and its complications. The successful end-point was defined as the cessation of clinical seizures for at least 12 h within 24 h after randomization. The frequency, duration and type of seizures were recorded by the nursing attendants. Phenobarbitone was administered as a slow i.v. bolus of 20 mg/kg, followed by a further 10 mg/kg if seizures persisted beyond 6 h. Sodium valproate was administered as a slow i.v. bolus of 20 mg/kg repeated after 6 h if seizures persisted. This dosage was based upon pilot data derived from pretrial studies (unpublished). Maintenance treatment was at the prescriber's discretion. If the trial drug was considered unsuccessful, it was concluded that the trial was a failure and second-line drugs were prescribed. Outcome measures were recorded for the whole study population. Results of routine investigations were abstracted from the clinical notes. Serum concentrations of trial drugs were measured after 24 h to ensure that target concentrations had been achieved.

Data were encoded for computer analysis using the SPSS PC+ statistical software package. The trial has been approved by the District Ethical Committee.

Fourth international symposium on sodium valproate and epilepsy, edited by David Chadwick, 1989; Royal Society of Medicine Services International Congress and Symposium Series No. 152, published by Royal Society of Medicine Services Limited.

RESULTS

Twenty-six patients have been entered to date (13 in each group). Children receiving sodium valproate tended to be less mature and of lower birthweight than the phenobarbitone group (Table 1). Similar frequencies of hyaline membrane disease, septicaemia and infants who died were present in each group. More phenobarbitone-treated children had underlying periventricular haemorrhage and its complications and two sodium valproate treated children had culture-positive CSF infections (one child with ventriculitis and hydrocephalus; one with meningococcal meningitis). Seizures related to periventricular haemorrhage tended to be associated with acute ventricular dilatation due to haemorrhage or cerebro-spinal fluid obstruction.

Despite the group differences similar success rates were found in each group: seven (46.7%) phenobarbitone treated and eight (53.3%) sodium valproate treated children ceased having fits within 24 h. One child in each group had a recurrence of seizures on stopping the trial drug after the trial period. Success did not appear to be influenced by the underlying pathology or the seizure type (Table 2), and did not correlate with the dose or serum level of the drug.

Sodium valproate did not appear to offer any advantage in terms of lesser sedation during the first 24 h compared with phenobarbitone. No elevation of bilirubin or of liver enzymes was noted during the administration of either trial drug. One child in each group had persisting jaundice: that in the phenobarbitone group having a persisting mild elevation of

Table 1   *Study populations*

	Phenobarbitone group	Sodium valproate group
Age at trial entry (days)	9(0–35)	10 (0–26)
Birthweight (g)	1295 (864–2096)	984 (610–2910)
Gestation (weeks)	30 (24–38)	27 (24–40)
Died	2	3
Aetiology:		
Septicaemia	2	4
CSF infection		2
PVH[a]	9	4
Perinatal asphyxia	2	3
Major seizure type:		
Tonic/clonic	1	1
Generalized clonic	10	10
Focal clonic	—	2
Subtle	2	—

Results expressed as median (range) or number with condition as appropriate.
[a]Periventricular haemorrhage and its complications

Table 2   *Trial data*

	Phenobarbitone group	Sodium valproate group
Drug dose over 24 h (mg/kg)	18 (6–23)	41 (19–66)
Drug level at 24–96 h	38.5 (19–55)	71 (35–223)[b]
(µg/l)	(n = 12)	(n = 11)
Control at <24 h—all	7/13 (46.7%)	8/13 (53.3%)
Septicaemia	1/2 (50%)	3/4 (75%)
CSF infection		1/2 (50%)
PVH[a]	6/9 (70%)	3/4 (75%)
Perinatal asphyxia	0/2 (—)	1/3 (33%)
Platelet count <150×10^9/l)		
Before randomization	3/12	4/11
After randomization	7/12	6/12

[a]Periventricular haemorrhage and its complications. [b]Isolated high level, remainder below 126 µg/l.

liver enzymes and conjugated bilirubin usually associated with parenteral nutrition; that in the valproate group presenting with elevation of conjugated serum bilirubin without elevation of liver enzymes, and recovering slowly over the following months. Neither is typical of drug-induced hepatitis. Thrombocytopenia (platelet count $< 150 \times 10^9/l$) was present in six children prior to entry (Table 2). All continued to have low platelet counts during anticonvulsant treatment and thrombocytopenia was noted in a further four children in the phenobarbitone group and two children in the sodium valproate group. All counts eventually recovered and were associated with underlying septicaemia or progression of periventricular haemorrhage.

DISCUSSION

Seizures are common events in the neonatal period and a symptom of underlying metabolic or neurological disturbance. Clear precipitating factors were identified in all children, although many were sick with multisystem disease. Although the treatment of neonatal seizures was only possible with a single agent in one-half of all cases, sodium valproate appeared to be as effective as phenobarbitone in this task. A few children who were classified as failures were switched to the opposite trial arm with success in some cases. In the main, however, diazepam and phenytoin were the second-line drugs chosen.

One of the major criticisms of phenobarbitone therapy in the newborn is the marked sedation that accompanies its use. The use of loading doses of sodium valproate did not appear to offer any advantage initially, but more rapid elimination characteristics mean that this does not persist. Although the non-persistence of sedation is felt to be an advantage clinically, there are as yet insufficient data to prove that this is so.

Sodium valproate is not normally recommended for use in the newborn because of the known immaturity of the hepatic enzyme systems and the association of the idiosyncratic hepatotoxicity with its use in younger children (2). Despite this, sodium valproate remains a popular drug for the treatment of convulsions in young children and its regular use in children under two years of age in Liverpool over many years appears to have been free of major complications to date. The inclusion of a control group gives important insight into the relationship between thrombo—cytopenia and sodium valproate, (3,4). Thrombocytopenia is a common finding in sick newborn infants and was found no more frequently with either drug. In this study no substantial differences could be detected between intravenous sodium valproate and phenobarbitone when used for the rapid control of neonatal seizures. In two years' use for newborn infants no significant complications of such therapy have been noted.

ACKNOWLEDGMENTS

Thanks are due to the Nursing Staff of the Mersey Regional Neonatal Intensive Care Unit for their diligent observations and record keeping.

REFERENCES

(1) Rochefort MJ, Wilkinson AR. Randomised trial of four anticonvulsants in the newborn. *Arch Dis Child* 1987; **62**: 646 (abstr).
(2) Brown JK. Valproate toxicity. *Dev Med Child Neurol* 1988; **30**: 121–5.
(3) Takebe Y, Haneda S, Koide N, *et al*. Pharmacokinetics and side effects of sodium valproate in neonatal convulsions. *Hirosaki Med J* 1983; **35**: 449–64.
(4) Nathan D, Guillon JL, Chevallier B, Gallet JP. Thrombopénie et erythroblastopénie chez un nourrisson d'un mois traité par valproate. *Ann Pediatr (Paris)* 1987; **34**: 149–50.

Discussion after Mr Price, Miss Moore and Dr Marlow

Interactive question from Dr Gram

If available to you would you consider the use of intravenous valproate?	Response
1 When oral therapy is temporarily impossible	52%
2 In the treatment of status epilepticus	15%
3 In both indications	33%

Dr Young *(Dundee, UK)*: Less than half of the children with convulsions have clinical manifestations and many of those who had apparent clinical control of the seizures continued to have electrophysiological evidence of seizures. No study should ignore electrophysiological monitoring. It has also been shown that the eventual neuro-developmental outcome is not very different in those in whom the convulsions were controlled and this raises some doubt about the use of potentially toxic agents in the small group with the haemorrhagic ischaemic aetiology.

Dr Marlow *(Bristol, UK)*: We are of course concerned about this, the point being that it was claimed that sodium valproate was much more effective than either phenobarbitone, phenytoin or clonazepam in the small study that was reported. If it is more effective in the rapid control of seizures then perhaps we should reappraise how we are using it. I take your point about EEG monitoring, but practically, in a very busy neonatal intensive care unit that is absolutely impossible. Most neonatal intensive care units in the UK do not have routine EEG monitoring and therefore we felt that it was justified to go ahead with a clinical trial rather than an EEG monitored trial.

Mr Briggs *(Oxford, UK)*: Could Mr Price explain why patients failed on diazepam?

Mr Price *(Leeds, UK)*: In our extensive care unit perhaps one in five of those that come into the hospital are in status epilepticus, and it is the diazepam-resistant group that reaches us. So this is a selected group of more difficult, or apparently more difficult, patients. I do not know how to answer the question. All I can say is that we have a group of patients who do not respond to boluses of diazepam.

Dr Jivani *(Blackburn, UK)*: Dr Marlow, do you think we can control neonatal seizures and should there be a controlled group without any medication to see whether we are benefiting these babies?

Dr Marlow: In many ways I feel that would be quite justified, but to get such a proposal passed by the ethical committee would be extremely difficult.

Dr Nielsen *(Denmark)*: What is known about the acute kinetics of valproate in brain and CSF? May that be a problem in treatment of status epilepticus?

Mr Price: We have always wanted information on brain levels and we did try about 10 years ago but had some difficulty in extracting the drug from the brain at that time so we gave it up. Perhaps we ought to try again because we talk about brain levels and yet we do not really know what is happening.

Dr Brodie (*Glasgow, UK*): We looked at CSF levels and free levels in the plasma following oral dosing in a number of patients going into neurosurgery and the concentrations in the CSF and the plasma were identical. It does, as you would expect, cross the blood brain barrier relatively quickly. How long it remains in the brain, of course, is another matter. I would like to make a contentious statement and ask a question. The contentious statement is, there is no therapeutic range for sodium valproate, although every speaker mentions it. The question is did your neonates show a placebo response?

Dr Marlow: It would be necessary to make the study blind in order to assess the sedative effects of these drugs. In our experience it is a very important aspect of our care. It is difficult to assess somebody who has major intracranial brain damage, which is easily detectable on ultrasound scanning when phenobarbitone levels are high and decay for 10 days to two weeks. In addition our ethical committee would be very unhappy with us not treating seizures.

Dr Eames (*Bristol, UK*): There is an impressive report from a rat model of brain injury and recovery demonstrating that a couple of induced seizures in rats by cortisol infusion approximately doubled the rate of recovery from the motor deficiency. This raises the interesting question of whether we should actually be preventing seizures in the first week after head injury for example, and perhaps in the first 24 h after neurosurgical injury.

Mr Price: Severe seizures and particularly status epilepticus, are known to have a bad effect on the brain because of the hypoxia that may develop and the metabolic problems within the brain. There have also been studies to suggest that if you can control early post-traumatic epilepsy then the chances of later epilepsy developing is less.

Interactive questions from Dr Gram

1. If available to you would you consider the use of intravenous valproate?   **Response**

    1 When oral therapy is impossible   32%
    2 In the treatment of status epilepticus   18%
    3 In both indications   50%

PREVIOUS VOTE TAKEN BEFORE THE SESSION

    1 When oral therapy is impossible   52%
    2 In the treatment of status epilepticus   15%
    3 In both indications   33%

2. Do you use valproate for indications other than epilepsy?   **Response**

    1 Yes   42%
    2 No   58%

3. If you use valproate in non-epileptic patients, do you use it for   **Response**

    1 Treatment of pain   56%
    2 In psychiatric disorders   28%
    3 In both indications   16%

Sodium valproate in the treatment of pain

K. Budd

The Royal Infirmary, Bradford, UK

Although antiepileptic drugs were first introduced into practice in the middle of the nineteenth century (1) and a connection made between epilepsy and certain episodic, painful conditions (2), it was not until nearly 100 years later in 1942 that the final juxtaposition between drug and condition was made when trigeminal neuralgia was found to respond to treatment with diphenylhydantoin (phenytoin) (3).

A further 20 years were to elapse before an improvement was seen through the introduction of carbamazepine (4). Thereafter, the treatment of trigeminal neuralgia was significantly diverted from surgery and alcohol injection, with all the manifest side effects, to the relatively harmless drug therapy which was broadened to include the palliation of other types of cranial and peripheral neuralgias (5).

Carbamazepine is now the accepted primary agent for the treatment of trigeminal and glossopharyngeal neuralgia and also for paroxysmal pain affecting other nerve distributions (6). Most patients will derive rapid and complete benefit but there remains a significant number in whom side-effects and the emergence of tolerance render alternative therapy necessary. There are also some patients who once well-established on therapy with carbamazepine, for no apparent reason exhibit 'breakthrough pain'. Intolerance and other problems may, in certain series, represent up to 40% (7).

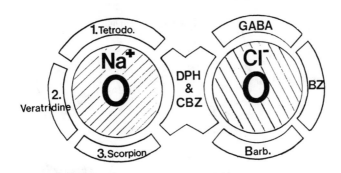

Figure 1 *GABA-A receptor complex*
Drug binding sites: *Naturally occurring neurotoxin binding sites:*
DPH—diphenylhydantoin   *1. Tetrodo—tetrodotoxin*
CBZ—carbamazepine   *2. Vera—veratridine*
BZ—Benzodiazepine   *3. Scorp—scorpion venom*
Barb—Barbiturate   *Na^+—sodium ion channel*
    Cl^-—chloride ion channel

Fourth international symposium on sodium valproate and epilepsy, edited by David Chadwick, 1989; Royal Society of Medicine Services International Congress and Symposium Series No. 152, published by Royal Society of Medicine Services Limited.

Because of this need for alternative therapy not dependent upon technical resources, there has emerged a group of therapeutic agents used to treat the neuralgias. These are:-

Hydantoins:	phenytoin
Benzodiazepines:	clonazepam, clobazam
Carboxylic acid:	sodium valproate
Iminostilbenes:	carbamazepine

Whilst the mode of action of all these agents may be loosely categorized as 'GABA agonists', the actual site and manner of their antinociceptive activity varies from group to group and, hence, their clinical usage and indications are not identical.

Carbamazepine and phenytoin both bind to specific 'phenytoin' receptors, (Fig. 1) causing voltage-sensitive sodium channel inactivation (9). This binding is enhanced in the presence of chloride ions and in high dosage will increase chloride permeability, stabilizing the cell near the resting membrane potential (8). Both agents are extensively used for the treatment of cranial nerve neuralgias together with some of the peripheral neuropathies (9). Phenytoin is usually the second choice for use if side-effects preclude continuation of use of carbamazepine.

The benzodiazepines bind with a dedicated receptor associated with the GABA-chloride ionophore complex, facilitating GABA-mediated transmission across synapses (10). Although not acting through the GABA-autoreceptor it does need the presence of GABA to be effective (Fig. 2).

Clonazepam is most valuable in the treatment of facial pain and some instances of post-traumatic neurogenic pain where anxiety plays a role in the generation of the symptom-complex. Clobazam, on the other hand, is more often used for the treatment of peripheral neurogenic and deafferentation pain especially when there is a marked psychogenic component in the patient's symptomatology. Sodium valproate possibly exerts some of its effect by augmenting post-synaptic GABA-mediated inhibition (11). The relatively low side-effect profile, especially when the dose is built-up gradually, renders it of increasing value not only in the neuralgias, neurogenic and deafferentation pain (12,13,14) but also in less obvious conditions such as tinnitus, Ekbom's syndrome and low back pain (15,16). A recent survey conducted into practice in Pain Relief Clinics throughout the UK, revealed

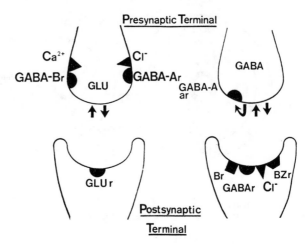

Figure 2 *GABA related synapses*
GABA. A ar—GABA-A antoreceptor
Br   —barbiturate receptor
Cl   —chloride ion channel
BZr   —benzodiazepine receptor
GABAr   —GABA-A receptor
GLU   —glutamate
GLUr   —glutamate receptor
GABA-Br   —GABA-B receptor

that the major areas of use of valproate were post-herpetic neuralgia, trigeminal neuralgia, phantom limb pain and low back pain.

Whilst the agent may be used as the sole therapeutic modality, a more profound effect is seen when it is prescribed in combination with a tricyclic antidepressant having an intact tertiary amine structure (amitriptyline, clomipramine) (17). The combination may, however, emphasize the central depressant effects of the drugs and drowsiness may be a problem, particularly in the elderly. This can be circumvented either by commencing medication with a single nocturnal dose followed by the gradual introduction of the remedy during the day until the optimal three-times-daily regimen is reached, or by the use of a less soporific tricyclic remedy such as nortriptyline.

In addition to the combination of valproate with tricyclic antidepressants, its therapeutic value may be enhanced when prescribed in conjunction with major tranquillizers such as perphenazine or pericyazine or with the butyrophenones haloperidol and droperidol. The analgesic effect and spectrum of activity may be increased by these combinations particularly when the pain is presenting in the face or neck.

In the implementation of treatment with valproate alone or in combination with other psychoactive agents, to ensure optimal results certain guidelines should be followed. These include:-

1. Commence the dose schedule at the lowest dose and increase at the rate of 100 mg per dose per week.
2. In elderly patients, the initial dose should be given at night time only for one week before introducing medication at the lowest possible dose during the day, initially once then twice daily plus the nocturnal dose.
3. Sufficient time on the medication must be allowed before evaluation is attempted. Consequently, patients should be encouraged to remain compliant and not to expect rapid analgesia; at least one month of therapy should be allowed at any starting dose before assessment.
4. Choice of additional therapy should be made with care, especially when specific combination therapy is contemplated.
5. Potential side-effects should be discussed with the patient as well as the likelihood that any drowsiness will diminish rapidly provided the patient remains on treatment. Persistent, marked drowsiness must be reported immediately to the physician.

In the prescription of valproate, certain pre-existing conditions should indicate the need for caution in either dose, frequency, rate of increase of medication or even whether to medicate or not. These include:-

1. Advanced age.
2. Medication with CNS depressants, e.g. barbiturates, benzodiazepines.
3. Medication with opioid analgesic agents.
4. Medication with some secondary analgesic agents.
5. Pre-existing thrombocytopenia, anaemia or leucopenia.
6. Previous allergy or serious side-effects with anticonvulsant drug.

Prolonged therapy with valproate may well induce initial hair loss about which patients, particularly female, should be warned and reassured. Weight gain may also be seen particularly when therapy is in combination with a tricyclic antidepressant which promotes water retention, e.g. amitriptyline.

CONCLUSION

Sodium valproate has been shown to be an excellent analgesic agent in a variety of painful syndromes of the neurogenic and autonomically mediated variety. Its efficacy across a wide spectrum of pathologies together with its favourable side-effect profile has meant that it has replaced other anticonvulsants and some physical techniques in the treatment of chronic pain (18).

REFERENCES

(1) Locock C. Discussion on Sieveking EH, Analysis of fifty-two cases of epilepsy observed by the author. *Lancet* 1857; i: 528.
(2) Trousseau A. In: *Clin Med Hotel Dieu*. TOME 1885; **2**: 156-65.
(3) Bergouignan M. Cures heureuses de nevralgies faciales essentielles par le diphenyl-hydantoinate de soude. *Rev Laryngol* 1942; **63**: 34-41.
(4) Blom S. Trigeminal neuralgia. Its treatment with a new anticonvulsive drug (G32883). *Lancet* 1962; i: 839-40.
(5) Crill WE. Carbamazepine. *Ann Int Med* 1973;**79**: 844-7.
(6) Anthony M. Relief of facial pain. *Drugs* 1979; **18**: 122-9.
(7) Rall TW, Schleiffer LS. Drugs effective in the therapy of the epilepsies.In: Goodman LS, Gillman AG, Gillman A, eds. *The pharmacological basis of therapeutics*, 6th ed. London: Macmillan, 1980: 448-74.
(8) Casey KL. Towards a rationale for the treatment of painful neuropathies. In: Dubner R, Gebhart GF, Bond MR, eds. *VIth World Congress on Pain*. Amsterdam: Elsevier, 1988: 165-74.
(9) Willow M. Pharmacology of diphenylhydantoin and carbamazepine action on voltage sensitive sodium channels. *Trends Neurosci* 1986; **9**: 147-9.
(10) Suria A, Costa E. Evidence fo GABA involvement in the action of diazepam on presynaptic nerve terminals in bullfrog sympathetic ganglia. *Adv Biochem Psychopharmacol* 1975; **14**: 103-12.
(11) Macdonald RL, Bergey GK. Valproic acid augments GABA-mediated post-synaptic inhibition in cultured mammalian neurones. *Brain Res* 1979; **170**: 558-62.
(12) Swerdlow M. The treatment of shooting pain. *Postgrad Med J* 1980; **56**: 159-61.
(13) Watkins PJ. Pain and diabetic neuropathy. *Br Med J* 1984; **288**: 168-9.
(14) Bhala BB, Ramamoorthy C, Bowsher D, Yelnorker KN. Shingles and post-herpetic neuralgia. *Clin Pain* 1988; **4**: 169-74.
(15) Tinnitus [Editorial]. *Lancet* 1984; i: 543-5.
(16) Budd K. Non-analgesic drugs in pain management. In: Lipton S, Miles J, eds. *Persistent pain*, vol 3. London: Academic Press, 1981: 223-40.
(17) Budd K. The pain clinic—chronic pain. In: Nunn JF, Utting JE, Brown BR, eds. *General anaesthesia*, 5th ed. London: Butterworths, 1989: 1349-70.
(18) Budd K. Recent advances in the treatment of chronic pain. *Br J Anaesth* 1989; **63**: 207-12.

Valproate and mania

H. M. Emrich and R. Wolf

Max Planck Institute for Psychiatry, Munich, Federal Republic of Germany

INTRODUCTION

Mania is a psychiatric syndrome which may appear to be far apart from epileptic disorders. Historically, however, new therapeutic approaches to the treatment of epileptic psychoses with affective symptoms have contributed much to the development of new treatments of endogenous affective disorders. For example, the work of Takezaki and Hanaoka in 1971 (1) using carbamazepine in epileptic patients with symptomatology suggesting hypermania, led to the question as to whether patients with endogenous mania might also profit from such a therapy, and indeed these authors, and subsequently Okuma et al. (2) demonstrated such a therapeutic effect with carbamazepine.

In the case of valproate the first studies in endogenous affective disorders were not performed with valproate itself, but its amidation product dipropylacetamide (valpromide). These investigations were performed by Lambert et al. as early as 1966 (3). The authors observed—as well as the anticonvulsant efficacy—psychotropic effects in non-psychotic disturbances of mood, especially affective lability, impulsiveness, irritability etc. In 1968, Lambert et al. (4) described therapeutic effects of valpromide in patients with bipolar manic depression. However, it was not until 1975 (5) that a more detailed description of the effects of valpromide in patients with affective disorders was given. It became apparent that valpromide had a mild antimanic, a slight antidepressant, and—especially in combination with low doses of lithium—a mood stabilizing effect in bipolar patients.

In 1984 Lambert et al. (6) described 108 cases of cyclothymia and 20 cases of mania and hypomania in a mixed group of 244 cases with affective disorders. The 128 cases described were treated with dipropylacetamide, with good or very good effects in 45 cases of cyclothymia and acceptable results in 39 cases; 24 of the cyclothymic patients showed no therapeutic effect. In the 20 cases of pure mania or hypomania, seven patients showed a good or very good response, nine a medium response, and four had no benefit from the treatment. Puzynski and Klosiewicz (7) described 10 bipolar cases and five schizoaffective cases treated with valpromide. The prophylactic effect of valpromide was especially noticeable with regard to manic phases, where a total reduction in the order of magnitude of 50% was observed. McElroy et al. (8) published a comprehensive overview of the use of valproate and valpromide in psychiatric disorders. These authors came to the conclusion that valproate represents a valuable addition to the therapeutic arsenal in the pharmacotherapy of affective disorders. In their studies they demonstrated an acute effect of valproate in mania in more than 75% of 17 bipolar cases.

ACUTE EFFECTS OF VALPROATE IN MANIA

At the Max Planck Institute in Munich our interest in the acute therapeutic effect of the GABAergic anticonvulsant valproate was raised from pharmacopsychiatric investigations pointing to the view that mania results from a dysfunction of inhibitory monotransmitters

Fourth international symposium on sodium valproate and epilepsy, edited by David Chadwick, 1989; Royal Society of Medicine Services International Congress and Symposium Series No. 152, published by Royal Society of Medicine Services Limited.

Table 1 *Acute effects of valproate*

Case	Age (yr)	Sex	Diagnosis (ICD–9)	Maximal dosage (mg/d)	Initial IMPS value (%)	Mean IMPS value at maximal dosage (%)	Change (%)
1	21	F	295.7	1800	27.1	3.4	87.5
2	23	M	296.3	3800	40.7	19.8	51.4
3	31	F	296.3	2700	23.1	13.6	41.1
4	18	F	296.3	1800	24.6	6.2	74.8
5	53	F	296.3	3000	15.7	16.8	−7.0
					$\bar{x}$ 26.2	12.0	49.6[a]
					± 9.1	7.0	36.6

[a] $p < 0.05$ *(Wilcoxon-test, one-tailed).*

in the CNS. GABA (gamma amino butyric acid) was an extremely challenging candidate in this regard. It was shown, using a double-blind ABA design, that high dosage propranolol exerts a rather specific antimanic action (9). Interestingly, it was possible to demonstrate that this effect is not mediated by beta-receptor blockade, since the d-stereoisomer, which is devoid of beta-receptor blocking properties, also has similar antimanic effects (10). The therapeutic action had been postulated by Delini-Stula, from animal experiments, to be mediated by a GABAergic component of the propranolol molecule (11). In line with this, Bernasconi *et al.* (12) demonstrated an indirect GABAergic effect of high-dosage propranolol *in vivo*. For that reason, we looked for other compounds which could clinically be applied to exert GABAergic effects in man. The first candidate was sodium valproate, a substance which is assumed to exert its anticonvulsant effect mainly via an indirect GABAergic mode of action.

We treated with valproate those patients who had a manic psychosis, using a double-blind, placebo-controlled, variable ABA design (A=placebo, B=active substance). The length of each treatment phase was unknown to the patient and to the psychiatrist performing the psychopathological evaluation. Informed consent was obtained from both the patients themselves and their close relatives prior to commencement of the trial. Psychopathological evaluation was performed by a physician using the Inpatient Multidimensional Psychiatric Scale (IMPS: 14). Five of the 12 IMPS subscales (EXC, HOS, GRN, MTR, CNP) were summed to form a score reflecting the patient's manic symptomatology. An extensive physical and neurological examination was performed in all patients prior to initiation of the trial. X-ray examinations were performed prior to onset of medication. Thrombocyte count and bleeding time, in particular, were controlled both before and during the course of medication. The therapeutic effect of valproate is represented in Table 1. The maximum dosage ranged from 1.8 to 3.8 g/day. An average reduction of the initial IMPS values by 49.6±36.6% resulted from this therapy (significant at the 5% level, Wilcoxon-test, one-tailed).

This therapeutic effect is in line with findings published by Brennan *et al.* (15).

PROPHYLACTIC EFFECTS OF VALPROATE

Long-term prophylactic medication with valproate (in one case with dipropylacetamide (DPA)) was given to 12 lithium non-responders, in 11 of them in combination with low doses of lithium (serum levels of 0.4–0.8 mmol/l); in one case, discontinuation of the lithium treatment for some time was necessary owing to the occurrence of severe lithium side-effects. The clinical course of these outpatients was evaluated by a trained psychiatrist (open study), using the VBS (Verlaufs-Beurteilungs-Skala, i.e. course-assessment scale), a self-constructed scale with eight degrees of intensity, adapted here to reflect the global impression of 'manic behaviour' and 'depression' (cf. 16).

The clinical course of patients under long-term valproate therapy (mostly in combination with low lithium dosage) is represented in Table 2. The patients included in this long-term prospective investigation belong to a group of 'problem cases' who did not respond

Table 2   *Clinical course of patients under long-term valproate/DPA therapy*

Case	Age (yr)	Sex	Diagnosis (ICD-9)	Average interval between phases during the last 5 years before treatment (months)	Duration of therapy (yr)	Number of relapses of the affective disorder during therapy	Improvement ratio (r)
Valproate (+ low-dosage lithium)							
S.W.	51	M	296.3	9	6.5	0	8.7
S.A.	37	M	295.7	10	6	3[a]	2.4
H.W.	42	M	295.7	5	5.5	0	13.2
B.W.	59	M	296.3	10	4.5	0	5.4
R.R.	36	F	295.7	19	4	2	1.3
S.M.	27	F	295.7	12	4	0	4.0
S.I.	63	F	296.1	7	3.5	0	6.0
H.H.	36	F	296.3	11	1.5[b]	0	1.6
L.H-P.	28	M	295.7	12	2.5	0	2.5
K.L.	28	M	295.7	15	1.5[b]	0	1.2
L.M.	29	M	296.3	3	2.5	0	10.0
DPA (+low-dosage lithium)							
L.H-W.	59	M	296.2	7	4	0	6.9
							$\bar{x}$ 5.3
							$\pm$ 3.9

[a]*Relapses only of schizophrenic symptoms.* [b]*Discontinuation of therapy after 1.5 years due to non-compliance.*

adequately to lithium. The average interval between phases over the five years preceding valproate/DPA treatment ranged from three to 19 months, whereas the relapse-free time during this treatment has ranged (up to the present) from 18 to 78 months. The most impressive therapeutic effects of valproate, used as an adjunct to the lowered dosages of lithium, continuously applied to the patients, is also apparent from Figs. 1–3, which represent the phase-charts of selected patients. If the 'improvement ratio' r is defined as

$$r = \frac{\text{average phase interval (months) after treatment}}{\text{average phase interval (months) before treatment}}$$

r=1 would mean no effect; r<1 deterioration; r>1 improvement; r=2 improvement by a factor of 2; r=3 improvement by a factor of 3, etc.

In the 12 cases examined, the average improvement ratio is 5.3 ± 3.9 (comparing the course of the illness during valproate/DPA prophylaxis with prior lithium prophylaxis).

A statistical analysis can be performed by a comparison of the average mean phase interval before valproate/DPA medication with the relapse-free time during this treatment (Table 3). The average values are: $\bar{x} = 10.0 \pm 4.3$ months before and $\bar{x} = 41.2 \pm 18.5$ months during treatment. The difference is highly significant ($p < 0.005$, Wilcoxon Test, two-tailed).

MODE OF ACTION OF VALPROATE

The most often cited hypothesis on the mechanism of action of valproate originated with Godin *et al*. (17) and suggests that valproate augments neuronal inhibition by increasing brain levels of GABA via an inhibition of the GABA—degrading enzyme GABA-transaminase. However, several objections to the increased-GABA-level hypothesis have been made: (a) the concentrations of valproate used by several authors were many times higher than the range of the therapeutic level for humans; (b) there was only a poor correlation between valproate-induced GABA levels in animal brain and the protection against chemically or electrically induced seizures (18,19); (c) it is not clear whether enhanced synaptic GABA concentrations lead to an increased GABA release into the synaptic cleft which might be necessary for enhanced GABAergic transmission; (d) recently, concentrations of valproate up to 10 mM were shown to have no inhibitory effect on GABA-T (20).

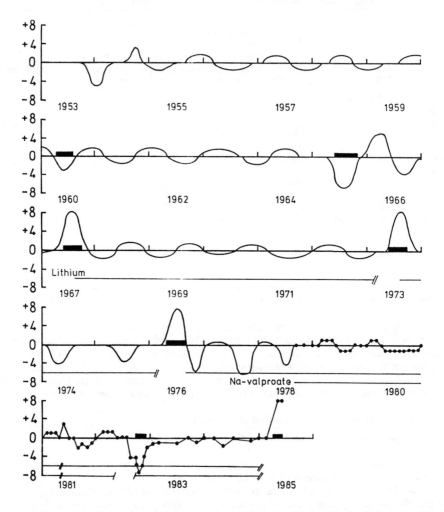

Figure 1 *Time course of the psychopathology of a patient with bipolar affective disorder (ICD–9, No. 296.3), represented by the use of the VBS (Verlaufs-Beurteilungs-Skala, i.e. course assessment scale; cf. 16) under prophylactic long-term medication with valproate in combination with low doses of lithium.* Symbols: *Heavy bars: hospitalization; $+8=$maximal mania; $-8=$maximal depression.*

A second hypothesis was proposed by Macdonald and Bergey in 1979 (21), who demonstrated an enhanced responsiveness of cultured spinal cord neurons to iontophoretically applied GABA. Recently, also direct membrane effects of valproate have been reported (22).

It was therefore of interest to investigate the action of valproate in therapeutic and higher concentrations on synaptic GABA release, utilizing the push-pull-cannula technique, a method of focal *in vivo* perfusion of brain structures, in unanaesthetized, freely moving rats. We chose the ovariectomized rat as an animal model in order to get an oestrogen cycle independent feedback situation of the hypothalamic-pituitary axis, and tried to reveal the effect of preoptically applied valproate on this neuroendocrine network, since there seem to be several interrelations between valproate, GABA, and neuroendocrine functions.

Preoptically applied sodium valproate, in a concentration range from 40 to 1600 µg/ml CSF, differentially affected the local release of GABA into the push-pull perfusate. Local

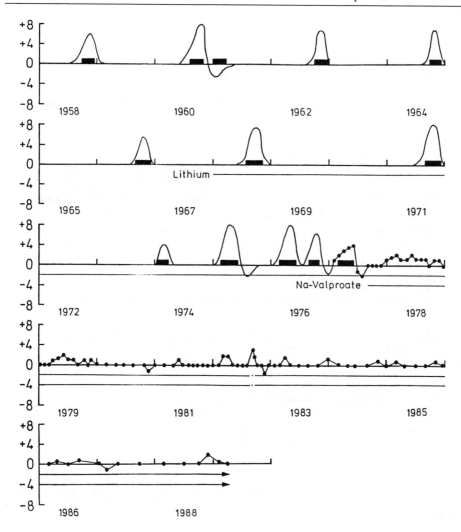

Figure 2 *Time course of the psychopathology of a patient with bipolar affective disorder (ICD–9, No. 296.3). Symbols as in Fig. 1.*

treatment with 40, 80, 100, and 200 µg/ml perfusion medium induced a highly significant decrease in preoptic GABA release (Fig. 4). After return to valproate-free medium this effect was reversible. A rapid onset and termination of the valproate effect within 5 min could be observed. With increased valproate concentrations the suppressive effect became less and at supra-therapeutic valproate levels of 1600 µg/ml CSF an increase in GABA release could be observed in four out of eight animals. This dose response relationship points to a biphasic effect of valproate on the available amount of GABA in the synaptic cleft, which may be produced by at least two different dose-dependent mechanisms of action. The present results indicate that the action of therapeutic concentrations of valproate involves an alteration of GABAergic transmission different from increasing synaptic GABA release. The data are consistent with the hypothesis that valproate action, at least at the level of the preoptic area, involves an enhancement of GABAergic transmission and causes—via a negative feedback mechanism—a suppression of GABA release into the synaptic cleft (23). This view is supported by further experiments from our laboratory, showing that perfusion of the preoptic area with valproate simultaneously caused a decrease

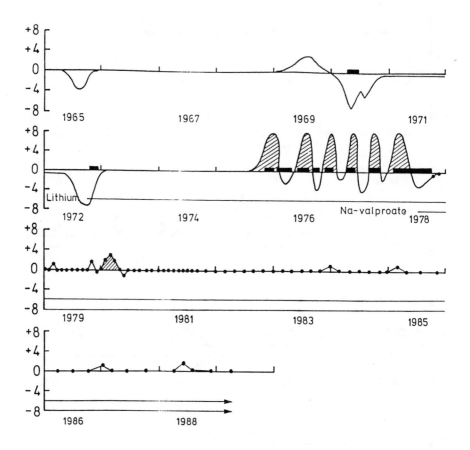

Figure 3 *Time course of the psychopathology of a patient with schizoaffective psychosis (ICD–9, No. 295.7). Symbols as in Fig. 1. Cross-hatched areas represent episode with admixture of schizophrenic symptoms.*

Table 3 *Statistics (valproate/DPA prophylaxis)*

Phase interval prior to treatment (months)	Relapse-free time during treatment (months)
9	78
10	32
5	66
10	54
19	30
12	48
7	42
11	18
12	30
15	18
3	30
7	48
x̄ 10.0	41.2
± 4.3	18.5

p < 0.005 (Wilcoxon, 2-tailed).

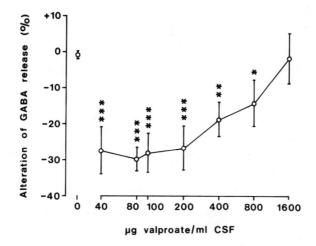

Figure 4 *Dose response relationship derived from a total of 51 rats, perfused with valproate at different concentrations (number of rats in parentheses): 0 (8), 40 (4), 80 (8), 100 (5), 200 (6), 400 (6), 800 (6), 1600 (8)* μg/ml CSF, respectively. Ordinate: *Mean percentage of intraindividual alteration of GABA release between the period under treatment (n = 8 fractions) compared with the period before treatment (n = 8 fractions). Mean values as circles with SEM as vertical bars are given.* Abscissa *(logarithmic scale): Concentrations of valproate per ml CSF.* Asterisks: *** $p < 0.001$, ** $p < 0.01$, * $p < 0.05$ *vs control group.*

in local GABA release and a suppression in pituitary LH secretion. These data can be explained by an enhancement of GABAergic transmission. Thus, the drug may exert its GABA-synergistic or -mimetic effect by direct inhibitory postsynaptic action on LHRH cell bodies, causing a suppression of LH secretion. Simultaneously, as a consequence of negative feedback interactions of valproate via the pre- and/or the postsynaptic membrane, the GABA release into the synaptic cleft is reduced.

SUMMARY

Valproate can be used as an effective sole therapeutic agent in acute mania as well as an adjunct to the lithium treatment. Furthermore, valproate can be used as a prophylactic agent in cyclothymia, especially with pronounced manic phases. It can also be shown that a combination of valproate with lithium is effective in 'problem cases' who respond insufficiently to lithium prophylaxis. The mode of action of valproate appears to be related to an increase in GABAergic transmission.

REFERENCES

(1) Takezaki H, Hanaoka M. The use of carbamazepine (Tegretol) in the control of manic-depressive psychosis and other manic-depressive states. *Clin Psychiat* 1971; **13**: 173–83.
(2) Okuma T, Kishimoto A, Inoue K, Matsumoto H, Ogura A, Matsushita T, Nakao T, Ogura C. Antimanic and prophylactic effects of carbamazepine (Tegretol) on manic depressive psychoses. A preliminary report. *Fol Psychiat Neurol Jpn* 1973; **27**: 283–97.
(3) Lambert PA, Carraz G, Borselli S, Carrel S. Action neuropsychotrope d'un nouvel antiépileptique: le Dépamide. *Ann Med Psychol (Paris)* 1966; **1**: 707–10.
(4) Lambert PA, Borselli S, Midenet J, Baudrand C, Marcou G, Bouchardy M. L'action favorable du Dépamide sur l'évolution à long terme des psychoses maniaco-dépressives. *Comptes Rendu du Congrés de Psychiatrie et de Neurologie de langue Française. 66eme session. Clermont-Ferrand, 16–21 Septembre, 1968*: 489–93.
(5) Lambert PA, Carraz G, Borselli S, Bouchardy M. Le dipropylacétamide dans le traitement de la psychose maniaco-dépressive. *L'Encephale* 1979; **1**: 25–31.

(6) Lambert PA. Acute and prophylactic therapies of patients with affective disorders using valpromide (dipropylacetamide). In: Emrich HM, Okuma T, Müller AA, eds. *Anticonvulsants in affective disorders.* Amsterdam: Excerpta Medica, 1984: 33–44.

(7) Puzynski S, Klosiewicz L. Valproic acid amide in the treatment of affective and schizoaffective disorders. *J Affect Dis* 1984; **6**: 115–21.

(8) McElroy S, Keck PE Jr, Pope HG Jr. Sodium valproate: Its use in primary psychiatric disorders. *J Clin Psychopharmacol* 1987; **7**: 16–24.

(9) Rackensperger W, Fritsch W, Schwarz D, Stutte KH, von Zerssen D. Die Wirkung des Beta-Rezeptoren-Blockers Propranolol auf Manien. *Arch Psychiat Nervenkr* 1976; **222**: 223–43.

(10) Emrich HM, von Zerssen D, Möller HJ, Kissling W, Cording C, Schietsch HJ, Riedel E. Action of propranolol in mania—Comparison of effects of the d- and the l-stereoisomer. *Pharmakopsychiatrie* 1979; **12**: 295–304.

(11) Vassout A, Delini-Stula A. Effects of β-bloquers (propranolol et oxprénolol et du diazepam sur differents modeles d'aggressivite chez le rat. *J Pharmacol (Paris)* 1977; **8**: 5–14.

(12) Bernasconi R. The GABA hypothesis of affective illness—Influence of clinically effective antimanic drugs on GABA turnover. In: Emrich HM, Aldenhoff JB, Lux HD, eds. *Basic mechanisms in the action of lithium.* Amsterdam: Excerpta Medica, 1982: 183–92.

(13) Bernasconi R, Hauser K, Martin P, Schmutz M. Biochemical aspects of the mechanism of action of valproate. In: Emrich HM, Okuma T, Müller AA, eds. *Anticonvulsants in affective disorders.* Amsterdam: Excerpta Medica, 1984: 14–32.

(14) Lorr M, Klett CJ,McNair DM, Lasky JJ. *Inpatient multidimensional psychiatric scale.* Palo Alto, CA: Consulting Psychologists Press, 1962.

(15) Brennan MJW, Sandyk R, Borsock D. Use of sodium valproate in the management of affective disorders—Basic and clinical aspects. In: Emrich HM, Okuma T, Müller AA, eds. *Anticonvulsants in affective disorders.* Amsterdam: Excerpta Medica, 1984: 56–65.

(16) Emrich HM, Cording C, Piree S, Kölling A, von Zerssen D, Herz A. Indication of an antipsychotic action of the opiate antagonist naloxone. *Pharmakopsychiatrie* 1977; **10**: 265–70.

(17) Godin Y, Heiner L, Mark J, Mandel P. Effects of di-n-propylacetate, an anticonvulsive compound, on GABA metabolism. *J Neurochem* 1969; **16**: 869–73.

(18) Schmutz M, Olpe H-R, Koella W. Central actions of valproate sodium. *J Pharm Pharmacol* 1979; **31**: 413–4.

(19) Kerwin RW, Olpe H-R, Schmutz M. The effect of sodium-n-dipropylacetate on gamma-aminobutyric acid-dependent inhibition in the rat cortex and substantia nigra in relation to its anticonvulsant activity. *Br J Pharmacol* 1980; **71**: 545–51.

(20) Löscher W. Effect of inhibitors of GABA transaminase on the synthesis, binding, uptake, and metabolism of GABA. *J Neurochem* 1980; **34**: 1603–8.

(21) Macdonald RL, Bergey GK. Valproic acid augments GABA-mediated post-synaptic inhibition in cultured mammalian neurons. *Brain Res* 1979; **170**: 558–62.

(22) Slater GE, Johnston D. Sodium valproate increases potassium conductance in *Aplysia* neurons. *Epilepsia* 1978; **19**: 379–84.

(23) Wolf R, Tscherne U, Emrich HM. Suppression of preoptic GABA release caused by push-pull-perfusion with sodium valproate. *Naunyn-Schmiedeberg's Arch Pharmacol* 1988; **338**: 658–63.

Discussion after Dr Budd and Professor Emrich

Dr Duncan *(London, UK)*: Could Dr Budd give us some facts and figures on how efficacious sodium valproate is in patients with pain?

Dr Budd *(Bradford, UK)*: There is very little published evidence about the efficacy and this is one of the reasons that a current study is under way to compare valproate with carbamazepine in many indications. The other problem is that by and large the patients that come to most pain relief services have had a plethora of drugs and other treatments by the time they reach us, and may have been on one or more of the anticonvulsants already. It does tend to bias one towards the agents that have not been tried. However, the global results from the study that I mentioned would indicate that in the patients who have failed on other anti-convulsant therapy one will get a 40% improvement which will range from patients saying that they have less pain, to those who are completely pain free.

Dr Binnie *(London, UK)*: Professor Emrich, you mentioned valpromide which has been marketed as a psychotropic drug although there seems to be some uncertainty as to whether any valpromide is absorbed into the body, other than as valproate. Are you aware of any studies that indicate a difference in the psychotropic actions of valproate and valpromide?

Professor Emrich *(Munich, West Germany)*: It is correct to say that within minutes valpromide in the body is transformed into valproate, so from the clinical profile of action there is no difference between valproate and valpromide.

Dr Abraham *(London, UK)*: Dr Budd, in my own experience using valproate there have been occasions when patients have found pain relief, but what criteria do you use, and how do you reach a level of 6 g? Have you had patients who show dramatic improvement with such high doses?

Dr Budd: In the survey, one centre was using up to that level but one does not necessarily need to go outside the normally accepted dose range. I would echo the comments made earlier, what is the dose range for valproate? I think we tend to limit ourselves unnecessarily.

Dr Abraham: What sort of programme do you have say, for somebody with atypical facial pain that has not responded to other drugs? Do you start with carbamazepine first and then tricyclics or valproate?

Dr Budd: It depends what other treatment they have had, but certainly my line of approach would be to start them on a combination of nortriptyline and valproate at a gradually increasing dose level for three months before one can assess them adequately. At that stage if there has been no response, then they will be switched over to amitriptyline and probably carbamazepine if they have not already had it. More recently we have adopted a slightly different technique in that patients that are started on psychotropic mixtures, usually nortriptyline and valproate will also get aspirin transdermally, and this is providing us with an interesting treatment for post herpetic neuralgia.

Dr Abraham: And for the trigeminal neuralgias?

Dr Budd: Again much depends on what other agents they have had previously. Normally we start off on 200 mg three times a day and moved up fairly rapidly to about 1200 mg twice or three times a day to see if we can get an effect. And if at that level there is no significant beneficial effect to their pain we will move over to a physical form of treatment.

Dr Gram *(Dianalund, Denmark):* This next question is a repeat of the one I asked before the session began.

Interactive question from Dr Gram

Would you consider the use of valproate for	**Response**
1 The treatment of pain	56%
2 In psychiatric disorders	28%
3 In both indications	16%
PREVIOUS ANSWER	
1 The treatment of pain	58%
2 In psychiatric disorders	28%
3 In both indications	16%

Interactive question from Professor Emrich

If you are using valproate for psychological disorder do you use it as	**Response**
1 Tranquillizer	8%
2 Mood stabilizer	73%
3 Other	19%

SESSION VI

PATIENT LIFESTYLE

Chairman: P. Fenwick

INTRODUCTION

Welcome to the sixth and penultimate session, dealing with cognitive behaviour, mind and sexual functioning. Cognitive behaviour has become more important recently and our awareness of the cognitive problems that patients with epilepsy have been continually growing. Sexual functioning is still the 'Cinderella' of epilepsy. The Scandinavians were one of the first groups to publish the early definitive papers on sexual functioning, and this was taken up by our Group and fortunately others have followed, but more data are needed.

In the first part of the symposium we are going to look at sexual functioning. Dr Brodie would like to begin with a question, and ask it again after his presentation.

Concerning sexual functioning in epileptic patients, choose one option	Response
1 The topic should be mentioned only by the patient and not by the doctor	8%
2 Patients should be encouraged to discuss any sexual problems	60%
3 Patients should be asked specifically about sexual arousal, performance and satisfaction	32%

Anticonvulsants and sexual function

M. J. Brodie

Clinical Pharmacology Unit, University Department of Medicine, Western Infirmary, Glasgow, UK

INTRODUCTION

There is much clinical evidence to support a relationship between treated epilepsy and hyposexuality both in men and women (1–4). A reduction in sexual interest, awareness and activity is particularly evident in patients with temporal lobe seizures (5–10). Is the sexual dysfunction a consequence of the seizure disorder, a function of its treatment or both? Does polypharmacy contribute to the problem? Are any individual anticonvulsants more or less likely to interfere with libido and performance?

HYPOTHALAMO-PITUITARY-GONADAL AXIS

Evidence is slowly accumulating that long term treatment with anticonvulsant drugs can have an adverse influence on the hypothalamo-pituitary-gonadal axis (1,2,11). In 1975, Christiansen and his colleagues (12) reported reduced urinary excretion of androsterone and dehydroepiandrosterone in male epileptic patients receiving anticonvulsant drugs. Shortly after, raised levels of sex hormone binding globulin (SHBG) were noted in both sexes (13–15). This led to the appreciation that although total circulating testosterone concentrations remained unaltered in treated male epileptics, free (unbound) testosterone, the active moiety, was reduced (10,16–18), particularly if more than one anticonvulsant drug was being taken (18,19). The premise that these changes are a consequence of enzyme induction is supported by a similar increase in SHBG produced by the antimicrobial inducer rifampicin (20) and by an acute reduction in free testosterone following carbamazepine ingestion in healthy volunteers (21) (Fig. 1). Low free testosterone levels provoke the release of luteinizing hormone from the anterior pituitary by negative feedback (15,18,22,23). The persisting depression of free testosterone despite luteinizing hormone stimulation implies an inability of the testicular Leydig cells to incease synthesis further. This may result from exhaustion (19) or from a direct toxic effect of anticonvulsant drugs on the testes (1).

Most studies of sex hormones have been performed in males. Because of the complexity of the menstrual cycle, data on hormone levels in female epileptics are sparse. Backstrom and Sodegard (24), however, have reported elevated SHGB and reduced percentage free testosterone at mid-cycle in six treated patients.

Evidence of central hormonal dysfunction in epileptic patients is conflicting and the balance is against an important direct influence of anticonvulsant drugs on the hypothalamo-pituitary axis (1,2).

PROLACTIN

The contributory role of prolactin to male hyposexuality is unclear. Hyperprolactinaemia is undoubtedly associated with impotence (25) and elevated prolactin levels appear to reduce

Fourth international symposium on sodium valproate and epilepsy, edited by David Chadwick, 1989; Royal Society of Medicine Services International Congress and Symposium Series No. 152, published by Royal Society of Medicine Services Limited.

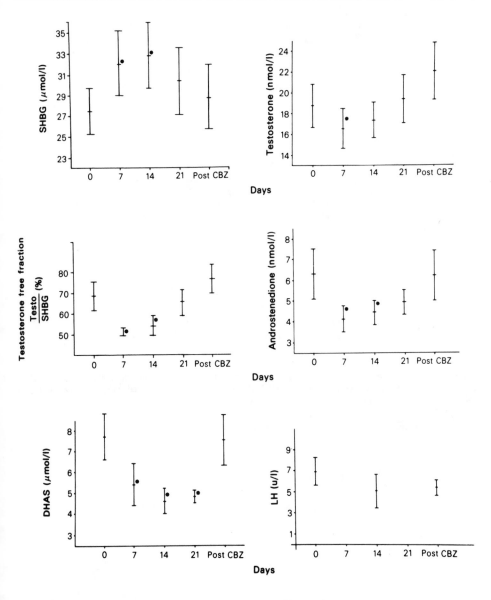

Figure 1   *Changes (mean ± s.e.m.) in sex hormone binding globulin (SHBG), testosterone, free testosterone fraction, androstenedione, dehydroepiandrosterone sulphate (DHAS) and luteinising hormone during carbamazepine therapy in 6 healthy male subjects (taken from reference 21—with permission).*

testosterone concentrations (26), perhaps by interfering with negative feedback control of gonadotrophin secretion (27). Generalized tonic-clonic seizures are often accompanied by a postictal rise in prolactin (28) that may persist for some hours (29). Complex partial seizures cause a smaller rise but these electrical events may be more frequent and are often subclinical (30,31). In addition, mean nocturnal plasma prolactin concentrations may be higher in epileptic patients than in non-epileptic control subjects (32). Elevated levels of basal prolactin have been noted in some patients treated with multiple antiepileptic drugs (17,18). These changes are modest in comparison with prolactin levels found in patients with pituitary disorders. Nevertheless, prolactin release could be a contributory factor to hyposexuality in susceptible patients.

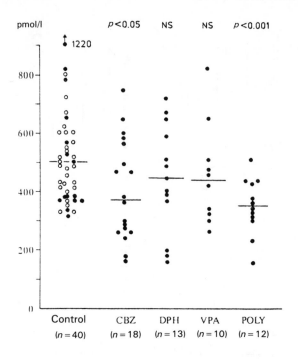

Figure 2 *Free testosterone concentrations in 53 male epileptic patients receiving carbamazepine (CBZ), phenytoin (PHT), sodium valproate (VPA) or combination (POLY) therapy and in 14 untreated epileptic patients (shaded) and 26 healthy controls (unshaded) (taken from reference 18—with permission).*

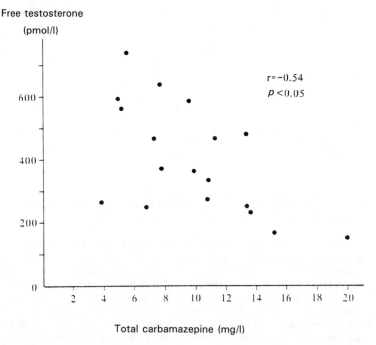

Figure 3 *Relationship between total plasma carbamazepine concentration and free testosterone in 18 male epileptic patients receiving the drug as monotherapy (taken from reference 18—with permission).*

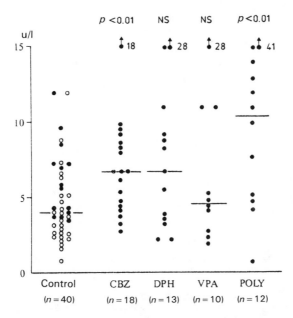

Figure 4 *Basal luteinizing hormone concentrations in 53 male epileptic patients receiving carbamazepine (CBZ), phenytoin (PHT), sodium valproate (VPA) or combination (POLY) therapy and in 14 untreated epileptic patients (shaded) and 26 healthy controls (unshaded) (taken from reference 18—with permission).*

INDIVIDUAL ANTICONVULSANTS

The fall in free testosterone during anticonvulsant therapy occurs partly as a result of enzyme induction with accelerated metabolism of the hormone and partly as a consequence of raised SHBG capacity which is also likely to be a product of metabolic induction. If this is so, variation in the extent of this process can be expected in individual patients treated with different anticonvulsant inducers which themselves do not produce identical effects on hepatic monooxygenase enzymes (33,34). Additionally, sodium valproate, which does not induce hepatic mixed function oxidase activity (35), may have a sparing effect on circulating sex hormones.

In a recent study in young male epileptic patients, treatment with carbamazepine was associated with low free testosterone (Fig. 2) which was concentration-related (Fig. 3) and accompanied by elevated basal levels of luteinizing hormone (18) (Fig. 4). Phenytoin monotherapy increased only SHBG synthesis ($p < 0.01$). Sodium valproate did not appear to influence any of the hormones measured. In this study basal prolactin concentrations were elevated in the carbamazepine-treated patients, a finding which confirmed a previous observation in smaller numbers of male epileptic patients (23).

SEXUAL EXPERIENCE SCALES

Despite substantial variations and deficiencies in design, most studies report findings consistent with hyposexuality in epileptic patients. The factors contributing to this important observation remain unclear, partly because no standardized approach to investigation of sexual function has been devised and partly because only a few studies have contained control data on sexual activity in healthy adults (1).

We have employed a computerized questionnaire devised and validated in the Netherlands by Frenken and Vennix (36). Four Sexuality Experience Scales (SES) have been produced comprising 83 self-report items with fixed response categories. The four scales give a score for sexual morality (SES1), acceptance of psychosexual stimulation (SES2),

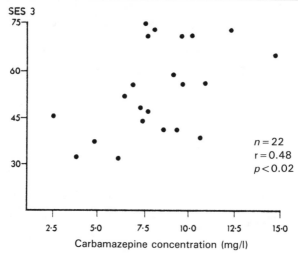

Figure 5 *Relationship between circulating carbamazepine concentration and sexual motivation scores in 22 young male epileptics receiving the drug as monotherapy. The higher the score the lower is the sexual appetite.*

sexual motivation (SES3) and attraction to one's own marriage (SES4). SES1 and 2 are administered to patients without a current sexual partner. All four scores are completed by patients entered into a stable heterosexual relationship.

The battery of questions is applied by an Amstrad CPC 6128 micro-computer with keyboard and joystick controls. A few extra specific enquiries e.g. morning erections, extramarital relationships etc. have been incorporated. Each patient takes around 20 min to complete the protocol. Blood is withdrawn at the same visit for circulating anticonvulsant and hormone concentrations. When possible, antipyrine 600 mg is administered and the patient collects saliva samples on six occasions over the next 32 h. Antipyrine kinetics are employed as a measure of enzyme induction.

Currently 129 men (27 healthy controls) and 131 women (20 healthy controls) have been recruited into the study. Preliminary analysis suggests that male epileptic patients ($n=97$) have more restrictive morality ($p<0.06$), accept less sexual stimulation ($p<0.0001$) and report a lower sexual appetite ($p<0.06$) than healthy controls ($n=26$). More schooling ($p<0.05$) and further education ($p<0.005$) were associated with lower morality scores in the epileptic patients ($n=89$). A negative correlation was obtained between circulating carbamazepine concentration and sexual appetite in 22 young men receiving the drug as monotherapy (Fig. 5).

Female patients ($n=97$) reported more restrictive morality ($p=0.08$) and accepted less sexual stimulation ($p<0.01$) than healthy controls ($n=19$). Treated epileptics ($n=80$) demonstrated more restrictive morality ($p<0.05$), admitted to a lower sexual appetite ($p<0.02$) and showed less attraction to marriage ($p<0.05$) then untreated patients ($n=17$). There was no correlation between age and morality or attraction to marriage but a negative relationship was obtained between duration of epilepsy and restrictive morality ($n=90$; $r=0.36$, $p<0.01$) and attraction to marriage ($n=40$; $r=0.47$, $p<0.01$). Again, more schooling ($p<0.05$), further education ($p<0.001$) and current employment ($p<0.002$) were associated with reduced morality scores. Patients receiving further education ($p<0.005$) and in current employment ($p<0.001$) allowed more sexual stimulation.

Male and female patients receiving phenytoin monotherapy ($n=25$) had lower sexual appetites and revealed a lesser attraction to marriage (both $p<0.05$) than those treated with carbamazepine ($n=46$).

CONCLUSION

All studies have reported hyposexuality in epileptic patients (1–4). It seems likely that the seizure disorder itself contributes to this impairment of sexual function particularly in patients with partial epilepsy arising from a focus in one or other temporal lobe (11).

Although the role of anticonvulsant medication has not been fully elucidated, the enzyme-inducing anticonvulsants carbamazepine, phenytoin, phenobarbitone and primidone (metabolized in part to phenobarbitone) probably exacerbate the problem in some susceptible individuals. These drugs have been shown in a number of studies to reduce free testosterone concentration by increasing its turnover and stimulating the production of the binding protein. A compensatory rise in luteinizing hormone suggests that these changes can have physiological consequences. As testosterone concentrations do not appear to return to normal despite pituitary-mediated stimulation, these drugs may precipitate testicular failure in young epileptic men with little leeway for response (17). This may result in reduced libido and sexual drive. A clear relationship has been reported between testosterone levels and nocturnal penile tumescence (37). Testosterone is essential also for normal spermatogenesis (38) and there is one report, so far unconfirmed, of abnormal sperm morphology and motility in treated epileptic patients (12).

The situation in epileptic women is less clear-cut. Fewer studies have been performed but hyposexuality in this population also seems likely (3,4). Sex hormone patterns have been little investigated but reduced free testosterone concentrations have been reported (24). Female sexual drive is thought to correlate highly with free testosterone levels at mid-cycle.

The extent of sexual impairment in the epileptic population is not entirely known: 44% of patients in the David Lewis Centre for Epilepsy claimed never to have had an orgasm (10). In the Veterans Administration study, 11% of patients receiving phenytoin, 13% on carbamazepine, 16% on phenobarbitone and 22% treated with primidone complained of sexual dysfunction (39).

It is possible that not all anticonvulsant drugs share the same propensity for sexual impairment. In particular, sodium valproate, may have a sparing effect on circulating sex hormones and, pragmatically, may represent an acceptable alternative in patients reporting sexual dysfunction. Unfortunately, a valproate-treated group was not included in the Veterans study. It is not certain, either, that all enzyme-inducing anticonvulsants have an identical influence on the hormonal milieu. Carbamazepine is a particularly effective inducer of steroid hormone catabolism.

Patients with epilepsy bear a heavy burden. They carry the stigma of a misunderstood disorder. They have difficulties with education and employment. They take anticonvulsant drugs which may interfere with their memory and concentration, alter their mood and sap their drive and will. It is likely that many are also hyposexual. We need to know the contributory factors so that affected individuals can be identified and appropriate treatment can be devised.

Specific enquiry should be made of all patients regarding libido and sexual performance before and after initiation of anticonvulsant therapy. A computerized questionnaire can take the embarrassment out of such an interview allowing patients to answer freely the most intimate questions. Such an approach is under way in the Epilepsy Clinic at the Western Infirmary, Glasgow, using a modification of the validated Sexual Experience Scales (36). A large number of non-epileptic individuals are being recruited to provide a firm data base for normal sexuality. Preliminary results suggest differences in sexuality between epileptic patients and healthy controls and hint at subtle differences between individual anticonvulsant drugs.

ACKNOWLEDGMENT

My grateful thanks go to Anne Somers for expert secretarial assistance.

REFERENCES

(1) Toone BK. Sexual disorders in epilepsy. In: Pedley TA, Meldrum BS, eds. *Recent advances in epilepsy* 3. Edinburgh: Churchill Livingstone, 1986: 233–60.

(2) Mattson R, Cramer JA. Epilepsy, sex hormones and anti-epileptic drugs. *Epilepsia* 1985; **26** (suppl 1): 240–51.

(3) Rust J, Golombok S. The validation of the Golombok Rust Inventory of Sexual Satisfaction. *Br J Clin Psychol* 1985; **24**: 63–4.

(4) Ndegwa D, Rust J, Golombok S, Fenwick P. Sexual problems in epileptic women. *Sex Marit Ther* 1986; **1**: 175–7

(5) Gastaut H, Collomb N. Etude du comportement sexual chez les epileptiques psychomoteurs. *Ann Medico-Physiol* 1954; **112**: 657–96.

(6) Taylor D. Sexual behaviour and temporal lobe epilepsy. *Arch Neurol* 1969; **21**: 510–6.

(7) Saunders M, Rawson M. Sexuality in male epileptics. *J Neurol Sci* 1970; **10**: 577–83.

(8) Shukla G, Srivastava O, Katiyar B. Sexual disturbance in temporal lobe epilepsy: a controlled study. *Br J Psych* 1979; **134**: 288–92.

(9) Pritchard PB. Hyposexuality: a complication of complex partial epilepsy. *Trans J Am Psych Assoc* 1980; **105**: 193–5.

(10) Fenwick PBC, Toone BK, Wheeler MJ, Nanjee MN, Grant R, Brown D. Sexual behaviour in a centre for epilepsy. *Acta Neurol Scand* 1985; **7**: 428–35.

(11) Herzog AG. A hypothesis to integrate partial seizures of temporal lobe origin and reproductive endocrine disorders. *Epilepsy Res* 1989; **3**: 151–9.

(12) Christiansen P, Degaard J, Lund M. Potency, fertility and sexual hormones in young male epileptics. *Ugeskr Laeger* 1975; **137**: 242–5.

(13) Victor A, Lundberg PO, Johansson EDM. Induction of sex hormone binding globulin by phenytoin. *Br Med J* 1977; **2**: 934–5.

(14) Barragy JM, Makin HLT, Trafford BJH, Scott DF. Effect of anticonvulsants on plasma testosterone and sex hormone binding globulin levels. *J Neurol Neurosurg Psych* 1978; **41**: 913–4.

(15) Toone BK, Wheeler M, Fenwick PBC. Sex hormone changes in male epileptics. *Clin Endocrinol* 1980; **12**: 391–5.

(16) Dana-Haeri J, Oxley J, Richens A. Reduction of free testosterone by antiepileptic drugs. *Br Med J* 1982; **1**: 85–6.

(17) Toone BK, Wheeler M, Nanjee M, Fenwick PBC, Grant R. Sex hormones, sexual activity and plasma anticonvulsant levels in male epileptics. *J Neurol Neurosurg Psych* 1983; **46**: 824–6.

(18) MacPhee GJA, Larkin JG, Butler E, Beastall GH, Brodie MJ. Circulating hormones and pituitary responsiveness in young epileptic men receiving long-term antiepileptic medication. *Epilepsia* 1988; **29**: 468–75.

(19) Rodin E, Subramanian MG, Schmaltz S, Gilroy J. Testosterone levels in adult male epileptic patients. *Neurology* 1987; **3**: 706–8.

(20) Brodie MJ, Boobis AR, Gill M, Mashiter K. Does rifampicin increase serum levels of testosterone and oestradiol by inducing sex hormone binding globulin capacity? *Br J Clin Pharmacol* 1981; **12**: 431–2.

(21) Connell JMC, Rapeport WG, Beastall GH, Brodie MJ. Changes in circulating androgens during short term carbamazepine therapy. *Br J Clin Pharmacol* 1984; **17**: 347–51.

(22) Hoffman H, Kahlert T. The effects of prolonged anticonvulsant treatment on the sexual hormones of male epileptic patients. *Nervenazt* 1981; **52**: 715–7.

(23) Rodin E, Subramanian MG, Gilroy J. Investigation of sex hormones in male epileptic patients. *Epilepsia* 1984; **25**: 690–4.

(24) Backstrom C, Sodegard R. Testosterone-oestradiol-binding globulin, unbound and total oestradiol and testosterone, and total progesterone during the menstrual cycle in women with epilepsy taking antiepileptic drugs. *J Endocr Invest* 1979; **2**: 359–66.

(25) Cooper AJ. Advances in the assessment of organic causes of impotence. *Br J Hosp Med* 1986; **36**: 186–92.

(26) Vermeulen A. The androgens. In: Gray CH, James VHT, eds. *Hormones in epilepsy.* London: Academic Press, 1979: 356–416.

(27) Franks S, Jacobs HS, Martin N, Nabarro JDN. Hyperprolactinaemia and impotence. *Clin Endocrinol* 1978; **8**: 277–87.

(28) Trimble MR. Serum prolactin in epilepsy and hysteria. *Br Med J* 1978; **2**: 1682.

(29) Abbott RJ, Browning MCK, Davidson DLW. Serum prolactin and cortisol concentrations after grand mal seizures. *J Neurol Neurosurg Psych* 1980; **43**: 163–7.

(30) Pritchard PB, Wannamaker BB, Sagel J, Nair R, DeVillier C. Endocrine function follow complex partial seizures. *Ann Neurol* 1983; **14**: 27–32.

(31) Yerby MS, Van Belle G, Friel PN, Wilensky AJ. Serum prolactins in the diagnosis of epilepsy: sensitivity, specificity and predictive value. *Neurology* 1987; **3**: 1224–6.

(32) Molaie M, Culebras A, Miller M. Nocturnal plasma prolactin and cortisol levels in epileptics with complex partial seizures and primary generalised seizures. *Arch Neurol* 1987; **44**: 699–702.

(33) Boobis AR, Davies DS. Human cyochromes P-450. *Xenobiotica* 1984; **14**: 151–85.
(34) McInnes GT, Brodie MJ. Drug interactions that matter: a critical reappraisal. *Drugs* 1988; **36**: 83–110.
(35) Perucca E, Hedges AM, Makki K, Ruprah M, Wilson JF, Richens A. A comparative study of the relative enzyme inducing properties of anticonvulsant drugs in epileptic patients. *Br J Clin Pharmacol* 1984; **18**: 401–10.
(36) Frenken J, Vennix P. *Sexuality experience scales*. Amsterdam: Swets and Zeitlinger, 1978.
(37) Fenwick PBC, Mercer S, Grant R, *et al*. Nocturnal penile tumescence and serum testosterone levels. *Arch Sex Behav* 1986; **15**: 13–21.
(38) Sharpe RM. Testosterone and spermatogenesis. *J Endocrinol* 1987; **113**: 1–2.
(39) Mattson R, Cramer JA, Collins JF, *et al*. Comparison of carbamazepine, phenobarbital, phenytoin and primidone in partial and secondarily generalised tonic-clonic seizures. *N Engl J Med* 1985; **313**: 145–51.

Oral contraceptive steroid therapy in patients taking anticonvulsant drugs

M. Orme[1], D. J. Back[1] P. Crawford[3], A. Bowden[2], P. Cleland[4], D. J. Chadwick[2], J. Tjia[1] and C. Martin[1]

[1]Department of Pharmacology and Therapeutics, University of Liverpool;
[2]Regional Neurosciences Unit, Walton Hospital, Liverpool;
[3]Atkinson Morley's Hospital, Wimbledon, London
and [4]Sunderland District General Hospital, UK

INTRODUCTION

A wide variety of anti-convulsant drugs have been implicated as causing failure of contraception or breakthrough bleeding in women taking long term oral contraceptive steroid (OCS) therapy. This was first reported in 1972 by Kenyon (1) but other cases and series have been reported. Coulam and Annegers (2) reviewed the literature in 1979 and provided four new cases of contraceptive failure. The drugs implicated include phenytoin, phenobarbitone, methyl-phenobarbitone, primidone, carbamazepine and ethosuximide. Phenytoin appears to be the most commonly implicated anticonvulsant and this is born out by recent data from the Committee on Safety of Medicine (CSM). Back and his colleagues showed in 1988 (3) that a total of 43 cases of contraceptive failure in women taking anticonvulsants with their OCS therapy had been reported to the CSM in the years 1973–1984. Phenytoin accounted for 25 of these cases, phenobarbitone for 20, with relatively smaller numbers for primidone, carbamazepine, ethosuximide and sodium valproate.

There is a plethora of data in animals (4) and in man (5) demonstrating the enzyme inducing ability of phenobarbitone, and primidone is reported to be a more potent enzyme inducing agent in man than phenytoin or phenobarbitone (6). However sodium valproate and ethosuximide are not known to be enzyme inducing agents in man. We have, therefore, conducted a series of studies to examine the potential interaction between OCS and anticonvulsants.

MATERIALS AND METHODS

Long term studies

The initial study conducted was with the anticonvulsant phenobarbitone given in doses of 30 mg b.d. to four young women with epilepsy (7). They were followed over a complete cycle of OCS use before phenobarbitone was started and then for two cycles after phenobarbitone was started. The women were aged 23 to 34 years, were in good general health and taking the contraceptive preparation Minovlar® (containing $50\,\mu g$ ethinyloestradiol (EE_2) and 1 mg of norethisterone acetate (N)). Blood samples were taken 12 h after the daily dose of Minovlar on days 11, 14, 16, 18 and 21 of the contraceptive cycle. Blood concentrations of EE_2 (8) and N (9) were measured by specific and sensitive radioimmunoassays (RIA). Phenobarbitone concentrations were measured by high pressure

Fourth international symposium on sodium valproate and epilepsy, edited by David Chadwick, 1989; Royal Society of Medicine Services International Congress and Symposium Series No. 152, published by Royal Society of Medicine Services Limited.

liquid chromatography and progesterone concentrations were measured by RIA in the samples taken on days 18 and 21 to assess whether failure of ovulation had occurred. Sex hormone binding globulin capacity (SHBG) was also measured by RIA (7).

Single dose studies

The other anticonvulsants were studied in single dose studies because of the difficulty in recruiting women in whom it was ethical to leave them for a month before starting anticonvulsant therapy. In the single dose studies women aged 16–37 were given a single dose of Eugynon 50 (containing 50 μg EE_2 and 250 μg of levonorgestrel (1Ng) prior to and 8–12 weeks after starting anticonvulsant therapy for tonic clonic seizures. Blood samples were taken prior to dosing and at 1, 2, 3, 4, 6, 8, 11, 14 and 24 h after dosing with Eugynon 50®. Plasma was assayed for EE_2 (8) and 1Ng (10) by radioimmunoassay. Six patients were studied before and during sodium valproate therapy (200 mg b.d.); five patients were studied before and during phenytoin therapy (200–300 mg/day) and four patients were studied before and during carbamazepine therapy (300–600 mg/day). Plasma concentrations of the various anticonvulsants were measured by high pressure liquid chromatography. The area under the plasma concentration versus time curve (AUC) to 24 h was measured by the trapezoidal rule, and statistical analysis was performed in all cases using Students' t test for paired samples.

RESULTS

Oral contraceptives and phenobarbitone

The results of the study with phenobarbitone are shown in Tables 1 and 2. The plasma concentrations of EE_2 and N are shown for cycle 1—the control pre-phenobarbitone values

Table 1 *Plasma concentrations of ethinyloestradiol (EE₂) and phenobarbitone in four women taking 30 mg twice daily of phenobarbitone and 50 μg daily of EE₂. Mean ± S.E.*

Patient no.	Plasma ethinyloestradiol concentration pg/ml		Plasma phenobarbitone concentration μg/ml
	Cycle 1	Cycle 2	Cycle 3
1	43.4±6.4	52.0±13.7	8
2	104.8±13.4	47.7±13.9[a]	6.5
3	125.6±23.8	50.3±4.7[a]	6
4	71.7±2.8	69.0±9.6	8.5
Mean±S.E.	86.4±18.1	54.7±4.8	7.25±0.6

[a]$p<0.05$

Table 2 *Plasma concentrations of norethisterone and sex hormone binding globulin (SHBG) in three women taking phenobarbitone 30 mg b.d. Mean ± S.E.*

Patient no.	Plasma norethisterone concentration ng/ml		Sex hormone binding globulin nmoles/1	
	Cycle 1	Cycle 2	Cycle 1	Cycle 2
1	2.0±0.4	1.2±0.1	156.8±12.6	234.0±6.7[a]
2	6.6±0.6	7.1±0.1	285.4±18.3	363.9±11.6[a]
3	4.6±0.2	4.4±0.7	320.2±4.3	369.2±14.3[a]
Mean±S.E.	4.4±1.3	4.2±1.7		

[a]$p<0.05$

and for cycle 3—the second cycle of use of phenobarbitone. There was no overall significant fall in the plasma EE_2 concentration in the four women (Table 1) but in patients 2 and 3 individually, significant falls in the plasma EE_2 concentration were seen from 104.8 ± 13.4 pg/ml to 47.7 ± 13.9 pg/ml and from 125.6 ± 23.8 pg/ml to 50.3 ± 4.7 pg/ml. Both women had breakthrough bleeding in their phenobarbitone cycles but no significant changes in plasma progesterone concentrations were seen.

There was no significant change in the plasma concentration of norethisterone in the women studied (Table 2). There were however significant increases in SHBG capacity in the women. Sex hormone binding globulin is increased by EE_2 and also by conventional enzyme inducing agents such as phenobarbitone. SHBG binds progestagens such as norethisterone thus effectively reducing the free concentration of norethisterone and further reducing the efficacy of the OCS.

Oral contraceptives and phenytoin

The results in five patients taking phenytoin are shown in Table 3. All five patients had their tonic clonic fits controlled by the dose of phenytoin shown in Table 3 in spite of the relatively low plasma concentrations that were achieved. There was no consistent pattern in the effects of phenytoin on ethinyloestradiol or levonorgestrel kinetics. Although four out of the five patients showed marked falls in the AUC of both steroids, because a slight rise was seen in one patient there was no significant effect overall. This lack of significant effect is partly due to the small number of patients studied, and partly due to the relatively low concentrations of phenytoin in the patients' plasma.

Table 3 *Area under the plasma concentration versus time curve for ethinyloestradiol and levonorgestrel in patients taking phenytoin*

Patients no	Daily phenytoin dose (mg)	Phenytoin concentration μg/ml	Ethinyloestradiol AUC pg/ml×h		Levonorgestrel ng/ml×h	
			Control	Treatment	Control	Treatment
1	250	1.0	641	303	41.8	22.6
2	200	3.5	956	326	23.1	17.2
3	200	7.0	944	234	10.5	13.7
4	200	3.0	785	1060	18.9	5.9
5	300	11.5	770	332	46.7	25.4
Mean±S.D.			819 ± 132	451 ± 343	28.2 ± 15.5	16.9 ± 7.7

Oral contraceptives and carbamazepine

The results in the four patients taking carbamazepine are shown in Table 4. All four patients had falls in the AUC of both EE_2 and 1Ng when they were taking carbamazepine and in some of these the falls were very considerable. The AUC of EE_2 fell significantly from 1163 ± 466 pg/ml×h to 672 ± 211 pg/ml×h ($p < 0.05$) while the AUC of 1Ng fell significantly during carbamazepine therapy from 22.9 ± 9.4 ng/ml×h to 13.8 ± 5.8 ng/ml×h ($p < 0.05$). All four patients had plasma concentrations of carbamazepine in or very close to the therapeutic range (4–8μg/ml).

Table 4 *Area under the plasma concentration versus time curve (AUC) for ethinyloestradiol and levonorgestrel in patients taking carbamazepine*

Patient no.	Daily carbamazepine dose (mg)	Carbamazepine plasma concentration (μg/ml)	Ethinyloestradiol AUC pg/ml×h		Levonorgestrel AUC ng/ml×h	
			Control	Treatment	Control	Treatment
1	400	8.0	1833	630	14.9	10.5
2	300	3.5	1024	960	20.2	8.7
3	600	8	750	451	20.1	14.3
4	600	4.5	1047	648	36.6	21.9
Mean±S.D.			1163 ± 466	672 ± 211	22.9 ± 9.4	13.8 ± 5.8
				$p < 0.05$		$p < 0.05$

Oral contraceptives and sodium valproate

The results in the six patients who were treated with sodium valproate 200 mg b.d. are shown in Table 5. Although the dose of sodium valproate was low, all six patients had their fits completely controlled. The plasma concentration of sodium valproate varied considerably between the six patients and was in general below the accepted range although the therapeutic range is not well established for this drug. There was no significant change in the AUC of ethinyloestradiol or levonorgestrel during sodium valproate treatment.

Table 5 *Area under the plasma concentration versus time curve (AUC) for ethinyloestradiol and levonorgestrel in patients taking sodium valproate 200 mg b.d.*

Patient no.	Sodium valproate concentration (μg/ml)	Ethinyloestradiol AUC pg/ml×h		Levonorgestrel AUC ng/ml×h	
		Control	Treatment	Control	Treatment
1	21	788	964	35.2	28.1
2	13	969	1075	20.9	31.5
3	45	981	873	26.4	33.1
4	17	758	1112	25.9	25.3
5	5	1339	1399	—	—
6	27	542	441	—	—
Mean±S.E.		880±109	977±130	29.1±2.9	29.2±1.9

DISCUSSION

These various studies have shown a fairly consistent pattern in the effect of anticonvulsant drugs on OCS therapy. Phenobarbitone had a significant effect in two of the four women studied to lower the plasma concentration of EE_2. The dose of phenobarbitone was low and it is likely with a larger dose that a higher proportion of patients would be affected. The lack of reduction of norethisterone concentrations was surprising but the initial metabolic step with norethisterone is a reductive step which is not inducible by standard enzyme inducers. In addition, the free concentration of norethisterone in plasma would be reduced by the increased binding of the drug to SHBG. In the phenobarbitone study, although no patient ovulated, as judged by a lack of increase in progesterone concentrations on day 21, two of the women did have breakthrough bleeding which is a sign of relative oestrogenic deficiency. Thus we feel that phenobarbitone is likely to interfere with OCS therapy, as born out by the CSM data. Women who are taking phenobarbitone will need to take an increased dose of OCS for effective contraceptive control. We suggest that they are started on a pill containing 50 μg EE_2 and the dose can be further increased if breakthrough bleeding occurs to 80 μg or even 100 μg EE_2 daily with a corresponding increase in the progestagen dose.

In the single dose studies with phenytoin, carbamazepine and sodium valproate it is not possible to tell what is happening to the pharmacodynamics of the OCS but on ethical grounds we felt we could not wait a month before starting the relevant anticonvulsant. The phenobarbitone studies were done in 1979 while the other anticonvulsants were studied much later when ethical matters were of greater importance. Nevertheless the degree of change of the AUC allows certain conclusions to be drawn. In the case of carbamazepine all the patients had a fall of the AUC for EE_2 and 1Ng which in some cases was quite marked. Carbamazepine is a potent enzyme-inducing agent in man (5) and would affect progestagen only pills as well as the more usual combined OCS preparations. The degree of change of AUC seen in this study would be expected to produce contraceptive failure in women on long term OCS from our previous studies in the field. Thus women taking carbamazepine should use higher doses of OCS if they wish to rely for contraception on their OCS preparation.

The situation with phenytoin is more confused. Although phenytoin is most commonly implicated in the CSM data as a cause of failure of OCS therapy, phenytoin is less commonly given to young women because of its cosmetic side effects—acne, greasy skin, hirsutism etc.

Nevertheless, young women are prescribed phenytoin and may be also taking OCS. Our data show no statistically significant affect of phenytoin on the kinetics of EE_2 or 1Ng; however the AUC of each drug is reduced by almost 50% for each drug. We believe that this trend is of clinical relevance and the lack of statistical significance is due to a type 2 error (too few patients studied). Further patients are being studied at the present time. In the meantime we believe that women taking phenytoin should use increased doses of OCS (at least 50 μg EE_2) in order to have effective contraception from their OCS.

Sodium valproate, in contrast to the other three anticonvulsant drugs, had no detectable effect on the kinetics of EE_2 or 1Ng. Sodium valproate is not known to be an enzyme inducer in man (5) and these data fit with the paucity of reported data to the CSM (3). We have shown that sodium valproate does not affect the kinetics of EE_2 or 1Ng and although we have not studied the pharmacodynamics of this interaction we believe that it is very unlikely that there would be a dynamic interaction. Women taking sodium valproate can rely on conventional low dose OCS preparations for contraceptive control.

ACKNOWLEDGMENTS

We wish to acknowledge financial support in these studies from the Mersey Regional Health Authority, the Medical Research Council, The World Health Organisation, the British Epilepsy Association, Ciba Geigy Pharmaceuticals, Labaz (Sanofi), Parke Davies and Co. Ltd. and Schering AG.

REFERENCES

(1) Kenyon TE. Unplanned pregnancy in an epileptic. *Br Med J* 1972; **i**: 686–7.
(2) Coulam CB, Annegers JF. Do anticonvulsants reduce the efficacy of oral contraceptives? *Epilepsia* 1979; **20**: 519–26.
(3) Back DJ, Grimmer SFM, Orme ML'E, Proudlove C, Mann RD, Breckenridge AM. Evaluation of Committee on Safety of Medicines Yellow Card reports on oral contraceptive-drug interactions with anticonvulsants and antibiotics. *Br J Clin Pharmacol* 1988; **25**: 527–32.
(4) Conney AH. Pharmacological implications of microsomal enzyme induction. *Pharmacol Revs* 1967; **19**: 317–66.
(5) Park BK, Breckenridge AM. Clinical implications of enzyme induction and enzyme inhibition. *Clin Pharmacokin* 1981; **6**: 1–24.
(6) Latham AN, Millbank L, Richens A, Rowe DJF. Liver enzyme induction by anticonvulsant drugs and its relationship to disturbed calcium and folic acid metabolism. *J Clin Pharmacol* 1973; **13**: 337–42.
(7) Back DJ, Bates M, Bowden A, *et al*. The interaction of phenobarbital and other anticonvulsants with oral contraceptive steroid therapy. *Contraception* 1980; **22**: 495–503.
(8) Back DJ, Breckenridge AM, Crawford FE, *et al*. An investigation of the pharmacokinetics of ethynylestradiol in women using radio-immunoassay. *Contraception* 1979; **20**: 263–73.
(9) Back DJ, Breckenridge AM, Crawford FE, *et al*. The pharmacokinetics of norethindrone in women d(1) Radioimmunoassay and concentrations during multiple dosing. *Clin Pharmacol Ther* 1978; **24**: 439–46.
(10) Back DJ, Bates M, Breckenridge AM, *et al*. The phamacokinetics of levonorgestrel and ethinyloestradiol in women—studies with Ovran and Ovranette. *Contraception* 1981; **23**: 229–39.
(11) Back DJ, Breckenridge AM, Crawford FE, *et al*. The effect of rifampicin on the pharmacokinetics of ethinyloestradiol in women. *Contraception* 1980; **21**: 135–43.

Discussion after Dr Brodie and Professor Orme

Dr Price (*Swindon, UK*): Can I ask Dr Brodie how his free testosterone was calculated. Was it a direct measurement or a calculated measurement based upon the total testosterone and SHBG and if the latter, how was the calculation made?

Dr Brodie (*Glasgow, UK*): It was a calculated measure which was published in Nanjee and Wheeler (*Ann Clin Biochem* 1985; **22**: 287–390). The derived figure correlated almost exactly with free measurement.

Dr Hoare (*Edinburgh, UK*): There is a definite relationship between affective disorder and hyposexuality; might this be the possible explanation for some of Dr Brodie's findings with relation to hyposexuality?

Dr Brodie: All hyposexuality problems are extremely complex. These were our 'normal' epilepsy out-patients. Although we have no data for degree of depression, I doubt whether they would differ substantially from normal controls. There are so many factors that you cannot control for, that I think we are going to have to do more studies! I do not believe that affective disorder is an important contribution to this form of hyposexuality, whereas probably reduction in sex hormones are. We have not yet looked at whether the levels in our patients correlate with hyposexuality. This is something we will do when we have greater numbers. It is important at this stage to acknoweldge that these early data are intriguing. These are not institutionalized patients, but walking, working, 'healthy' epileptics. We need to set up a substantial database to look statistically at all the factors that might be relevant.

Professor Mattson (*Connecticut, USA*): We have seen clear indications of hyposexuality on antiepileptic drugs and significantly more with primidone. This gave us the opportunity to look at the mechanism in a limited way because when we crossed over the patients who failed the drug because of sexual complaints, from primidone to either phenytoin or carbamazepine, the problem disappeared, and these were under blinded conditions. I think there is a specific drug relationship, probably above and beyond the enzyme-induced decrease in testosterone. The differences that you have reported and that we have also observed in free testosterone correlate rather poorly with libido in most endocrine studies.

Dr Brodie (*Glasgow, UK*): As a clinical pharmacologist, I would like to think that this is a very complicated drug-related situation! Enzyme-inducers do not have identical effects in different individuals. Professor Orme's data show that. There is some suggestion that if the free testosterone concentration is low, this related to impaired libido, and Dr Fenwick has done some work which seems to support this. The numbers, of course, are small and that is always going to be a problem. Perhaps there is also a toxic effect on the testes which can vary with different drugs. You have certainly demonstrated that primidone is probably the most 'toxic' of the five major drugs used in adults. As there are clear-cut differences between the drugs, maybe we will be able to say to a patient, 'Your hyposexuality is due to this drug, and if I switch you to another one, sexual function will return'.

Dr Fenwick (*London, UK*): We have some new data which have not yet been published. We used tritiated testosterone to study metabolic turnover of testosterone and test the enzyme hypothesis. We have also looked at pituitary function so that we could see whether the pituitary was disordered or not, and at testicular function. Those data are yet to be published, but they show that metabolism is not increased, so although enzyme induction is important in the short term, it may not be quite so important in the long term. The pituitary part of the cycle is not affected. What is affected are the testes. We do not have any specific answers with regard to different drugs. There are two actions, one, enzyme induction which by increasing SHBG indirectly lowers testosterone levels and so increases the LH drive on the testes to produce testosterone and two, by poisoning the testis with anticonvulsant drugs leads to a further reduction in testosterone. Those two factors seem to finally lead to testicular testosterone secretion failure. It is still a complex question but the current research emphasis is shifting a little bit away from enzyme induction and more to how we are directly interfering with testicular function with our drugs. Sodium valproate may be the least involved.

This question repeats the one asked at the start of Dr Brodie's talk:

Interactive question from Dr Brodie

Concerning sexual functioning in epileptic patients, choose one option		**Response**
		(No.)
1 The topic should be mentioned only by patients and not by the doctor		
	(Neurologist)	58
	(Other)	26
2 Patients should be particularly encouraged to discuss any sexual problems		
	(Neurologist)	64
	(Other)	28
3 Patients should be asked specifically about sexual arousal, performance and satisfaction		
	(Neurologist)	64
	(Other)	70

Interactive question from Professor Orme

Patients taking most anticonvulsant drugs should		**Response**
		(No.)
1 Not rely completely on oral contraceptive steroids for contraception		
	(Neurologist)	70
	(Other)	46
2 Oral contraceptive steroids are fully effective in patients with anticonvulsant drugs with appropriate dosage adjustment		
	(Neurologist)	100
	(Other)	60
3 Sodium valproate is the only anticonvulsant drug not to interact with oral contraceptive steroids		
	(Neurologist)	18
	(Other)	24

Professor Orme (*Liverpool, UK*): An interesting difference between the neurologists' response and the others, but in actual fact one can legitimately answer yes to all three.

Education: A review

G. Stores

Department of Psychiatry, University of Oxford, Oxford, UK

INTRODUCTION

Educational aspects of epilepsy are many and wide-ranging from the learning process itself to the social implications of educational policy and practice. The purpose of this account is to comment briefly on selected aspects that appear to be of particular clinical importance and which have been the subject of important recent research.

Pronouncements (almost wholly negative) about the effects of epilepsy on the capacity to learn date from very early times (1). Particularly pessimistic views were expressed last century, even by otherwise enlightened observers, such as the reforming psychiatrist Esquirol (2), based on experience with very unrepresentative groups of patients.

More scientific and discriminating approaches have indicated that children with epilepsy are at special risk of educational problems (3). However they have also demonstrated the falsehood (and the harm) of generalizing about 'epilepsy' as if it were one condition, and have pointed out the preventive and therapeutic possibilities that exist in the minority of children affected this way.

Understanding of the factors which can place children (and also adults) with epilepsy at special risk of education difficulties is far from complete and fundamental issues remain concerning educational measurements, for example. As can be judged from the two books recently published on the topic (4,5), there is much current interest in educational aspects of epilepsy and it is increasingly possible to identify various biological and psychosocial factors which should be considered when attempting to explain educational problems in the individual child.

SUBTLE SEIZURE DISCHARGE

The effects of brief bursts of 'subclinical' seizure discharge on performance and possibly on educational attainments have been studied experimentally since the 1930s. Much interesting information has accumulated concerning the most disruptive type of seizure discharge although differences between individuals (and even within one individual at different times) are prominent. Complexity of the task is an additional important consideration (6). These relatively subtle effects of epileptic activity need to be considered, along with other possibilities, especially in the child whose educational abilities decline.

In considering the psychological effects of subtle seizure discharge it is useful to define such discharge according to its duration (7). The types traditionally studied are of brief duration i.e. more than 3 s and up to perhaps several minutes. Discharges shorter than this are often seen in the EEGs of people with epilepsy but traditionally have been considered as clinically insignificant. However, recent findings suggest that even very brief discharges are capable in some patients of causing 'transient cognitive impairment' and reduced educational attainments, the extent and type of which bears some relationship to the frequency and site of origin of the discharges (8,9).

Fourth international symposium on sodium valproate and epilepsy, edited by David Chadwick, 1989; Royal Society of Medicine Services International Congress and Symposium Series No. 152, published by Royal Society of Medicine Services Limited.

At the other extreme, seizure discharge (usually generalized in distribution) can continue for hours, days, weeks or even longer ('non-convulsive status epilepticus'). The effect of this type of discharge on behaviour is variable ranging from striking confusional, demented or stuporose states (although often not recognized as epilepsy) to very subtle changes which are only detectable by special observation and yet which can be sufficient to impair learning ability (10). A variation on this theme is the occurrence of 'electrical status during sleep' (11).

There is evidence from various sources that repeated prolonged exposure to nonconvulsive seizure discharge might have a serious and possible permanent deleterious effect on brain function (10). If this is so it needs to be treated with much more vigour than is usually the case.

ANTIEPILEPTIC DRUGS

The study of the possible psychological effects of antiepileptic drug treatment (including educational consequences) has become a very popular pursuit over the last 10 years or so. These investigations have been interesting but more instructive about the difficulties of conducting relevant research on this topic than about the precise risk of psychological effects in the individual patient. Various problems are encountered in relating published accounts to everyday paediatric practice (12). These problems include:
1. Ethical constraints on research methodology especially concerning controls.
2. The relevance to children with epilepsy of findings on adult patients or normal volunteers.
3. Polypharmacy, variable drug dosage, mixed intelligence and age levels in the subjects studied.
4. Prominent individual differences in reactions to drug treatment.
5. Questionable relevance to everyday behaviour of many of the psychological measures used.

Although some studies have suggested that certain antiepileptic drugs tend to have adverse effects on learning and behaviour, and that these effects are often dose-related, the precise impact of these findings on prescribing for the individual patient is likely to be limited because of the inconsistent, marginal or very general results.

Because of the difficulties in this area of research special efforts are required to keep in touch with everyday clinical reality and to achieve a balanced view. This has been the intention in a controlled study of our own concerning the psychological effects, in newly diagnosed cases of childhood epilepsy, of valproate or carbamazepine given at the modest dosage usually required in paediatric practice (Stores, Williams & Styles, unpublished observations). All children in the study were attending normal school. In this non-specialist setting no adverse effect on various measures of cognition and behaviour (including educational attainments) were seen with either drug when pre-treatment scores were compared with those obtained after 12 months' treatment.

SLEEP AND AROUSAL DISORDERS

Missing from the usual lists of reasons for poor educational progress in children with epilepsy is any reference to sleep disorders. This is curious as some children with epilepsy might well be expected to be predisposed to sleep problems (for example because of emotional upset or treatment effects) and sleep problems might well affect daytime behaviour including performance at school.

Recent preliminary studies have been carried out in an attempt to correct this omission (13). The first consisted of a questionnaire survey in which parents were asked about various sleep problems in their epileptic children. Compared with a group of controls children with epilepsy had significantly more sleep problems and these were significantly associated with daytime psychological difficulties.

'Unrefreshing' sleep was prominent among these reported problems. In order to explore the physiological accompaniments of this complaint, a second study was carried out in which home sleep recordings were performed on a group of epileptic children said to have unrefreshing sleep. No differences in conventionally assessed sleep structure were seen between these children and a non-epileptic group of controls, but when assessments were made of physiological changes of the 'microarousal' type (not recognized in conventional sleep staging and not usually associated with clinical awakening), a different pattern of occurrence was seen in the epileptic children.

These findings raise the possibility of an arousal disorder associated with at least some forms of childhood epilepsy with possible adverse effects on daytime functioning. The results suggest one possible explanation for the frequent complaint that children with epilepsy are less alert, even those with good attainments (14), or for the paradoxical alerting effects in such children of sensory stimulation which acts as a distraction in normal children (15).

ATTITUDES

Biological factors appear still to attract most research attention. Interesting as they are (and important in selected cases), it is likely that psychosocial factors make a numerically greater contribution to the learning and other psychological difficulties of children with epilepsy. The stated reasons for referral to our own Special Epilepsy Centre for Children are overwhelmingly neurological in nature. However review of such children on admission reveals that the majority have serious educational, behavioural and family problems which are often the result not so much of biological influences as unhelpful and inappropriate attitudes on the part of those responsible for the children's welfare (16).

Children with epilepsy appear to be at special risk of educational problems but those who care for such children often have 'educational' problems of their own in that they have not been given enough information about the condition. As a result, they frequently adopt too pessimistic a view about the child's future. In this modified sense the negative attitude of 19th century observers, to which reference was made at the start, still exists.

Our own experience in providing a special epilepsy service strongly suggests that parents, doctors, teachers and others are often ill-informed or misinformed about the childhood epilepsies and their consequences for educational achievement and general development. Especially when the child incorporates the negative views of others into his or her own self image, the prophecy of poor attainments readily fulfills itself.

CONCLUSIONS

The most pressing educational issue concerning epilepsy is the need for better education all round. A most important challenge is how to achieve comprehensive and up to date coverage of the epilepsies in undergraduate and postgraduate medical teaching programmes, and how better to educate the public including parents, teachers and prospective employers. There is also a considerable need to educate affected children themselves about their condition in order to prevent mistaken notions from developing or to correct inappropriate ideas. Education of parents and children is needed across the whole socioeconomic range. It is disturbing to find a bias towards middle class families in referrals to our own NHS Special Centre (16) suggesting that many children of lower socioeconomic origins may well be deprived of special help and advice.

Research into the effects of biological factors is obviously scientifically more appealing but unless similar attention is paid to psychosocial factors, including educating the public and the professions, the prospects in life of many children with epilepsy will remain severely limited.

REFERENCES

(1) Temkin D. *The falling sickness*, 2nd ed. Baltimore: Johns Hopkins Press, 1971.
(2) Esquirol JED. *Mental maladies. A treatise on insanity*, trans, Hunt EK, 1845. Philadelphia: Lea and Blanchard, 1838.

(3) Stores G. Learning and emotional problems in children with epilepsy. In: Reynolds EH, Trimble MR, eds. *Epilepsy and psychiatry*. London: Churchill Livingstone 1981: 33–48.

(4) Aldenkamp AP, Alpherts WCJ, Meinardi H, Stores G, eds. *Education and epilepsy*. Amsterdam: Swets and Zeitlinger, 1987.

(5) Oxley J, Stores G, eds. *Epilepsy and education*. London: Medical Tribune Group, 1987.

(6) Stores G. Studies of attention and seizure disorders. *Dev Med Child Neurol* 1973; **15**: 376–82.

(7) Stores G. Effects on learning of 'subclinical' seizure discharge. In: Aldenkamp AP, Alpherts WCJ, Meinardi H, Stores G, eds. *Education and epilepsy*. Amsterdam: Swets and Zeitlinger 1987: 14–20.

(8) Kasteleijn-Nolst Trenite DGA, Barker DJ, Binnie CD, Buerman A, Van Raaij M. Psychological effects of subclinical epileptiform EEG discharges. I. Scholastic skills. *Epilepsy Research* 1988; **2**: 111–116.

(9) Siebelink BM, Barker DJ, Binnie CD, Kasteleijn-Nolst Trenite DGA. Psychological effects of subclinical epileptiform EEG discharges. II. General intelligence tests. *Epilepsy Research* 1988; **2**, 117–21.

(10) Stores G. Psychological aspects of nonconvulsive status epilepticus in children. *J Child Psychol Psychiat* 1986; **27**: 575–582.

(11) Tassinari CA, Bureau M, Dravet C, Dalla Bernadina B, Roger J. Epilepsy with continuous spikes and waves during slow sleep. In: Roger J, *et al.* eds. *Epileptic syndromes in infancy, childhood and adolescence*. London: John Libbey Eurotext 1985: 194–204.

(12) Stores G. Antiepileptic drugs. In: Aman MG, Singh NN eds. *Psychopharmacology of the developmental disabilities*. New York: Springer-Verlag 1988: 101–118.

(13) Zaiwalla Z. Sleep abnormalities in children with epilepsy [abstract]. *Electroenceph Clin Neurophysiol* 1989; **72**: 29P.

(14) Bennett-Levy J, Stores G. The nature of cognitive dysfunction in schoolchildren with epilepsy. *Acta Neurol Scand* 1984; **69** (Suppl 99): 79–82.

(15) Stores G, Hart JA, Piran N. Inattentiveness in schoolchildren with epilepsy. *Epilepsia* 1978; **19**: 169–75.

(16) Stores G. Children with epilepsy in need of long-term multi-disciplinary care. In: Parsonage M, Grant RHE, Craig AG, Ward AA, eds. *Advances in epileptology, XIVth epilepsy international symposium*. New York: Raven Press 1983: 229–32.

Psychomotor and cognitive function in antiepileptic monotherapy

R. A. Gillham

Department of Clinical Psychology, Institute of Neurological Sciences,
Southern General Hospital, Glasgow, UK

INTRODUCTION

It is generally accepted that antiepileptic drugs (AEDs) can produce cognitive side effects. However, research studies aiming to specify and quantify these are beset with methodological problems. The main difficulty comes from the fact that drugs are not the only factor causing cognitive impairment in people with epilepsy. Seizures, psychosocial factors and the cerebral pathology underlying the epilepsy also affect cognitive function and the relationship between these various agents is complex (Fig. 1).

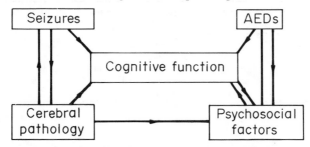

Figure 1 *Diagram showing interrelationships between factors affecting cognitive function in epilepsy.*

There are a number of possible experimental paradigms which control for some of these variables but most have major limitations. For example, specific effects of sodium valproate (VPA) have been demonstrated in normal volunteers, but results are conflicting; some showing improvement in alertness and reaction time (1, 2) and others demonstrating sedation (3) and impaired decision times (4). Volunteer studies, although unconfounded by the effects of seizures and other epilepsy-related factors, may overestimate cognitive side-effects by failing to measure the effect of the disorder of epilepsy itself on function, the long term changes in performance as tolerance of the drug and its effects develops, and the beneficial effect of improved seizure control.

A methodologically sound experiment is to measure performance of patients with epilepsy when on a high dose of an AED and when on a low dose. This is usually done blind and in a cross-over design; Amann *et al.* (5), show a deterioration with increasing dose of VPA on four psychomotor tasks and Trimble and Thompson (6) found five differences all indicating greater impairment with the higher dose of the drug. Such an experiment may well detect small decrements in performance but the relative importance of these compared to the effect of seizure variables cannot be demonstrated. Within-subject designs, whether high dose/low dose comparisons, or drug/placebo comparisons have many advantages since they avoid the practical difficulties of attempting to match groups of subjects and they

Fourth international symposium on sodium valproate and epilepsy, edited by David Chadwick, 1989; Royal Society of Medicine Services International Congress and Symposium Series No. 152, published by Royal Society of Medicine Services Limited.

cut down on error variance attributable to unmeasured or non-specific differences between the groups. Yet such studies have not established beyond doubt the specific effect of VPA on cognitive and psychomotor function. Sommerbeck et al. (7) for example, show increased reaction time, while Harding et al. (8) show decreased reaction time. Again this type of paradigm does not allow the measurement of long-term changes in intellectual performance brought about by improved seizure control and increasing tolerance of the drug or its effects.

Another major problem contributing to the inconsistency of findings across studies is the lack of standardization of method. Although reliability and validity have been established for most cognitive tests, the diversity of these tools makes study comparisons hazardous. One of the simplest tests, reaction time, for example, has many different versions.

This study attempts to overcome some of the difficulties in earlier work. The purpose was to show the precise aspect of cognitive function affected by a particular drug, and to show the relative significance of the deficit compared to disabilities caused by other factors.

METHODS

Patients

There were five groups of patients (see Table 1).

Table 1 *Characteristics of patient groups*

	Age	Sex		Seizure type		Duration	Seizures month
CBZ ($n=35$)	27 yrs	16 m	19 f	15^a	20^b	12 yrs	7
VPA ($n=26$)	36 yrs	10 m	16 f	12^a	14^b	13 yrs	6
PHT ($n=19$)	34 yrs	9 m	10 f	8^a	11^b	14 yrs	4
Untreated ($n=26$)	27 yrs	12 m	14 f	12^a	14^b	6 yrs	2
Non-epileptic ($n=24$)	36 yrs	9 m	15 f				

Values are means.
[a]Generalized tonic-clonic
[b]Complex partial

The treated patients were all well established on a single anticonvulsant. The untreated patients were studied after a single seizure or at least six months after a trial of drug withdrawal. The non-epileptic subjects were individuals who had been referred to a psychology clinic with no known neurological disorder, and who, on assessment, were judged not to require treatment.

There were no statistically significant differences between the groups of patients in age, years in secondary education, or Performance IQ. There were no differences between the

Table 2

Psychomotor	Decision Time[a]
	Choice Reaction Time[a]
	Finger Tapping Rate
	Threshold Detection[b]
	Movement Detection[b]
Memory	Forward Digit Span[c]
	Backward Digit Span[c]
	Paired Associate Learning[c]
	Visual Span[b]
Side effect rating scales	Side Effect Scale
	Sedation Score

[a]Leeds Psychomotor Tester
[b]Developed in Psychology Dept. University of Stirling.
[c]Wechsler Memory Scale

treated groups in duration of epilepsy, seizure frequency and time since last seizure. VPA is more commonly prescribed for patients with generalized seizures than for patients with partial seizures. Amann *et al.* (5) have shown that children with generalized seizures tend to perform better on some cognitive tests than those with partial seizures. Care was taken to match the groups of treated patients for seizure type to avoid any bias.

Neuropsychological assessment

A battery of 12 neuropsychological tests was used in the assessment of psychomotor and cognitive function (Table 2). This battery has been developed by our group over a series of studies, and its reliability and sensitivity to the effect of AEDs on function has been established (9, 10, 11, 12).

RESULTS

Analysis of variance showed that none of the individual psychometric tests discriminated between the five patient groups. Paired comparisons showed significant differences between the worst and best group on three tests: the VPA group performed significantly better than the PHT group on the Finger Tapping test, the non-epileptic group performed better than the CBZ group on the Threshold Detection task, and the VPA group performed better than the PHT group on the Paired Associate Learning task, $p < 0.05$ in each case. However the validity of such comparisons is doubtful since they are only three out of a possible 120 and the risk of type I error is high.

Each set of test scores was then converted to a standard scale with a mean of 0 and standard deviation of 1. It was thus possible to summate the 5 psychomotor tests to get an overall 'psychomotor' score, similarly the four memory tests and the two side-effect scales.

Figs. 2, 3 and 4 show the effect of the three drugs on these three modalities, relative to the untreated and non-epileptic groups.

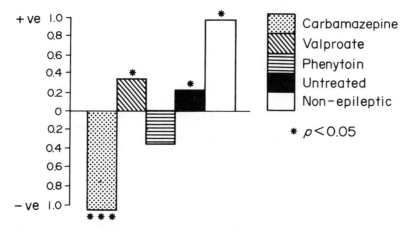

Figure 2 *Comparison of five patient groups on psychomotor composite score.*

The CBZ group performance significantly worse on the psychomotor scale than the VPA group.

The PHT group performed significantly worse on the memory scale and the VPA group. There is a large difference between the untreated and non-epileptic group. This gives an indication of the relative amount of impairment caused by the disorder itself. The CBZ mean score is virtually identical to the untreated score so it might be concluded that CBZ causes no memory impairment. But on the other hand the VPA group are superior to the untreated group, suggesting, since the groups were matched for age, general intelligence,

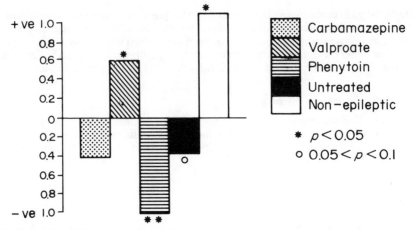

Figure 3 *Comparison of five patient groups on memory composite score.*

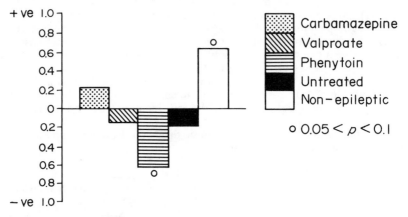

Figure 4 *Comparison of five patient groups on side-effect composite score.*

educational level and seizure variables, that this drug somehow produces an improved performance, perhaps by increasing alertness as suggested by previous studies (2).

Phenytoin seems to cause more subjective side-effects than the other drugs although the difference is not significant. The CBZ group appear to feel better than the untreated group. Again this is consistent with previous research showing that CBZ has an antidepressant effect.

DISCUSSION

In general the differences between the non-epileptic group and the untreated group give some indication of the effect of the disorder itself on cognitive function. The use of both these control groups allows evaluation of the relative significance of the additional impairment produced by each AED. Thus although the CBZ group, and the PHT group perform more poorly on memory tests than the normal group, the CBZ composite score is virtually identical to that of the untreated group, showing that the drug has not produced any additional impairment, and that the additional impairment produced by PHT may not necessarily be of great clinical significance.

The untreated group had a lower seizure frequency than the treated groups but in a multi-group study where more than one comparison is being made this is not necessarily a problem. For example, if it was known only that the CBZ group had a lower psychomotor score than the untreated group it would not be possible to say whether this was due to the drug effect, or to the effect of the additional seizures. But if it is also demonstrated that the VPA group perform as well as the untreated group, despite the higher frequency, and that they perform better than the CBZ group even though seizure frequency in these two groups is the same, then it can be concluded with some confidence that the poor psychomotor performance in the CBZ group is attributable to a specific drug effect.

Finally some conclusions may be drawn, bearing in mind firstly that although the battery included tests of a wide range of aspects of memory and psychomotor function, many types of intellectual performance were not assessed, and secondly that although the sample size was larger than in many previous studies it was not so large as to allow generalizations to be made as to matters of fact without further investigation and replication.

CONCLUSIONS

1. AED induced cognitive impairment is subtle relative to impairment caused by the disorder of epilepsy itself.
2. CBZ was associated with more psychomotor impairment than VPA and more than the disorder itself.
3. PHT was associated with more memory impairment than VPA but not significantly more than the disorder itself.
4. VPA was not associated with significant impairment relative to the non-epileptic group in this sample.

It appears, then, that individual AEDs have their own pattern of effect on cognitive function and that this can be distinguished from effects produced by seizure variables, such as type and frequency. Chadwick (13), in a recent review, concluded that 'VPA is at least as effective as PHT and CBZ in the treatment of generalized and partial seizures. Given the similar efficacy other factors . . . . may therefore determine anticonvulsant selection for monotherapy.' Clinicians should target the choice of anticonvulsant for the individual patient so that any unwanted side-effects are those which interfere least with his or her life-style.

REFERENCES

(1) Harding G, Pullen JJ. The effect of sodium valproate on the EEG, the photosensitive range, the CNV and reaction time. Electroencephalogr. *Clin Neurophysiol* 1977; **43**: 465.
(2) Betts TA, Crowe A, Alford C. Psychotropic effects of sodium valproate. *Br J Clin Pract* 1982; **18**: 145–6.
(3) Boxer CM, Herzberg JL, Scott DF. Has sodium valproate hypnotic effects? *Epilepsia* 1976; **17**: 367–70.
(4) Thompson PJ, Trimble MR. Sodium valproate and cognitive functioning in normal volunteers. *Br J Clin Pharmacol 1981*; **12**: 818–24.
(5) Amman MG, Werry JS, Paxton JW, Turbott SH. Effect of sodium valproate on psychomotor performance in children as a function of dose, fluctuations in concentration and diagnosis. Epilepsia 1987; **28**: 115–24.
(6) Trimble MR, Thompson PJ. Sodium valproate and cognitive function. *Epilepsia 1984*; **25** (suppl): S60–4.
(7) Sommerbeck KW, Theilgaard A, Rasmussen KE, Lohren G, Gram L, Wulff K. Valproate sodium: evaluation of so-called psychotropic effect. A controlled study. *Epilepsia* 1977; **18**: 159–67.
(8) Harding GFA, Pullen JJ, Drasdo N. The effect of sodium valproate and other anticonvulsants on performance of children and adolescents. In: Parsonage MJ, Caldwell ADS, eds. *The place of sodium valproate in the treatment of epilepsy*. London: Academic Press, 1980: 61–7.
(9) Macphee GJA, Goldie C, Roulston D, Potter L, Agnew E, Brodie MJ. Effect of carbamazepine on psychomotor function in naive subjects. *Eur J Clin Pharmacol* 1986; **30**: 37–42.
(10) Macphee GJA, McPhail EM, Butler E, Brodie MJ. Controlled evaluation of a supplementary dose of carbamazepine on psychomotor function in epileptic patients. *Eur J Clin Pharmacol* 1986; **30**: 37–42.

(11) Brodie MJ, McPhail E, Macphee GJA, Larkin JG, Gray JMB. Psychomotor impairment and anticonvulsant therapy in adult epileptic patients. *Eur J Clin Pharmacol* 1987; **31**: 655–660.
(12) Gillham RA, Williams N, Larkin J, Butler E, Wiedman K, Brodie MJ. Concentration–effect relationships with carbamazepine and its epoxide on psychomotor and cognitive function in epileptic patients. *J Neurol Neurosurg Psychiat* 1988; **51**: 929–33.
(13) Chadwick DW. Valproate monotherapy in the management of generalised and partial seizures. *Epilepsia* 1987; **28** (suppl 2): S12–17.

Epilepsy and mental disability

J. A. Corbett

University of Birmingham, Birmingham, UK

Sir Leonard Cheshire and his wife Baroness Ryder in their Stevens Lecture to the Royal Society of Medicine (1) on 'The hope of the disabled' summed this issue up by emphasizing that the overwhelming wish of people with a disability is the freedom to choose where they live, who they live with and for a meaningful role in society achieved primarily through satisfying work.

Because of the nature of the disease, its mystique, and the need for dependent social relationships this is not easily achieved by many people with epilepsy but must remain their aspiration if the disability is to be conquered.

The World Health Organisation (2) has proposed that a distinction should be made between impairment, disability and handicap. Impairment is defined as the loss or abnormality of psychological, physiological or anatomical structure or function. Transient interruption of consciousness associated with epileptic seizures, disordered behaviour or cognitive failure would thus encompass the most common forms of mental impairment.

Disability is the restriction or lack (resulting from impairment) of ability to perform an activity. Using this definition mental retardation (developmental cognitive failure), psychiatric illness arising in adult life and epilepsy (defined as recurrent seizures) are the predominant forms of mental disability. As such they may substantially interfere with such aspects of day to day life as the ability to live independently or engage in work and social relationships.

These disabilities only become handicapping when they limit or prevent fulfilment of a role in life that is regarded as normal for an individual and require special services.

A widely quoted estimate suggests that in 50% of people with epilepsy, seizures will be controlled by medication and that 80% of people with seizure disorders are able to work independently. The converse of this is that half those with epilepsy are recurrently impaired and a substantial minority disabled or handicapped by their seizure disorder. It is currently most acceptable to talk with our patients about disability rather than impairment or handicap and much of our recent social legislation and benefit system now uses this term. There is less certainty about what qualifies as a disability for a given individual and some overcome the most severe disability which to another person might result in a severe handicap. Much will also depend on the social context in which disability occurs—the level of employment, community support and acceptance and availability of services.

A recent MORI poll in this country suggests that 10% of the population regard themselves as disabled in one way or another but there have been few studies of disability which have used relevant measures, such as the ability to work or live independently. Most epidemiological studies have excluded those who are mentally disabled as a result of psychiatric illness or mental handicap. Epilepsy, in common with mental disability, is less visible than physical handicap and presents particular difficulties in measurement.

Disability is not directly related, in most cases, to the severity of the primary impairment but more to the individual's perception and ability to live with the underlying impairment. The perception may be related to feeling of stigmatization. Ryan et al. (3) in a study of nearly 500 adults with epilepsy found that there was no universal feeling of

Fourth international symposium on sodium valproate and epilepsy, edited by David Chadwick, 1989; Royal Society of Medicine Services International Congress and Symposium Series No. 152, published by Royal Society of Medicine Services Limited.

Table 1 *Prevalence of epilepsy in children and young people*

National Child Development Studies	0.7–0.4%
(Cooper 1965, Ross & Peckham 1983)	
Febrile convulsions without epileptic sequelae	2.2%
Epilepsy in children with mild mental retardation IQ 50–70	3–6%
Lifelong seizures in children with severe mental retardation IQ 50	32–44%
(Corbett *et al.* 1975, Richardson *et al.* 1981)	
Lifelong history of seizures in children with profound mental retardation IQ 20	50%
History of seizures in previous year in children with severe mental retardation IQ 50	19%
Children with severe mental retardation IQ 50 receiving anticonvulsants	20%
People with severe mental retardation aged 14–28 years suffering from epilepsy	28%

being stigmatized. The perception depended less on the severity of the seizures than on educational attainment, limitations imposed by the disorder and the realization that there might be discrimination when seeking employment.

The prevention and amelioration of mental disability associated with epilepsy may be most fruitfully examined in childhood although similar principles apply in adult life when acquired brain damage and psychiatric disorder are associated with epilepsy.

Until recently reports of the prevalence of epilepsy in normal children and those with developmental disability have been based on selected populations most of whom have been institutionalized or attending special clinics.

Over the past twenty years epidemiological studies of cohorts of children representative of the general population, who have been followed up into adult life, have avoided the biases inherent in earlier studies.

The estimates for normal children in Table 1 are taken from the British National Child Development studies (4,5) while those for children with developmental disability are based on case register studies from Aberdeen in Scotland (6) and Camberwell in South London (7). In both cases the children have been followed up into adult life.

While most cases of mild mental retardation are of multifactorial origin, representing the lower end of the normal distribution of intelligence the increased prevalence of seizures in this group gives an indication of the contribution of brain damage or dysfunction to mild learning difficulties. There is a very considerable increase in seizures in severely and profoundly mentally disabled children, most of whom have neurological evidence of brain damage.

In both the Camberwell and Aberdeen studies there was a tendency for seizures to be of early onset and for them to remit to some extent in later childhood, although they were still much more persistent than in non-handicapped people. There was a further peak of onset in adolescence or early adult life so that the overall prevalence remained the same with around 20% of people with severe mental handicap having a history of one or more seizures in the past year and requiring continuous medication. Thus although there is a greater vulnerability of the damaged brain to seizure discharge it seems that this is still susceptible to genetically determined developmental processes accounting for the bimodal distribution.

Epileptic seizures and severe learning disability are both epiphenomena denoting underlying brain dysfunction in this population. Because seizures are usually associated with transient impairment in cognitive function and thus learning and because they occur most frequently in the developmental period it is possible that they may be implicated in the aetiology of learning disability but such a causal relationship does not usually account for the strong association between epilepsy and mental retardation.

Although mild learning difficulty in children with epilepsy is not uncommon most people with epilepsy do not suffer from serious mental deterioration and seizures may be very frequent without resulting deterioration.

The relationship is more subtle and complex and account has to be taken of other social and psychological factors to which people with epilepsy are vulnerable. These include interruption or restriction of school work, stigmatization, role failure and added psychiatric disorder. It is also necessary to consider the long term consequences of anticonvulsants and other psychotropic medication on the developing brain. In seeking to account for the severe intellectual deterioration which is seen in a small number of people usually with

Table 2 *Aetiology of severe mental retardation IQ 50 and epilepsy in Camberwell children aged 0–14 years n = 140*

	Number	%
Infections	23	34
Trauma and other physical agents	9	33
Metabolic	6	51
Gross brain disease (e.g. phakomatoses)	8	100
Perinatal adversity	16	41
Major chromosomal abnormalities	35	16
Others with a family history	13	23
Others with no family history	30	30

complicated epilepsy dating from childhood all these factors need to be taken into account and it is also necessary to consider the effect of such factors as recurrent head injury due to astatic myoclonic seizures and exclude the many individually rare neurodegenerative disorders which are associated with epilepsy in childhood.

Whether or not epilepsy occurs in a particular condition depends largely on the nature and site of the cerebral insult and the age at which it operates.

Table 2 shows the prevalence of seizures in various situations associated with mental retardation. Epilepsy is particularly common for example in the phakomatoses such as tuberous sclerosis and the Sturge Weber syndrome. It seems to be almost inevitable if the person is severely retarded and this may be related to the extent of the brain involvement. The type of epilepsy however is largely age dependent so that tuberous sclerosis not infrequently presents with infantile spasms while myoclonic astatic attacks symptomatic of Lennox Gastaut syndrome may be seen if the onset is later and the child is walking.

Another way of looking at the relationship between epilepsy and disability is to examine the prevalence of epilepsy in various handicapping conditions.

The data in Table 3 are taken from studies of school children on the Isle of Wight (8).

The handicaps may be divided into those with neurological abnormality (distinguishing between conditions associated with lesions above and below the brain stem) and chronic physical conditions which do not affect the nervous system directly such as asthma or diabetes.

The relationship between the various disabilities can then be examined by comparing the association between psychiatric disorders in children whose disability is associated with epilepsy and those in whom it is not and as might be expected there is a descending order of frequency with the highest prevalence of psychiatric disorders being found in those with brain damage above the brain stem associated with epilepsy.

The type of secondary handicap associated with mental retardation has important relationships with the seizure disorder.

Epilepsy is particularly frequent in spastic cerebral palsy where seizures occurred in over 60% of children with severe mental retardation in the Camberwell study (7). It was less frequent in those with perceptual handicaps such as deafness and blindness. In mental retardation associated with psychiatric disorders which comprise the commonest secondary handicap, seizures were most frequent in those with hyperkinetic disorders and with pervasive developmental disorders. This latter group includes the continuum of autistic disorders seen in childhood and while early onset seizures are less common in this condition it is very common for autistic impairments to follow infantile spasms. Generalized seizures

Table 3 *Relationship between handicapping conditions in children and psychiatric disorder*

Handicapping condition	Psychiatric disorder %
General population 9–11 year olds	6.6
Physical disorders not affecting the nervous system	10.3
Neurological disorders at or below the brain stem	13.3
Uncomplicated epilepsy	28.6
Lesions about the brain stem without seizures	37.5
Lesions above the brain stem associated with seizures	58.3
Temporal lobe epilepsy	90.9

occur more commonly for the first time in adolescence in autism and this is seen in around 30% of cases and is more frequent when there is intellectual retardation.

Often there is an isolated generalized tonic clonic seizure which may have been precipitated by the use of epileptogenic psychotropic medication such as chlorpromazine given to control behaviour but sometimes persistent complex partial seizures occur and the onset of epilepsy may be associated with regression in behaviour and deterioration in cognitive ability.

The general principles of diagnosis and treatment of epilepsy in people with mental disability are similar to those in people who are not disabled but a number of general and specific points do need to be borne in mind.

In the past health and social services for people with mental retardation were provided separately from mainstream services and there was also a tendency to label people as mentally retarded in a similar fashion to the labelling of people as epileptics rather than as people first.

A major consequence has been that people with mental handicap and epilepsy have tended to be denied access to specialized services for the investigation and treatment of epilepsy. This situation was compounded by the tendency to base specialized services for people with mental handicap in institutions which became their only home.

With an increasing move towards community care there is a recognition of the need to improve access of people with a mental disability to generic services. In spite of this recognition of need there is still strong evidence that people with epilepsy associated with mental disability who are living in the community still have difficulty in obtaining access to specialized services for epilepsy.

Recent evidence from epidemiological studies of people in contact with services for mental handicap in Birmingham suggest that in a significant proportion of those receiving long term psychotropic or anticonvulsant medication this is still inadequately supervised (9) and that when people are discharged from institutional care adequate plans are often not made for supervision of their medication so that prescription, often of multiple drugs, is continued routinely, without the person even being seen by their general practitioner (10). It also seems that while children with mental disability growing up in the community may receive adequate supervision of their epilepsy while they are of school age, this often does not continue with a carefully planned transfer to adult services when they get older.

I believe that the solution to this problem is not to set up separate services for people with a mental disability who happen to have epilepsy; and that the situation will only be improved by education of those working in primary health care and community mental handicap teams about both epilepsy and mental handicap; and improving the access of people with a mental handicap to epilepsy services.

Greatest importance will be attached to the taking of a careful developmental history and a description of the person's skills, behaviour and additional handicaps in interview with the parents or carer.

Accounts from those whose observing seizures take on particular importance in view of the difficulty which the mentally disabled patient might have in describing subjective experiences associated with seizures.

It must be remembered that many seizure disorders in people with mental retardation may comprise isolated attacks or be self limiting. In each case a careful judgement needs to be made between the advantages of early treatment limiting recurrence with reduction in parent or staff anxiety and the disadvantages of committing a person who already has learning difficulties to treatment which may further impair learning or behaviour. It is always necessary to consider alternative or additional strategies of management which will reduce the need to depend totally on pharmacological treatments.

First and most essential is the reduction of anxiety in the person's caring network and a realization that the arrival of the handicapped child will have been experienced as a partial bereavement which will have been compounded by the onset of the epilepsy. A parent may take a handicapped child into their own bed for fear that they will not wake when seizures occur at night and this will lead to increased anxiety when the child's dependency needs cannot be met. This may engender fear in the child and contribute to an increase in seizure frequency and then to a demand for yet more medication. These anxieties need to be weighed against the fact that seizures are now the main cause for the increased mortality in severely and profoundly handicapped children.

Such considerations will extend to the handicapped person's total caring network of dependent relationships and care staff and teachers are understandably reluctant to allow the person the dignity of taking reasonable risks in day to day life.

In conclusion I hope I have said sufficient to indicate some of the complex relationships between disability, particularly mental disability, and epilepsy and the need for close and continuing dialogue between the team dealing with the disability and the doctor treating the epilepsy if the disability is to be minimized and more major handicap prevented.

REFERENCES

(1) Ryder S, Cheshire L. The hope of the disabled person. London: *Royal Society of Medicine*, 1983; 19.

(2) World Health Organisation. *International classification of handicaps, disabilities and impairments*. Geneva: World Health Organisation, 1980.

(3) Ryan R, Kempner K, Emlen AC. The stigma of epilepsy as a self concept. *Epilepsia* 1980; **21**: 433–44.

(4) Cooper JE. Epilepsy in a longitudinal study of 5,000 children. *Br Med J* 1965; **1**: 1020–2.

(5) Ross EM, Peckham CS. School children with epilepsy. In: Parsonage M, Grant RHE, Craig AG, Ward AA, eds. *Advances in epileptology—the XIVth Epilepsy international symposium*. New York: Raven Press, 1983; 215–20.

(6) Richardson SA, Koller H, Katz M, McLaren J. Seizures and epilepsy in a mentally retarded population over the first 22 years of life. *Appl Res Mental Retard* 1980; **1**: 123–38.

(7) Corbett JA. Epilepsy and mental retardation—a follow up study. In: Parsonage M, Grant RHE, Craig AG, Ward AA, eds. *Advances in epileptology—the XIVth Epilepsy international symposium*. New York: Raven Press, 1983; 203–14.

(8) Rutter M, Graham P, Yule W. A neuropsychiatric study in childhood. *Clinics in developmental medicine*. London: Heinemann, 1970: 35–6.

(9) Clarke DJ, Kelley S, Thinn K, Corbett JA. Disabilities, drugs & mental retardation. 1. Disabilities and the prescription of drugs for behaviour in three residential settings. 1989; (In press).

(10) Thinn K, Clarke DJ, Corbett J. Disabilities, drugs and mental retardation. 2. A comparison of antipsychotic drug use before and after discharge from hospital to community. 1989; (In press).

Discussion after Drs Stores and Gillham and Professor Corbett

Interactive question from Dr Fenwick

How many of you thought about a disorder of sleep structure producing a disability in cognitive function during the day in epileptic patients?		**Response (No.)**
1 Considered it	(Neurologist)	128
	(Other)	64
2 Not considered it	(Neurologist)	58
	(Other)	56

Dr Brown *(Cheshire, UK):* Over the last 10 years there has been a lot of interest in putting patients in front of microcomputers and measuring their reaction times in milliseconds under the effect of different drugs. A number of test batteries have been established and there are others growing up. I am a little concerned because most of my patients do not live in a laboratory and one millisecond is not going to make much difference to them. Is it not about time that we also looked at the influence of drugs on everyday life and the pattern of living. What difficulties do patients have at home getting up in the morning and getting to work; do their friends and relatives notice that they forget things; whether they fall asleep in front of the television at night, and what happens when they go to bed, and, take the studies out of the laboratory.

Dr Gillham *(Glasgow, UK):* I absolutely agree with you and one of my long term aims is to find a test that can be done quickly and conveniently in the clinic, is scientifically proven to be reliable and valid, but which also relates well to problems of everyday life. But what you are suggesting is something for the future and we are not really ready to go into that until we find what precisely we are looking for in a well controlled laboratory setting.

Dr Stores *(Oxford, UK):* I take a rather different view. I think some appropriate measures of clinical value are already available. There has been some work done in recent years to develop memory tests for example, that are to do with everyday memorising and there are parent teacher rating scales concerned with real life behaviour that relate very closely to the kind of information one would normally want to collect in the clinic. For those reasons we have emphasised this kind of assessment. They are subject to certain methodological shortcomings but on balance I do believe there is more value in clinical measures than purely laboratory findings, interesting as those might be.

Professor Corbett *(Birmingham, UK):* The Rivermead test which was developed in Oxford by Dr Barbara Wilson looks at function in day to day life situations, and seems to be particularly useful.

Dr Besag *(Surrey, UK):* The Medical Research Council is helping us with a major project comparing both normal children and children with epilepsy on the Rivermead Behavioural

Memory Test. We are able to compare this, which is a memory test based on very practical tasks, with other tests of cognitive function and other tests of behaviour. Unfortunately I cannot report any results, the preliminary results were discussed only last week and it will probably be a year or two before they are available.

Dr Hosking *(Sheffield, UK):* I am interested that a number of studies have concluded by saying that we must give certain information to teachers, social workers and anybody else who is prepared to listen. What concerns me is whether we are neglecting an area of research in this field, if we take children with learning difficulties and epilepsy. Little research has been undertaken on the problems that teachers and social workers should be told. I wonder if we should not be entering another phase of enquiry and supporting that to a greater extent that hitherto.

Dr Stores: There is no doubt that very basic information about the epilepsies is lacking in many groups and that should be corrected as a matter of some urgency. But I would agree it would be best done in the light of the particular problems faced by these groups. I think that the two approaches complement each other.

Dr Gillham: The Rivermead test is a test battery with a great many uses, but my own experience of it is that you need to have a very poor memory indeed before you begin to fail, and its major use is with quite severe head injured patients. In the kind of patient group that I was looking at, although they were all reporting poor memory, they are not going to show differences on something as general as the Rivermead and you need to have very sensitive psychometric tests before you show differences. These differences are very subtle, compared to the possible impairment produced by the disorder itself, or by the subjective feeling of poor memory that patients have.

Dr Stores: I would be interested in the reactions of two groups—those who consider themselves epileptologists, and those who do not—to the following question

---

Interactive question fom Dr Stores

Considering the frequency with which doctors encounter patients with epilepsy and the time constraints in teaching programmes do you believe that epilepsy: **Response**

1 Receives too much attention in undergraduate and post-graduate courses compared with other topics		(No.)
	(Epileptologists)	1
	(Not epileptologists)	1
2 Is covered adequately		
	(Epileptologists)	70
	(Not epileptologists)	1
3 It is not given anything like as much attention as it deserves		
	(Epileptologists)	110
	(Not epileptologists)	120

Dr Stores: Neurologists have realised that it is not given as much attention as it deserves, but a fair number think it is covered adequately. That is interesting because it seems to conflict with my own experience in terms of results. For those who think it is not covered adequately, the great problem now is how do you correct that deficiency; who is going to teach these various groups about epilepsy adequately, how is one going to gain access to teaching programmes? That is quite a challenge.

CLOSING SESSION

Chairman: D. Chadwick

Epilepsy genes: a molecular approach to familial epilepsy

J. Poulton

University Department of Paediatrics, John Radcliffe Hospital, Oxford, UK

SOME LANDMARKS OF THE NEW GENETICS

'We wish to suggest a structure for the salt of deoxyribose nucleic acid (DNA). This structure has novel features which are of considerable biological interest. . . . It has not escaped our notice that the specific pairing we have postulated immediately suggests a possible copying mechanism for the genetic material'. With these words (1), Watson and Crick launched an era in which genetics would be transformed out of all recognition. The role of messenger RNA in transcription, the translation into proteins and the elucidation of the genetic code followed in quick succession. Hamilton Smith's discovery of restriction enzymes (2), which recognise and cut DNA at specific sequences, enabled the development of restriction mapping and cloning. Sequencing of DNA bases enabled prediction of protein sequences from cloned genes (3), and is now a routine procedure in molecular biological research. The term, 'The new genetics' was coined as the application of these techniques to medicine became apparent (4). DNA segments from thousands of different regions of the human genome have been cloned, and the chromosomal location of very many have been identified. This has resulted in the recent announcement of a map of polymorphic DNA markers covering the entire human genome (5), enabling gene localisation, which makes subsequent identification of genes responsible for inherited disorders a real possibility. The technique of locating genes using linkage analysis will be discussed later in this essay. Its application has resulted in advances in antenatal diagnosis and detection of carriers of genetic diseases such as Duchenne muscular dystrophy, and diagnosis of presymptomatic patients in diseases with a variable age of onset such as Huntington's Chorea.

Once a gene has been located, 'reverse genetics' can be used to analyse DNA from diseased individuals and identify the defective protein in diseases whose biochemical basis is completely obscure, and may ultimately suggest new therapeutic possibilities. An exciting example of this was the identification of the gene responsible for Duchenne muscular dystrophy. Cytogenetic analysis revealed that a proportion of patients had large deletions, and localized the gene to a region of the X chromosome. DNA analysis mapped its location more closely, and ultimately showed that the gene spanned a few percent of the X chromosome, which is an enormous length. The protein encoded by the gene was entirely unknown. Once the gene had been cloned, the protein was identified within months as a high molecular weight molecule found in association with triads of sarcoplasmic reticulum and with tubules of the T system, and may be responsible for linking these membranes to the contractile proteins (6). Before 'reverse genetics' can be used, the gene must be located, for instance using linkage analysis. If these two approaches are combined, identifying the genes and characterising the defective proteins causing epilepsy is a real possibility. Although potential applications include antenatal diagnosis and selective abortion of affected fetuses for severe phenotypes, the exciting possibility of understanding disease pathogenesis and therapeutic possibilities of even more compelling.

Fourth international symposium on sodium valproate and epilepsy, edited by David Chadwick, 1989; Royal Society of Medicine Services International Congress and Symposium Series No. 152, published by Royal Society of Medicine Services Limited.

How far can these astonishing advances help epilepsy sufferers? This essay will first establish that many of the epilepsies are genetic diseases, and then describe three possible genetic experimental approaches.

EPILEPSY AND GENETICS

Three main lines of evidence that some of the epilepsies are genetic disorders will be presented: clinical studies, animal models and inference from knowledge of cell biochemistry and physiology.

Clinical studies

Epilepsy has been defined as a paroxysmal and recurring disorder in which there are disturbances of consciousness, sensation or behaviour of any sort which are caused primarily by cerebral disturbances (7). This immediately suggests that this is a group rather than a single disorder, with a range of aetiologies. However it might not be an enormous exaggeration to state that although the medical classification of seizures has grown complex, the assignation of the common syndromes into aetiological categories has not progressed much since the era of Hippocrates (8).

McKusick (9) now lists over a hundred probable single gene disorders in which epilepsy may be a feature, comprising about 1% of all epilepsies. In most there are several other features, and in some the biochemical defect has been identified. As this essay is concerned primarily with those syndromes in whom seizures are the prime feature, these will not be discussed further. Similarly, although convulsions may be a feature of several different chromosomal anomalies, of which the best known is Down's syndrome, these will be omitted from the ensuing discussion.

Twin studies of epilepsy have usually been of insufficient size to attempt to subclassify cases by type of seizure. The average concordance rate for epilepsy in monozygotic twins is about 57% (range 40–90%) and for dizygotic twins 11% (5–20%). There is therefore clearly a genetic component at least some of the common syndromes. Interestingly, other attempts to document overall genetic risks in unclassified epilepsy have shown familial clustering, but with increased transmission by affected mothers compared to fathers. Careful epidemiological analysis (10) suggests that this is not a reporting bias, or an effect explained by differential fertility. Affected women really are about twice as likely to transmit epilepsy to their offspring as affected men. As sex incidence is reasonably equal, this cannot be X linked, and does not fit any single nuclear gene model. Possible explanations include a transplacental or intrauterine factor, imprinting or involvement of maternally inherited mitochondrial DNA. An experimental approach to investigating this question is outlined later.

Probable single gene disorders (determined by a single major locus, although other minor loci have some influence on phenotype) include benign familial neonatal convulsions, benign rolandic epilepsy and juvenile myoclonic epilepsy. Commoner syndromes such as grand mal major motor seizures, absence epilepsy and febrile convulsions are more likely to be multifactorial (a number of genetic determinants are inherited independently, and other nongenetic factors may be involved in shaping the final phenotype). Studies of each of these groups will be discussed in turn.

Benign familial neonatal convulsions occur in the first three months of life, without any clear precipitating factor. The prognosis for normal neurological development is excellent, although a proportion continue to have seizures. Inheritance in 14 families was autosomal dominant (11). A recent study reveals linkage to DNA markers on the long arm of chromosome 20 (12).

Benign rolandic epilepsy (benign focal epilepsy) is also probably an autosomal dominant, comprising about 16% of all afebrile seizures with onset under 15 years of age. Bray and Wiser (13) studied 40 probands and their families. Centrotemporal spikes were evident in the electroencephalogram (EEG) in 30% of first degree relatives, supporing an autosomal dominant gene. This was confirmed by Heijbel et al. (14) in a smaller study of 19 cases. They found that of 34 siblings, 15% had seizures and rolandic discharges and 19% had

had rolandic discharge alone. Of 38 parents the corresponding figures were 11% and 3%. They concluded that there was age dependent penetrance.

In the past it has been stated that juvenile myoclonic epilepsy is an ideal candidate for linkage analysis (15) because the convulsive tendency persists into adult life so that three and four generation families may be available for study. Investigations of these families are already in progress. Disappointingly, this has turned out to be a heterogenous group so that the number of families required to investigate linkage is much higher than expected.

Grand mal epilepsy (generalized onset major motor seizures) comprises around 4–10% of all epilepsy. Its inheritance has been studied in some detail, in most cases excluding patients with any other neurological abnormality. Eisner et al. (16) showed that the risk to siblings increased with younger age of onset in the proband. Thus 7.5% of sibs would have had symptoms by aged 20 if the proband had seizures by aged four, but this fell to 4.3% if the proband's seizures started between four and 15 years.Metrakos and Metrakos (17) investigated 211 patients with either petit mal or grand mal epilepsy, and generalized spike and wave (GSW) on EEG. They found that the risk to sibs was 12.7% compared to 4.7% among siblings of controls. They also found that GSW occurred in an unusually high proportion of sibs. Furthermore, sibs who had a GSW pattern had a 25% chance of developing epilepsy. They concluded that GSW is inherited as an autosomal dominant disorder with age-specific penetrance. Tsuboi and Endo (18) studied offspring of patients with tonic-clonic seizures, and found that overall risks to siblings were 4.7% for seizures, 16.8% for febrile convulsions and 37.3% for an abnormal EEG pattern, lending some support to the view of Metrakos and Metrakos. However, none of these satisfactorily explained the maternal inheritance pattern. Andermann (19) has recently suggested that the data fit a polygenic model better.

Absence epilepsy comprises about 3–4% of all patients with epilepsy. Doose et al. (20) studied 250 children with absence seizures and found that 6.7% of sibs had seizures. Of the 242 sibs on whom EEG information was available, 22.3% had abnormalities including GSW or photoconvulsive reactivity.

The prevalence of febrile convulsions is about 2–5% in children between ages 1 and 5 in Europe and USA, but about 6.7% in Japan. Risk to siblings are 8.0% and 20.7% respectively (21). When interpreted as polygenic model, the proportion of the variation attributable to genetic factors is 60–80% in both cases (22). However, in families of probands with more than three febrile fits, Rich et al. suggested that the most parsimonious model is an autosomal dominant.

Animal models

The second piece of evidence that some of the epilepsies may be genetic comes from animal models. Several different single gene disorders are known to casue seizures with names as diverse as the shaker drosophila, the tottering mouse and the ether-a-gogo drosophila (23). Most of them are autosomal recessive, and in contrast to the human epilepsies discussed above are only one aspect of a complex neurological disease: for instance most of the mice models have an accompanying movement disorder. A few basic principles can be gleaned: mutations at any one of several unlinked loci can result in indistinguishable phenotypes: the phenotypic expression of the mutant gene may also be affected by minor unlinked loci. These findings are consistent with the clinical studies: genetic heterogeneity of clinical syndromes and polygenic inheritance are clearly problems to be taken seriously.

The most interesting aspect of animal models is their ability to suggest pathogenetic mechanisms and candidate genes for human disease. Two examples of these will be discussed. Electrophysiological measurements on afferent axons of the shaker Drosophila have revealed that the A current is prolonged (24). This is known to be mediated by voltage-sensitive potassium channels which control repolarization. It is therefore likely that the phenotype is caused by a defect in the structure or function of this protein complex.

For some time gamma aminobutyric acid (GABA)-mediated inhibition has been thought to be important to the mammalian central nervous system. There is some evidence that derangement of its functional pathway may result in seizure activity, and sodium valproate, a related compound is an effective anticonvulsant in many clinical syndromes. Studies on the seizure-susceptible Mongolian gerbil demonstrate a reduction in the number of GABA receptors (25). As genes for the GABA receptor (26) and for glutamic acid decarboxylase (27) which is involved in GABA synthesis have now been cloned, these could be used as candidate genes.

Inferences from cell biology

Factors which may be causes of epilepsy can be roughly grouped into three: those affecting the capacity of membranes in pacemaker neurons to develop intrinsic burst discharges, the presence of disinhibition and the presence of excitatory circuits (28). Membrane potentials could be influenced by defective receptors or iontophores: disinhibition could be caused by a deficiency of GABA or endorphins, for instance because of defective enzymes in their synthetic pathways or defective release. Mutations in any one of the genes encoding these proteins themselves or regulating their synthesis or function could possibly cause seizures.

In summary there is good clinical evidence that at least some epileptic syndromes have a genetic component. This is strengthened by the existence of animal models of epilepsy caused by single gene disorders, and by recognition of key elements in brain function in which mutations could cause malfunction likely to give rise to seizures.

EXPERIMENTAL APPROACHES

Although animal models of epilepsy have provided useful insights into possible mechanisms for human epilepsy, and candidate genes for molecular genetic studies, the definitive experiments must be done on humans. Therefore, this essay will emphasize approaches which apply these findings to humans, rather than extend them in animals.

Linkage analysis

Locating genes in the human genome responsible for epileptic syndromes is a formidable task. The diploid human genome comprises 6 000 000 000 base pairs, of which only about 10% is actually structural genes, the remainder being noncoding DNA. There are probably between 50 000 and 150 000 genes, of which only a few thousand have been cloned.

Linkage analysis depends on the cosegregation of disease phenotype with DNA markers. During meiosis crossing over occurs, so that DNA segments initially located on the same chromosome may not be co-inherited. The nearer the DNA segments, the more likely is co-inheritance. The proportion of meioses where recombination has occurred (recombination fraction) can thus be used as a measure of this distance. A recombination fraction of 50% implies that the markers are not linked and may lie on different chromosomes: no recombination implies close linkage: they may be only a few million bases apart.

Two parallel approaches to locating genes responsible for epileptic syndromes will be described, one involving linkage analysis with random DNA markers, and the other with candidate genes.

Linkage analysis with random DNA markers

Linkage analysis is an old technique which has been revolutionized by the new genetics. Instead of a few doze protein markers representing only a proportion of this enormous length of DNA, there are now thousands of polymorphic DNA markers fairly evenly spaced covering over 95% of the human genome. The recent discovery that each individual has a unique genetic 'fingerprint', a restriction pattern using the 'minisatellite' probe for repetitive so called satellite DNA (29), has enabled forensic identification of suspects and confirmation of paternity. The latter is as essential to the clinical scientist as to the CID, because in linkage studies a single case of nonpaternity can produce misleading results and might conceal linkage. Furthermore, clones of these highly variable regions (HVRs) can be used as highly polymorphic probes for linkage analysis. This is because each region of minisatellite DNA consists of a number of repeats which varies widely between individuals. It is unlikely that both alleles in any individual will each contain the same number of repeats. If restriction digests, Southern blotting and hybridization with the probe are carried out it is likely that he will have two different alleles which can be distinguished from each other, and are hence informative for linkage phase.

Linkage analysis with candidate genes

A second approach to linkage analysis is the use of candidate genes. Animal models of epilepsy suggest numerous possible functional groups of proteins which could be causative. Available clones include the alpha subunit of Na+K+ATPase, Ca++ATPase, Na+ channel protein Ca2+ cadmodulin kinase, protein C kinase, cAMP dependent protein kinase, GABA-benzodiazepine receptor and glutamic acid decarboxylase (15). A defect in any of these genes might demonstrate linkage. Linkage disequilibrium for a particular allele would suggest a recent mutation. Rearrangements such as small deletions might even be identified.

Problems associated with linkage analysis

The practical problems associated with linkage analysis have been recently reviewed (5). The most formidable one is probably the difficulties in obtaining pedigrees in whom the mode of inheritance is clear on which to work. As discussed above, the term 'epilepsy' includes a heterogenous group of conditions with perhaps an even larger number of causes. 'Phenocopies' are clinical syndromes caused by environmental factors which are indistinguishable from those caused by a genetic syndrome. This may make the mode of inheritance unclear. There may be not only allelic heterogeneity (more than one alternative alleles at a locus), but also genetic heterogeneity (more than one locus affecting a clinical phenotype). Most of the common disorders appear to be polygenic, and those which are clearly caused by single genes account for a tiny minority of patients. The problem of genetic heterogeneity can be overcome in part by using very large pedigrees or isolated communities. Even where the mode of inheritance has been identified with some certainty, penetrance is usually incomplete, and this makes heterogeneity hard to detect and linkage may be very difficult to ascertain. Before embarking on the common epilepsies, it would be beneficial to find more clinical markers for individual subgroups, and ways of identifying asymptomatic carriers. This approach has borne fruit in the search for the asthma gene (30). Inheritance of atopy was thought to be polygenic until it was found that there was an autosomal dominantly inherited ability to raise specific IgE, with 90% penetrance. The existence of a blood test to identify individuals no longer displaying clear atopic features made it possible to interpret pedigrees, and linkage has now been found. It would therefore seem reasonable to search harder for a similar feature, for instance physiological measures such as specific EEG changes in response to epileptogenic stimuli. Alternatively new subclassifications may be possible on the basis of emerging data such as that appearing from in situ hybridization.

Thus, in the presence of such additional information, it is possible that linkage analysis could be carried out not only on pedigrees of patients with probable single gene disorders such as benign familial neonatal convulsions and benign rolandic epilepsy, but also on the other conditions listed above. Approaches would include use of highly polymorphic DNA markers, such as those derived from HVRs as discussed above. There are now over 600 polymorphic DNA markers commercially available, and it has been estimated that 95% of the human genome has been covered by markers at intervals of about three centimorgans (5). Thus, if sufficient DNA samples could be obtained from homogenous large pedigrees there would be a good chance that linkage could be established.

Analysis of mitochondrial DNA

The evidence that epilepsy is more commonly inherited from the mother than the father is hard to explain on the basis of single nuclear gene disorders. Mitochondrial DNA is exclusively maternally inherited, and provides a possible explanation. The phenotype of a patient with a dominant gene for an epileptic syndrome whose penetrance is incomplete might depend on other genetic loci. If so, one of these could be a mitochondrial gene. Evidence that a phenotype may depend on the interaction between nuclear and mitochondrial gene products is the recent demonstration of a mitochondrial point mutation in patients with maternally inherited Leber's optic neuropathy (31). As all the offspring of a carrier mother have an identical mitochondrial DNA type, nuclear genes must be invoked to explain the excess of affected males over females. Furthermore, mitochondrial DNA deletions (32) and duplications (33) are probably both capable of causing mitochondrial myopathy, and some of these cases had convulsions.

Recombination of mitochondrial DNA has never been documented in man, and the accumulation of neutral mitochondrial mutations has been used b population geneticists as both a genetic clock, and a measure of genetic diversity (34). As a result, there is an extensive classification into mitochondrial types, based on polymorphisms. If a mitochondrial mutation were involved in the expression of epileptic phenotypes, it would probably be confined to one or a group of mitochondrial types or clans. This could easily be investigated by typing epileptic mother child paris, where both were affected. To do this, mitochondria must be isolated, either from placenta or from blood or cell lines.

The mitochondrial DNA is then digested with various restriction enzymes, the DNA fragments end labelled and electrophoresed and autoradiographed. This should be compared to the mitochondrial typing of patients who inherit their epilepsy from their father.

This approach could identify a group of patients with a single or few different mitochondrial types interacting with nuclear genes to result in epilepsy, but would not localise the defect. Sequencing one of them and comparing any base changes to the reference sequence and the others in the group might reveal the abnormality, and this might shed light on the major nuclear genes causing the primary disorder.

In situ hybridization

Tissue specific gene expression can be verified by RNA analysis. Animal models suggest candidate genes whose expression could be defective in epileptics, for example reduced numbers of GABA receptors in the seizure-susceptible Mongolian gerbil (25). This could be due to a mutation in the GABA receptor gene itself resulting in the production of a defective or unstable protein. Alternatively, gene expression might have been down regultaed by some alteration in other genes controlling it. If so, less of its specific RNA might be present in the affected cells, and if so, this should be detectable.

The technique of in situ hybridization allows identification of minute quantities of RNA in a tissue section. Probes can be radiolabelled antisense RNA or DNA oligonucleotides, both of which would be complementary to the species to be detected. After hybridization of one tissue slice with the radiolabelled probe, and a similar one with the control probe (complementary to the probe sequence) autoradiography is carried out. Microscopic comparison with the original tissue and the control identifies the tissue layers containing the RNA in question. Furthermore, the technique can be adapted for high resolution in order to identify the cells which express the gene.

This powerful technique provides information about tissue specific expression of candidate genes for epilepsy. One advantage is that it could pick up a deficiency due to the affected gene, or its regulators. It involves no assumptions about modes of inheritance, and does not require such large numbers of patients.

The final stage

Unfortunately, localizing and cloning the genes causing human epilepsies is not the final answer. It may be difficult to ascertain the function of a putative epilepsy gene identified by linkage analysis even after sequencing both wild and mutant alleles. Protein homology searches may provide clues, as may immunoblotting and *in situ* hybridisation. In the case of Duchenne muscular dystrophy, the uncertainty was solved within a few months.

CONCLUSION

Molecular genetics is now well able to begin the search for epilepsy genes. Animal work has provided candidate genes for investigation, and linkage analysis is now sophisticated and workable. Single gene disorders suitable for linkage analysis are in a minority, and problems of heterogeneity and incomplete penetrance prevent simple analysis of the common syndromes. As new information emerges, it may become possible to reclassify patients into homogenous groups more suitable for linkage studies. The doors will then be wide open for understanding the molecular basis of epilepsy and hence new therapeutic possibilities.

ACKNOWLEDGMENTS

I would like to thank Dr R. M. Gardiner for encouragement, Sanofi for providing the motivation, and my husband Dr I. S. McLean for support and proofreading.

REFERENCES

(1) Watson JD, Crick FHC. Molecular structure of nucleic acids. *Nature* 1953; **171**: 737–8.
(2) Watson J, Tooze J, Kurtz DT. *Recombinant DNA: a short course*. New York: Scientific American Books, 1983.
(3) Sanger F, Nicklen S. Coulsen AR. DNA sequencing with dideoxy terminating nucleotides. *Proc Natl Acad Sci USA* 1977; **74**: 5463–7.
(4) Comings D. In: Weatherall DJ, ed. *The new genetics and clinical practice*. Oxford University Press, 1982.
(5) Lander ES. Mapping complex genetic trials in humans. In: Davies KE, ed. *Genome analysis: a practical approach*. Oxford, Washington: IRL Press, 1988.
(6) Slater CR. Muscular dystrophy: the missing link in DMD? *Nature* 1987; **330**: 693–4.
(7) Williams D. Modern views on the classification of epilepsy. *Br Med J* 1958; **i**: 661–3.
(8) Temkin O. *The falling sickness*, 2nd ed. Baltimore, London: Johns Hopkins University Press, 1971.
(9) McKusick VA. *Mendelian inheritance in man*, 7th ed. Baltimore: Johns Hopkins University Press, 1986.
(10) Ottman R, Hauser WA, Susser M. Genetic and maternal influence on susceptibility to seizures. *J Epidemiol* 1985; **122**: 923–39.
(11) Plouin P. Benign neonatal convulsions. In: Roger J, Dravet C, Bureau M, Dreifuss FE, Wolf P, eds. *Epileptic syndromes in infancy, childhood and adolescence*. London, Paris; John Libbey, 1985.
(12) Leppart M, Anderson VE, Quattlebaum T, *et al*. Benign neonatal convulsions linked to genetic markers on chromosome 20. *Nature* 1989; **337**: 647–8.
(13) Bray PF, Wiser WV. Hereditary characteristics of familial tempero-central focal epilepsy. *Pediatrics* 1975; **36**: 207–11.
(14) Heijbel J, Blom S, Rasmusen M. Benign epilepsy of childhood with centro-temporal EEG foci: a genetic study. *Epilepsia* 1975; **16**: 285–93.
(15) Delgado-Escueta AV, Greenberg DA. Mapping genes in juvenile myoclonic epilepsy. *Rev Neurol (Paris)* 1987; **143**(5): 361–2.
(16) Eisner V, Paul LL, Livingston S. Hereditary aspects of epilepsy. *Johns Hopkins Hosp Bull* 1959; **105**: 245–71.
(17) Metrakos K, Metrakos JD. Genetics of convulsive disorders. *Neurology* 1960; **11**: 474–83.
(18) Tsuboi T, Endo S. Incidence of seizures and EEG abnormalities among offspring of epileptic patients. *Hum Genet* 1977; **36**: 173–89.
(19) Andermann E. In: Anderson VE, Hauser WA, Penry JK, Sing CF, eds. *Genetic basis of the epilepsies*. New York: Raven Press, 1982.
(20) Doose H, Gerken H, Leonhardt R, Volzke E, Volz C. Centrencephalic myoclonic astatic petit mal. *Neuropediatrie* 1970; **2**: 59–78.
(21) Anderson VE, Genetics in the epilepsies. *Trends Neurol Sci* 1985; **8**: 513–6.

(22) Rich SS, Annegers JF, Hauser WA, Anderson VE. Complex segregation analysis of febrile convulsions. *Am J Hum Genet* 1987; **41**: 249–57.
(23) Noebels JL. Isolating single genes of the inherited epilepsies. *Ann Neurol* 1984; **16**: S18–21.
(24) Noebels JL. Tracing the cellular expression of neuromodulatory genes. *TINS* 1985; **8**: 327–30.
(25) Olsen RW, Warnsley JK, Lee RJ, Lomax P. In: *Advances in Neurology*. Vol. 44. New York: Raven Press, 1986.
(26) Schofield PR, Darlison MG, Fujita N, *et al*. Sequence and functional expression of the $GABA_A$ receptor shows a ligand gated receptor superfamily. *Nature* 1987; **238**: 221–7.
(27) Banner C, Silverman S, Thomas JW, *et al*. Isolation of a human brain cDNA for glutamate dehydrogenase. *J Neurochem* 1987; **49**: 246–52.
(28) Delgado-Escueta AV. Summation of the workshops and discussion; the new wave of research in the epilepsies. *Ann Neurol* 1984; **16**: S145–58.
(29) Jeffreys AJ, Wilson V, Thein S. Hypervariable minisatellite regions in human DNA. *Nature* 1985; **314**: 67.
(30) Cookson WOCM, Hopkin JM. Linkage between immunoglobulin response underlying asthma and rhinitis and chromosome llq. *Lancet* 1989; **i**: 1292–5.
(31) Wallace DC, Singh G, Lott MT, *et al*. Mitochondrial DNA mutation associated with Leber's hereditary optic neuropathy. *Science* 1988; **242**: 1427–30.
(32) Holt I, Harding AE, Morgan-Hughes JA. Deletions of muscle mitochondrial DNA in patients with mitochondrial myopathies. *Nature* 1988; **331**: 717–9.
(33) Poulton J, Deadman ME, Gardiner RM. Duplications of mitochondrial DNA in mitochondrial myopathy. *Lancet* 1989; **i**: 236–40.
(34) Cann R, Stoneking M, Wilson AC. Mitochondrial DNA and human evolution. *Nature* 1987; **325**: 31–6.

Driving and epilepsy:
New draft EEC directive for a
common Community driving licence

J. Taylor

Department of Transport, London, UK

The First EEC Directive for a common Community licence came into force on 1 January 1983. Since that time the format of driving licences issued within the European Economic Community have had to conform and amongst other things the British driving licence has changed colour from green to pink. Recently the Community issued a Second Directive (1) in draft form which revises the basic medical standards for Community driving licence holders and applicants. So far as epilepsy is concerned, paragraph 12 of the new Draft Directive states—

'Epileptic seizures or other sudden disturbances of the state of consciousness constitute a serious danger to road safety if they occur to a person while driving a motor vehicle.'

For motorcars and motorcycles—'a driving licence may be issued or renewed subject to an examination by a competent Medical Authority and to regular medical check-ups. The Authority shall decide on the state of the epilepsy or other disturbances of consciousness, its clinical form and progress (no seizures in the last 2 years, for example) the treatment received and the results thereof'.

For goods vehicles and buses the Draft Directive requires that 'driving licences shall not be issued to or renewed for applicants or drivers suffering or liable to suffer from epileptic seizures or other sudden disturbances of the state of consciousness'.

1975 saw the First International Conference on Valproate at Nottingham. In that same year in the United States there were over 16 million motor vehicle accidents, 8600 pedestrians and 37 400 passengers and drivers were killed. In addition to the 46 000 killed, two million people were seriously injured. Road traffic accidents are the leading cause of death for people under 40 and cause more lost years of life than all forms of cancer put together. In 1975 the United States had the lowest road traffic accident fatality rate of any country per hundred million kilometres travelled. Road traffic accidents kill more Americans each year than were killed in the 10 years of the Vietnam War (2).

Japan has three times the United States fatality rate, Kenya has 22 times the United States rate. Table 1 shows the European league of deaths per hundred million kilometres travelled in 1983. Finland is top of the league with the lowest death rate equating to the United States and Great Britain comes second (3).

The World Health Organisation has described the road traffic accident epidemic as the primary public health problem of 20th Century.

On the spot studies in the United Kingdom and Indiana estimate that most road traffic acidents are multifactoral in aetiology and over 90% have human factor involvement (Fig. 1), (4,5). Acute collapse of drivers and riders has an incidence of approximately four per thousand serious road traffic accidents (6). Approximately 50% of acute collapses are due to epilepsy (7) (Fig. 2).

Fourth international symposium on sodium valproate and epilepsy, edited by David Chadwick, 1989; Royal Society of Medicine Services International Congress and Symposium Series No. 152, published by Royal Society of Medicine Services Limited.

Table 1 *European car user deaths
per 100 million car km in 1980*

Yugoslavia	11.0
Poland	7.0
Spain	6.5
Greece	4.6
Austria	4.3
Belgium	3.9
France	2.8
Holland	2.4
W. Germany	2.2
Italy	2.1
Eire	1.7
Denmark	1.4
Norway	1.3
Sweden	1.2
Hungary	1.1
Gt Britain	1.0
Finland	0.9

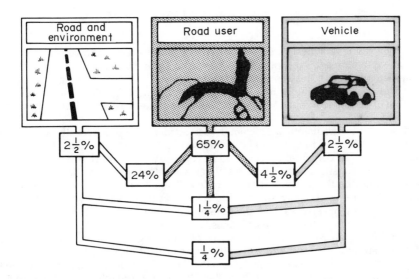

Figure 1 *Contributory factors in road accident interactions.*

Epilepsy is frequently a covert influence in road accidents and is rarely established as a cause of fatality because the only evidence in the case of a convulsion is molar teeth bites on the tongue. There are other forms of epilepsy apart from convulsions which are equally liable to cause accidents. Most road traffic accident fatalities have some element of brain trauma and who can say which came first, the accident or the fit? People with epilepsy suffer most from these accidents and approximately two-thirds are episodes involving single vehicles.

Between 1985 and 1988 the body fluids of 1273 people killed in British road accidents were quantitatively and qualitatively estimated (8). 1.3% (13) had anti-convulsants present. In all cases the anti-convulsants were in the prescribed dosage range. There was a bias in age towards the elderly, three fatalities were below the age of 40 years and nine over the age of 40 years. In terms of road user groups two were car drivers, two motorcyle riders, two were passengers and seven were pedestrians—there were no pedal cyclists. Only one of the pedestrians and one of the passengers had alcohol present over the British legal limit of 80 mg/100 ml. One of the pedestrians had alcohol present below that

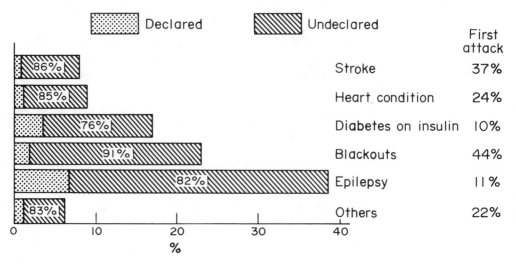

Figure 2 *Causes of 2000 road accidents involving collapse at wheel, based on reports by the police to the DVLC.*

level also. Of the 13 fatalities, three were receiving more than one anti-convulsant. In total six had phenytoin present, five phenobarbitone, three primidone, two carbamazepine and one valproate. Although this sample was small, drivers and riders taking anti-convulsants appeared to be approximately four times over-represented on the basis of the British population of people with epilepsy and the estimate of the number of British drivers with epilepsy (9).

Partial seizures are frequently a problem in road accidents. Typical recently was the young man who had attempted to join a motorway the wrong way up a slip-road. He was stopped by the Police and at consultation revealed his epilepsy and said that he never suffered from loss of consciousness during seizures; when asked to describe an attack, he was totally at a loss saying that the symptoms were 'indescribable'. This is not an uncommon and infrequent scenario in epilepsy and driving casework. Some years ago I used to try and entice a description of seizures from the patient but now I accept that inability to describe what happens implies altered consciousness and a complex partial seizure.

Dr Colin Binnie has reported that some people showing EEG spikes have difficulty in driving in a straight line and show cognitive impairment (10).

Many people with epilepsy conceal it from the Driver Licensing authorities. At the First Valproate International Symposium Prof. Van Der Lugt from Holland reported that only 14% of young Dutchmen declaring epilepsy to gain exemption from military service had declared it when applying for their driving licence (11). My 2000 Police-Reported Accidents-at-the Wheel Study showed that 70% of people who collapsed at the wheel on account of witnessed tonic-clonic seizures had failed to declare the condition to the Licensing Authorities even though they suffered more than one. There is a clear need for more research in relation to epilepsy and driving. We need to monitor the notification rate to the Licensing Authorities and look at different strategies to persuade better reporting. We need also to consider legislation and administrative rules to ensure that they are fair and just and are as far as possible scientifically validated. In an increasing number of countries there is a move to allow the clinician a discretion as to whether or not his patient can drive or not. Such a system does sometimes place an enormous burden on the patient-doctor relationship. There are many patients who are happy to abide by their doctor's decision but others challenge any recommendation against immediate driving. In Great Britain we have had the wisdom of an expert Panel who advised the Government to introduce a statutory bar which at the present time precludes driving if a person has had attacks awake within the last two years but which offers a concession to persons who have attacks confined to sleep for over three years (12). Currently our Panel is considering a proposal to reduce the period of waiting to one year and abolish the sleep concession except in the case of existing beneficiaries who would lose their right to drive should an attack awake supervene. Overall, my view is that a statutory bar period of freedom from epileptic attacks is more efficacious than a clinical discretion. This can lead the epileptologist into the double jeopardy of being blamed by his patient for being too strict and in the event of a disaster being subject to a civil law claim of negligence for being too permissive. In Britain recently there has been a substantial increase in the number of claims made against doctors for negligence. It is better that people with epilepsy should have their period of freedom from attacks before driving prescribed by Parliament so that they blame the law rather than their doctors.

Some years ago in the south of England a young man presented himself to his general practitioner for a medical examination for a heavy goods vehicle driver's licence. The first question on the form was 'Has the applicant suffered from any attack of Epilepsy since the age of 5 years?'. The doctor put the question to his patient who explained that he had had some fits at the age of 11, but he added 'Doctor, if you put that on the form I won't get a job.' Being a kind man as indeed are most doctors, the doctor obliged. Subsequently there was a catastrophe when the young man had a fit at the wheel of his goods vehicle and partially demolished a cottage. The cottage owner endeavoured to obtain the funds for the rebuilding of the cottage through her Insurers. They sought redress through the Third Party Motor Insurers who in turn refused to meet liability because they said that this was an epileptic attack and that the driver had not been negligent. Eventually, the cottage Insurers in making enquiries, interviewed the young man who explained that he had told his Doctor that he had epilepsy and yet in spite of that his doctor had not put it on the form. The end result was that the doctor's Insurer paid for the rebuilding of the cottage at substantial expense in an out of Court settlement.

REFERENCES

(1) Commission of the European Communities (COM (88) 705 Final) 'Proposal for a Council Directive on the Driving Licence' Annex III para 12–12.2. Brussels, 13 Jan 1989.
(2) Shinar D. *Psychology on the road, the human factor in traffic safety*. New York: John Wiley 1978: 102–3.
(3) Department of Transport Road Accidents Great Britain 1983. *The casualty report*. London: HMSO, 1984.
(4) Sabey BE, Staughton GC. Interacting roles of road environment, vehicle and road user in accidents. Paper presented at *5th International Conference of the International Association of Accident and Traffic Medicine*. London: September 1975.
(5) Treat JR, Tumbas NS, McDonald ST, *et al* Tri-level study of cause of traffic accidents. Report No. DOT-HS-034-3-5-35-77 (TAC), Indiana University, March 1988.
(6) Grattan E, Jeffcoate GO. Medical factors and road accidents. *Br Med J* 1968; **1**: 75.
(7) Taylor J. Medical fitness to drive. In: Harrington JM, ed. *Recent advances in occupational health*. Edinburgh: Churchill Livingstone, 1987: 103.
(8) Everest JT, Tonbridge RJ, Widdop B. Incidence of drugs in road traffic fatalities in England and Wales. *11th World Congress International Association for Accident and Traffic Medicine*. Dubrovnic: May 1988.
(9) Espir M. Medical aspects of fitness to drive. Ed. Andrew Raffle. 4 ed. 1985: 26. Medical Commission on Accident Prevention, 35–43 Lincoln's Inn Fields, London WC2A 3PN.
(10) Kasteleijn-Nolst Trenite DGA, Riemersma JBJ, Binnie CD, Smit AM, Meinardi H. *Electroencephalography and clinical neurophysiology*. Dublin: Elsevier Scientific Publishers Ireland, Ltd, 1978: 167–70.
(11) Van der Lugt PJM. Is an application form useful to select patients with epilepsy who may drive? *Epilepsia* 1975; **16**: 743–6.
(12) The Motor Vehicles (Driving Licences Regulations SI 1987/1378) Amendment 1989 SI 373. London: Her Majesty's Stationery Office.

DISCUSSION

Dr Chadwick *(Chairman):* Could I ask the audience a question using the interactive system.

Assuming that we retain a statutory limitation on driving would you:	Response
1 Be happy with a regulation which stipulated 1 years seizure free before driving was allowed	38%
2 Would prefer to maintain the current more complicated arrangement with its sleep provision	55%
3 Have no feelings either way	7%

Dr Fenwick *(London, UK):* I would be interested in your comments, first of all on the United States which uses a six month ban, and secondly on the Japanese whose laws are absolutely draconian—one fit and you never drive again. Where do you think the balance is and are you going to be happy with a year?

Dr Taylor *(London, UK):* We know from the last few years that medico-legal problems do arise when we make clinical decisions or undertake surgical procedures. The clinician is going to be open to a charge of negligence if subsequently the patient damages somebody else, or even themselves. I am in favour of a statutory period, but six months is a little short. We are waiting for the results of the MRC study of antiepileptic drug withdrawal. Looking at the proposal for a one year ban, Tony Johnson was, if anything, a little critical that one year was too far. As far as Japan is concerned, I have no comment.

Dr Poole *(Oxford, UK):* What is a sensible attack free period? We are arguing about an interval without knowing the common repetition interval which would allow us to say, if someone has had no seizures for 5 years, the risk is very small.

Dr Taylor: The answer to that is we need a lot more research. We need to know much more about people who have covert seizures with a positive EEG and we cannot yet answer the questions that you have just posed. At the moment the world is in total disarray as far as standardisation is concerned and it is very difficult for people who move from country to country, with these different proposals and rules. I welcome the time when research shows that after five years freedom from seizures we can say there is no further risk.

Lifestyle changes in epilepsy patients following treatment with valproate

R. H. Mattson, M. L. Prevey, J. A. Cramer, R. A. Novelly and C. T. Swick

Yale University School of Medicine, New Haven, CT, USA

Successful treatment of epilepsy is usually measured by a decrease in the number and/or severity of seizures. Freedom from adverse effects of antiepileptic drugs is also of great importance. Such outcomes can be quantitated to varying degrees (1). Perhaps the most important outcome is a favourable change in lifestyle usually expressed as psychosocial adjustment. For many reasons, few studies examine such results. Definition of favourable change in psychosocial function is, in part, a subjective issue. Paradoxically, a good seizure outcome actually can make life less satisfactory. For example, elimination of seizures might be assumed to be an advantageous result of treatment, but such control might result in loss of financial aid. Lifestyle changes also result from many influences other than seizure control and drug related adverse effects. Coexistent organic brain disease, personality type, societal or interpersonal interactions, education, and normal maturation, all are factors that influence lifestyle and psychosocial outcome (2). Recognizing the difficulties and limitations in attribution of psychosocial adjustment to changes in antiepileptic drug treatment, it nonetheless seemed worthwhile to examine the outcome of conversion of patients with generalized idiopathic epilepsy from a combination of antiepileptic drugs to valproate therapy. Measurable endpoints included the following: changes in seizures, adverse effects including neuropsychological function; and psychosocial adjustment as measured by employment, school performance, independent living, and motor vehicle driving.

METHODS OF STUDY

Sixty patients having idiopathic generalized epilepsy with uncontrolled tonic–clonic seizures were given valproate therapy and followed for 2–13 years (mean 8.5 years). Fifty five patients also had a history of absence and/or myoclonic seizures at some time. The age of onset of the epilepsy was in childhood or teens in all cases, although only three were still in the teens at last follow-up. All patients had an electroencephalogram (EEG) revealing generalized spike and wave discharges and no specific symptomatic cause for the epilepsy. All but one patient had normal intelligence. The patients had a mix of epilepsy syndromes, including juvenile absence epilepsy, juvenile myoclonic epilepsy, and grand mal epilepsy not included in the specific subgroups (3). Four patients may have had symptomatic localization related epilepsy. They had tonic–clonic seizures only and had generalized spike wave on EEG. A secondary bi-synchrony was possible, but this distinction could not be made with confidence.

Sixty patients were begun on valproate therapy beginning in 1976. Analysis was carried out only on patients entered by 1987 so the shortest period of follow-up was two years. After being placed on valproate therapy in addition to existing antiepileptic drugs, doses were adjusted to obtain optimal control and minimal side-effects. All patients were

Fourth international symposium on sodium valproate and epilepsy, edited by David Chadwick, 1989; Royal Society of Medicine Services International Congress and Symposium Series No. 152, published by Royal Society of Medicine Services Limited.

then crossed to monotherapy by tapering off other antiepileptic drug therapy (4). The results of treatment were analysed for several measures of outcome including seizure type, frequency and severity; systemic and neurotoxic side effects, neuropsychological changes (tested in two small subgroups); and changes in lifestyle as measured by employment, independent living, educational change and ability to drive a motor vehicle.

Seizure control

The numbers and frequency of seizures of myoclonic, absence, and tonic–clonic type were assessed. All patients had had tonic–clonic seizures at some time. The seizure frequencies were based on reports by the patients. An initial group of 11 patients also had 6 h EEG monitoring before treatment, during a placebo lead in and following three months of valproate therapy. The final 17 patients were studied in a clinical pharmacokinetic crossover protocol which also had pre- and post-EEG monitoring of outcome (5).

Adverse effects

Specific adverse effect frequency and severity was asked of all patients and tested at the clinic visits (1). These adverse effects were expressed as an occurrence at any time on drug as well as a time of last analysis.

NEUROPSYCHOLOGICAL TESTING

Reliable neuropsychological testing data were available from six patients prior to beginning therapy, after placebo, and after three months of VPA therapy. Tests included grip strength, index finger tapping, peg board, digit span, visual search, visual flicker fusion, trails B, digit symbol, and word fluency. In addition, eight of the 17 patients in the crossover trial (5) were available for neuropsychological testing before and after conversion to valproate monotherapy. Tests included two memory measures (Rey Osterrieth Complex Figure, Rey Auditory Verbal Learning Test) and a brief repeatable behavioural toxicity battery (finger tapping, Lafayette Peg board, word finding, paced auditory serial addition tests (PASAT) and Stroop colour naming. Alternate forms were administered in order to control for test–retest effects. The functions tested can be considered to sample memory, attention/concentration and motor skills. In addition, mood was assessed using the Profile of Mood States (POMS) (6).

Psychosocial/lifestyle function

Vocational Status was categorized as employed, unemployed or student. The employment was also divided into similar, improved, or worsened level of employment. Improvement was defined as at least a 25% increase in salary, change from part time to full time, and improved function from unskilled to skilled, or skilled to professional activity. Assumption of the full responsibilities as a housewife was also considered full employment.

School performance was compared before and after conversion to valproate monotherapy. Twenty-nine patients were students at the time of initiating treatment, 24 of whom completed schooling during the 13 years of observation. Those who continued to be in school were evaluated for whether their school performance became worse, remained the same, improved, or significantly improved. An improvement was considered movement from a special class to a regular class, or an increase in marks of a full grade point. A marked improvement indicated ability to attend school which was previously not possible, or graduation to higher level education and training.

Independent living

Patients were classified as needing total care, partial care, or being independent both before and following valproate treatment. Total care meant attendance by a family member or significant other was needed much of the time for medical and/or psychological help with activities of daily living. Partial care meant the patient was unable to live independently because some support was needed. In such instances the family or spouse had to attend a certain number of needs such as transportation, helping with meals, etc. Independent status meant the patient was able to live alone, or, if living with another, required no special support other than would be expected of a spouse or family member.

Motor vehicle licensure

Patients were categorized as follows: having a motor vehicle licence (with at least occasional use); qualified but not holding a motor vehicle for reasons of disinterest, a lack of necessity to drive, or unqualified for other than seizure related reasons; or unable to drive due to persistent seizures occurring with a frequency or timing to cause a risk.

RESULTS

Seizure control

Fifty seven of the 60 patients could be assessed for seizure control. All came under control for at least several months with addition of valproate (three patients of the 60 withdrew due to unacceptable side effects). Forty-five of the 57 patients (79%) seizures came under full control after conversion of monotherapy. Among this group, sporadic and infrequent seizures occurred when attempts were made to discontinue medications purposely by the medical team or the patient, when running out of medication on a few occasions or under multiple stresses including sleep deprivation and occasional excessive alcohol use. Three of the 45 patients who had come under complete control came off all treatment and have remained seizure free for more than four years. Twenty others who attempted withdrawal purposely or inadvertently, had recurrences. The recurrences following drug discontinuation occurred in eight of those patients despite being seizure free for at least three years on VPA monotherapy. The remaining 22 declined to attempt drug withdrawal due to a multiple year history of uncontrolled seizures continuing into adulthood. Twelve patients did not obtain full control of tonic–clonic seizures with valproate monotherapy, despite increasing the dosage to cause unacceptable sedation, tremor, hair loss, or weight gain. In 11 of the 12 patients with inability to maintain complete control of seizures, carbamazepine or phenytoin was added to the valproate therapy. In seven of the these patients tonic–clonic seizures were controlled, and in the remaining four full control was not possible despite maximal tolerated doses of medications. One patient changed to a different antiepileptic drug due to pregnancy plans.

Systemic side effects

Two-thirds of the patients experienced weight gain of >10% of their pre-valproate body weight that led two patients to stop taking VPA. These women had gained more than forty pounds. Over months and years most other patients gradually returned to near pretreatment weight. No significant liver disturbances was encountered other than occasional transient elevation of hepatic transaminases. Although mild thrombocytopenia occurred in many patients, this never required discontinuation of drug. Transient hair loss was observed in 11 patients, but returned with dose reduction in all but one patient. This patient who was lost to follow-up for a decade, had continued on high dose with associated tremor, weight gain, and hair loss. When seen in recent follow-up, the dose was reduced, but after three months no evidence of return of hair has been seen.

Neurological side effects

Sedation and ataxia were largely limited to start-up when valproate was administered with other antiepileptic drugs. This was a minor problem during long-term monotherapy after dose adjustment. Tremor occurred in 23 of 57 of patients followed long-term. After a decrease in dosage, minor action tremor was noted in some patients, but this had little effect on everyday function.

Neuropsychological effects

Valproate addition

Neuropsychological testing was performed in six patients treated with valproate as add-on after a placebo lead-in. No significant improvement was found on placebo. Improvement in index finger tapping, peg board, ($p<0.05$) and word fluency ($p<0.07$) was found after three months of valproate therapy.

Valproate monotherapy

Eight different patients who underwent conversion to valproate monotherapy showed statistically significant improvements in cognitive functioning (particularly concentration), motor speed and affective state (4).

Employment and schooling prior and after treatment

At last follow-up, 52 of 60 patients were employed, three unemployed, and five still in school. One patient is not having seizures, but is psychologically disabled. The other patient is in prison for theft. Of the 22 initially employed at the beginning of the treatment, six had a significant improvement in occupational status.

Twenty-nine patients were in school when valproate therapy was initiated (20 secondary school, three in elementary school, and six at a university). Twenty-four of the 29 patients completed school and all but one became fully employed. Of the five patients remaining in school, academic performance showed some improvement in four and remained the same for one student.

Independent living

At last follow-up all 60 patients were partly or fully independent. Thirty of the 60 patients had shown a significant improvement in level of independence. Twenty-five had moved from a level of partial care to full independence, for others went from total care to independence and two from total care to partial care.

Motor vehicle licensure

Thirteen patients held a motor vehicle licence prior to valproate therapy. Although seizures were not fully controlled on starting VPA, some had experienced earlier remission enabling them to obtain the licence. In others, the severity or timing of attacks (i.e. nocturnal or early morning occurrence) did not preclude some driving. At final assessment 47 of the 60 patients held a driver's licence and five others had sufficient control to qualify, but elected not to obtain a licence. Five patients continued to have seizures of a frequency and severity, despite addition of other drugs, to make them ineligible for licensure. Fifteen patients were too young to be eligible for driving at the time valproate was started and on final analysis three patients continued to be too young to drive.

DISCUSSION

Sixty patients with idiopathic generalized epilepsy and uncontrolled seizures were treated with valproate and followed long term. They were assessed for seizure control and adverse effects as well as psychosocial or lifestyle function as measured by employment, school performance, independent living, and ability to obtain a license to drive a motor vehicle. A major improvement was found in every category. A small number who remained in school showed improvement in this area also. The reasons for the improvement are complex and often multi factorial. The natural history of improvement or spontaneous remission of epilepsy must be considered one reason for favourable outcome. Four patients no longer take medication nor do they have seizures after many years off the drug. An unknown number of our patients who are fully controlled may also have spontaneously remitted, although at least 20 attempted and failed in efforts to come off drug therapy. Most of the patients had had uncontrolled seizures for many years prior to VPA therapy, putting them into a category in which spontaneous remission is relatively low.

The large percentage of patients employed at last follow-up in part can be explained by the increase in the number of patients who completed school and entered the workforce. It is impossible to know how many of these patients would have been able to find employment after completing school had they not been placed on valproate which provided full seizure control. One-third of patients of employment age were employed prior to VPA treatment. It might be assumed that the students completing school with uncontrolled seizures would have had a similar percent of unemployment. The importance of a relative decrease in side effects with valproate therapy is more difficult to assess. It may well have accounted for an improvement in school performance, and may have assisted in an increase in level of employment status, but it is impossible to separate this factor from control of seizures.

The neuropsychological assessment showed a tendency for improvement in test measures when valproate was added to other antiepileptic drugs. This effect was almost certainly due to a dramatic improvement in seizure control. The further significant improvement on psychological testing measures after conversion from polytherapy to monotherapy suggest that a decrease in side effects also plays a role in improvement in lifestyle (6,7).

Many factors interact to determine a patient's lifestyle and psychosocial adjustment. A clear determination of which factors play the most important role is difficult, if not impossible, to define.

SUMMARY AND CONCLUSIONS

A large group of patients with idiopathic generalized tonic–clonic and absence or myoclonic seizures after long term treatment with valproate can expect a very good prospect for a relatively normal psychosocial adjustment. Specifically there is a high probability of seizure control, minimal side effects, excellent potential for employment, the ability to operate a motor vehicle and to live independently.

The study also makes clear that psychosocial or lifestyle measures can be used to assess treatment outcome. Our study represents an effort in developing such methods, but more detailed validated and systematic approaches are needed.

REFERENCES

(1) Cramer JA, Smith DB, Mattson RH, Delgado Escueta A, et al. A method of quantification for the evaluation of antiepileptic drug therapy. Neurology 1983; 33 (suppl 1): 26–37.
(2) Augustine EA, Novelly RA, Mattson RH, et al. Occupational adjustment following neurosurgical treatment of epilepsy. Ann Neurol 1984; 15: 68–72.
(3) Commission on Classification and Terminology of the International League Against Epilepsy. Epilepsia 1989; 30 (suppl 4): 389–99.
(4) Mattson RH, Cramer JA. Crossover from polytherapy to monotherapy in primary generalized epilepsy. Am J Med 1988; 84 (suppl 1A): S23–S28.
(5) Mattson RH, Cramer JA. Disinduction of valproate metabolism: Timing and magnitude of change. (This publication.)
(6) Prevey ML, Mattson RH, Cramer JA. Improvement in cognitive functioning and mood state after conversion to valproate monotherapy. Neurology 1989 (in press).
(7) Trimble MR, Thompson PJ. Sodium valproate and cognitive function. Epilepsia 1984; 25 (suppl): S60–64.

DISCUSSION

Dr Nasar *(Bridlington, UK):* When you convert the patients from phenytoin and phenobarbitone to monotherapy how quickly do you do it, and how do you progress on the monotherapy.

Professor Mattson *(Connecticut, USA):* I usually reduce the phenobarbitone by about 30 mg every other week, and the phenytoin by 100 mg per week. I reduce carbamazepine by about 200 mg a week. There are a number of different studies that indicate that you probably can go faster than that, and it would not make a great deal of difference, but if you go too fast you will trigger seizures.

Dr Aicardi *(Paris, France):* Do you believe in withdrawal seizures, and what do you do when the patient has a seizure shortly after discontinuing treatment?

Professor Mattson: Yes I do believe in withdrawal seizures, certainly with the barbiturates, and that is why I proceed so slowly. If there seems to be a slight increase in the frequency or even the severity of the seizure on eliminating the phenobarbitone I try to wait several weeks before doing anything about it. If they are on phenytoin and phenobarbitone and they have more problems I increase the dose of phenytoin. It is not the optimal way of correcting a withdrawal effect, but it may attenuate the severity of the seizures.

Dr Poole *(Oxford, UK):* Is there a novelty effect in new medication whereby it might do better than an old one?

Professor Mattson: I am sure there is. In the first study I referred to, however, we had a placebo lead-in. I am not sure if you are asking whether one becomes tolerant to the antiepileptic drug, or whether you are talking about a placebo effect. Whether or not people become tolerant to the antiepileptic drugs, I cannot say. My feeling is they do not, but there are times when somebody goes back on a drug they have been off for a couple of years and it seems to work better than before. That clearly is an occasional anecdotal experience.

Concluding remarks

Dr David Chadwick

I intend to use the interactive system to assess how successful this conference has been and what people have got out of it. It was possible to attend seven sessions.

1. How many of the sessions have you attended?	Response
0	3%
1	0%
2	2%
3	2%
4	8%
5	45%
6	25%
7	15%

Well that is a skewed deviation but I am delighted to see that it skewed in the right direction. There may of course be a very significant selection bias here, in that those who did not attend are relatively unlikely to have voted!

2. Which of the sessions did you think was best?	Response
1 Aspects of management	4%
2 Childhood epilepsy	16%
3 Adult epilepsy	4%
4 Unwanted effects	6%
5 Recent developments with valproate	17%
6 Patient life-style	5%
7 Closing session	3%
8 Interactive case histories	40%
9 Don't know	5%

Unfortunately it is not possible to publish the case histories, because without the actual video the question and answer sessions would be meaningless to the reader. Nevertheless this response does illustrate how valuable those case histories were, and how much we appreciate all the work that went into them. Thank you to both Lennart Gram and Jørgen Alving for that.

Fourth international symposium on sodium valproate and epilepsy, edited by David Chadwick, 1989; Royal Society of Medicine Services International Congress and Symposium Series No. 152, published by Royal Society of Medicine Services Limited.

3.	Which session did you think was the worst?	Response
	1 Aspects of management	12%
	2 Childhood epilepsy	7%
	3 Adult epilepsy	6%
	4 Unwanted effects	7%
	5 Recent developments in valproate	18%
	6 Patient life-style	17%
	7 Closing session	17%
	8 Interactive case histories	1%
	9 Don't know	15%

4.	Do you regard the interactive system as	Response
	1 Worthwhile	40%
	2 Could have been worthwhile if used better	35%
	3 Don't know	25%

One very difficult aspect of organising these meetings is deciding how much time to allow for discussion and it is probably one of the things that causes the greatest contention.

5.	In this meeting would you say that the time for discussion has been	Response
	1 Too little	28%
	2 Just enough	70%
	3 Too much	2%

6.	The organisation of the symposium has been	Response
	1 First class	82%
	2 Acceptable	17%
	2 Poor	1%

This is obviously an opportune moment to thank Geoffrey Yaffé, both for the planning and the organization of the Symposium and all the members of staff of Sanofi UK Limited who have worked so hard throughout the Symposium to make sure everything ran smoothly. A particular vote of thanks for secretarial assistance to Mrs P. Castree.

One of the difficulties about meetings like this is getting the balance right between the social and scientific aspects.

7.	Has this meeting been	Response
	1 Too scientific	17%
	2 Just right	80%
	3 Too socially orientated	3%

8.	What do you think has been the main value of this meeting?	Response
	1 Educational content	38%
	2 Informal discussions	40%
	3 Other	20%

9.	How much have you really learned from this meeting?	Response
	1 A lot	5%
	2 Picked up some important points that will be of value in the future	90%
	3 Learned nothing from attendance from this meeting	5%

All that remains for me to do now is to thank you for coming along and making this a very enjoyable occasion, and of course to thank Sanofi UK Limited again for their financial support and organization of this meeting.